NUTRITION COUNSELING SKILLS

for Medical Nutrition Therapy

Linda G. Snetselaar, RD, PhD, LD
Chair of Preventive Nutrition Education
Associate Professor and Research Nutritionist
Department of Preventive Medicine
and Internal Medicine
University of Iowa
Iowa City, Iowa

AN ASPEN PUBLICATION®
Aspen Publishers, Inc.
Gaithersburg, Maryland
1997

Library of Congress Cataloging-in-Publication Data

Snetselaar, Linda G.
Nutrition counseling skills for medical nutrition therapy / Linda G. Snetselaar.
p. cm.
Includes bibliographical references and index.
ISBN 0-8342-0755-9 (hardbound)
1. Nutrition counseling. I. Title.
[DNLM: 1. Counseling—methods. 2. Nutrition. 3. Diet Therapy. 4. Food Habits.
QU 145 S671n 1997]
RM218.7.S66 1997
615.8'54—dc21

DNLM/DLC
for Library of Congress

96-53385
CIP

Orders: (800) 638-8437
Customer Service: (800) 234-1660

About Aspen Publishers • For more than 35 years, Aspen has been a leading professional
publisher in a variety of disciplines. Aspen's vast information resources are available in both
print and electronic formats. We are committed to providing the highest quality information
available in the most appropriate format for our customers. Visit Aspen's Internet site for
more information resources, directories, articles, and a searchable version of Aspen's full
catalog, including the most recent publications: **http://www.aspenpub.com**
Aspen Publishers, Inc. • The hallmark of quality in publishing
Member of the worldwide Wolters Kluwer group

Aspen Publishers, Inc., is not affiliated with
the American Society of Parenteral and Enteral Nutrition.

The author has made every effort to ensure the accuracy of the information herein. However, appropriate information sources should be consulted, especially for new or unfamiliar procedures. It is the
responsibility of every practitioner to evaluate the appropriateness of a particular opinion in the context of actual clinical situations and with due considerations to new developments. Authors, editors,
and the publisher cannot be held responsible for any typographical or other errors found in this book.

Editorial Resources: Ruth Bloom
Library of Congress Catalog Card Number: 96-53385
ISBN: 0-8342-0755-9

Printed in the United States of America

1 2 3 4 5

To
my husband,
Gary
and my children,
Tyler, Jordan, and Daniel

Table of Contents

Preface

This text in its third edition focuses on increasing the effectiveness of nutrition counselors as facilitators of behavioral change. This edition provides new and updated material to help nutrition counselors determine the client's readiness to change. The term "nutrition counselor" describes all health professionals involved in counseling clients or patients to provide dietary information or facilitate dietary adherence. Nutrition counselors may be registered dietitians or other health professionals—medical doctors, nurses, psychologists, or behavior therapists—who interact with registered dietitians.

Readers of this text will acquire or enhance the following abilities:

1. demonstrate effective use of tools for nutrition counseling and communication skills in medical nutrition therapy
2. select and apply appropriate strategies when presented with nutrition problems
3. evaluate progress, achievements, and failures in both clients and themselves
4. adapt counseling strategies based on self-evaluations and client evaluations.

Nutrition Counseling Skills for Medical Nutrition Therapy was written to supplement a major course in nutrition principles. It does not replace discussions on basic nutrition, and the information in the text will be most useful to readers with a thorough understanding of the subject as taught in a college curriculum. The intent of the text is to (1) apply communication and counseling skills and strategies to the discipline of nutrition and (2) provide for their practice in situations that require specific dietary modifications. Ideally, a course in counseling psychology will expand the knowledge and skills presented in this text.

Each chapter begins with objectives; reference lists at the end of each chapter are provided for further study. Part I covers basic theories on communication and counseling skills with an emphasis on identifying the client's readiness to change. Part II demonstrates how to use counseling skills and nutrition tools in specific nutrition situations in which eating behaviors may pose problems. Part III provides suggestions for evaluating and terminating counseling sessions.

The text frequently uses the term "eating pattern" in place of "diet." The rationale for this change in terminology is that "diet" tends to denote the following of an eating regimen for a short time with regression to old habits as an eventual outcome. In treating or preventing chronic disease, changes in eating behaviors are long term, and the nutrition counselor's goal is to assist the client or patient in maintaining change over time.

Linda G. Snetselaar

PART I

The Basics of Communication and Counseling Skills for Medical Nutrition Therapy

Part I covers basic theoretical aspects of communication and counseling skills in relation to medical nutrition therapy. The first chapter provides an historical perspective of counseling for medical nutritional therapy. Chapter 2 discusses basic communication skills that provide strategies to facilitate our interactions with clients. The third chapter focuses on the client's readiness to change as an essential element in dietary behavior modification. This chapter on motivational interviewing departs from assigning blame to the client for past adherence problems and focuses on constructive ways to provide the client with feedback that can result in positive dietary change.

CHAPTER 1

Overview of Nutrition Counseling

CHAPTER OBJECTIVES

1. Discuss the influence of counseling theory on the client.

2. Describe three theories that influence the nutrition counselor.

3. Discuss two ways in which counseling is important to the work of the nutrition counselor.

4. Identify the components of counseling skills.

5. Diagram the counseling spectrum.

DEFINITION OF NUTRITION COUNSELING IN MEDICAL NUTRITION THERAPY

Nutrition is both a science and an art. The nutrition counselor converts theory into practice and science into art. This ability requires both knowledge and skill.[1,2]

Nutrition counseling is a combination of nutrition expertise and psychological skill delivered by a trained nutrition counselor who understands how to work within the current medical setting. It focuses on both foods and the nutrients contained within them, emphasizing our feelings as we experience eating.

Nutrition counseling has moved from a brief encounter as the patient leaves the hospital with suitcase in hand to an in-depth session. Today nutrition counseling sessions include analysis of factors such as nutrition science, psychology and physiology, and an eventual negotiated treatment plan followed by an evaluation. Research has shown that this in-depth approach can produce excellent dietary compliance based on biological markers, even with complicated dietary regimens that are difficult to accommodate in the real world.[3,4]

HISTORY OF NUTRITION COUNSELING

Over the years nutrition advice has been a part of nearly every culture. Early Greek physicians recognized the role of food in the treatment of disease.[5] In the United States in the early 1800s, Thomas Jefferson described his eating habits in a letter to his doctor in what may be one of the first diet records (Exhibit 1–1).[6] After World War II, advances in chemical knowledge allowed nutrition researchers to define metabolic requirements.[7] This marked the beginning of the study of patterns of nutrients needed by all persons in relation to their age, sex, and activity. These patterns are vital to the assessment phase of counseling.

Selling and Ferraro, in discussing the psychology of diet and nutrition in 1945, recommended what at that time must have been an unconventional view:

1. knowing the client's personality
2. knowing the client's psychological surroundings
3. eliminating emotional tension
4. assisting the client in knowing his own limitations
5. arranging the diet so that it has the effect of encouraging the client
6. allowing for occasional cheating [on the diet][8]

Exhibit 1–1 A Colonial Era Diet Report

". . . I have lived temperately, eating little animal food, & that. . . as a condiment for the vegatables, which constitute my principal diet. I double however the doctor's glass and a half of wine."

From Thomas Jefferson
to his Doctor

Original in Jefferson Papers, Library of Congress, Washington, DC.

In 1945, the flood of scientific knowledge relating nutrition to disease obscured this advice. Nutrition counselors expended only minor efforts to put these critical ideas into practice.

Over the years the counselor's role has changed. In the past, the role fell more on the authoritarian side of a continuum; today a counselor must be able to function in all roles at appropriate times (Figure 1–1). Ivey et al. describe the role of counseling as knowing which strategy to use for which individual given specific conditions.[9]

Pioneers in the Field

In the early 1900s, Frances Stearn started a food clinic at the New England Medical Center. Her work continues today with dietitians who emphasize the counseling aspects of nutrition.

In 1973, Margaret Ohlson stressed the importance of creating an interviewing atmosphere in which the client can respond freely. Ohlson warned against a common problem in dietetic counseling sessions: speaking at the expense of missing important factors during the interview.[10]

Selling and Ferraro say that there no longer is any justification for prescribing a diet without also recognizing the psychological factors in a case. They recommend a diagnostic study to determine the right psychodietetic approach.[11] Indeed, the thrust in counseling today is matching the treatment to each individual case.[12]

THEORIES OF NUTRITION COUNSELING

Theories form the basis for developing counseling skills to change eating habits. Both clients and nutrition counselors use theories and beliefs in determining what will take place during an interview.

Theories Influence Clients

Clients approach nutrition counseling sessions with mind-sets about themselves and the world around them. They present "a history of being healed or hurt

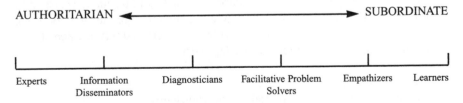

Figure 1–1 Roles of the Nutrition Counselor Today

by others, of being accepted or rejected, or of dominating others."[13] They come with a positive or negative self-image and a record of success or failure in diet modification. From this personal background stem their personal theories of what counseling is and should be.

Most nutrition counselors have faced a client who slouches down in the chair, slams a diet instruction sheet on the desk, and demands: "Well, what are you going to do to get me to follow this diet?" This client sees the counselor as an expert, the person with all of the answers—and an adversary. A second client may walk into the office, sit down, and speak only in response to direct questions. Still a third client may arrive commenting, "Well, how can we work out this problem I've been having with my diet?"

All three clients see the world through different eyes. The first does not want any responsibility. The second may be afraid of authority figures. The last sees the counselor as an advocate, as someone who can help increase self-directed solutions to dietary problems. Lorr lists five descriptors of clients' perceptions of counselors: (1) accepting, (2) understanding, (3) independence encouraging, (4) authoritarian, and (5) critical-hostile.[14]

Prior to the interview, clients may see the nutrition counselor as rejecting, dominating, or hostile. Consequently, they resort to behavior they have used in the past in dealing with an unapproachable person. Other clients, on the basis of past experience, see counselors as friendly, supportive, respectful, and positive. Both of these situations can create self-fulfilling prophecies. Counselors can become trapped into behaving in accordance with the clients' theory of the world. Thus, it is important to be open with a client and to discuss interpersonal factors that may influence both client and counselor. Gerber recommends discussing frankly and openly any interpersonal factors that may negatively affect counseling for dietary change.[15]

Clients also come to a nutrition counseling session with feelings about themselves. Some may want to succeed in changing yet seek to sabotage any efforts toward change so their routines will stay the same.[16] Clients may say, "New eating habits may be healthy, but what changes will they make in my family life?" A familiar image of themselves as overweight can give obese persons a sense of identity and security that they can lose when the pounds come off. A client may say, "Why should I change my feeling of security to a feeling of having to shape up to what people want me to be?" Clients may come to counselors feeling confused, disturbed, and self-defeated by new knowledge that their health is threatened.[17]

In summary, clients come to counseling with:

- attitudes and beliefs about people
- ideas and feelings about counselors and counseling
- self-images

- basic incongruities in desired outcomes:
  1. a desire to continue along a familiar course
  2. a desire to make changes to improve health and well-being[18]

Counseling is a skill that can correct or validate clients' preconceived beliefs. It enables counselors to behave as decent, empathic persons in spite of the "provocation to be less or the seduction to be more than they are."[19]

Theories Influence Counselors

Many theories influence the way a nutrition counselor conducts a session. Six specific theories are (1) person-centered therapy, (2) rational-emotive therapy (RET), (3) behavioral therapy, (4) Gestalt therapy, (5) family therapy and (6) self-management approach. An analysis of their characteristics as they apply to the nutrition counseling session follows. Many concepts within these theories overlap.

Person-Centered Therapy

Carl Rogers is the founder of person-centered therapy, originally client-centered therapy.[20] Three major concepts form the basis of this theory.

1. All individuals are a composite of their physical being, their thoughts, and their behaviors.
2. Individuals function as an organized system, so alterations in one part may produce changes in another part.
3. Individuals react to everything they perceive; this is their reality.

When counselors try to change dietary behaviors, they also must be concerned with clients' thoughts. Behavioral alterations may produce changes in the clients' physical being as well as the cognitive (thoughtful) being. Counselors must also assess client perceptions thoroughly because what clients perceive as reality influences their ability to follow an eating pattern. The skill of listening is very important to this therapy.

The goals of client-centered therapy include the following:

- promoting a more confident and self-directed person
- promoting a more realistic self-perception
- promoting a positive attitude about self [21]

Rogerian, person-centered therapy focuses on each person's worth and dignity. The emphasis is on the ability to direct one's own life and move toward self-actualization, growth, and health.[22]

Nutrition counselors can provide the tools to help clients solve their own problems by assessing their current dietary behavior and establishing realistic goals for change. Practitioners also can assess clients' thoughts about their body image and food behaviors. Changing thoughts from negative to positive is a first step toward the client's mastery of positive self-reinforcement skills.

Rational-Emotive Therapy

Rational-emotive therapy (RET) was developed by Albert Ellis. He determined that irrationality is the most frequent source of individuals' problems. Self-talk (the monologues individuals have with themselves) is the major cause of emotion-related difficulties.[23] The major purposes of RET are to demonstrate to clients that self-talk, the source of their problems, should be reevaluated and eliminated along with illogical ideas.[24] Clients' major goal in RET is to look to themselves for positive reinforcement for behaviors.

For example, in dietary counseling, a client with hyperlipidemia might say: "I knew I shouldn't eat that piece of cream pie, but I did. After eating it, I decided, well, what's the use, you've been such a bad person for eating it. You're just making yourself fat and ugly. It's no use. So I ate the entire pie."

The RET counselor in this case can help change self-talk to more positive thoughts: "I ate one piece. Even if it was high in fat, I don't need to feel guilty. I won't eat another piece and that's great. I'm really doing well. I feel better about myself."

Behavioral Therapy

Behavioral counseling, as described by Pavlov, Skinner, Wolpe, Krumboltz, and Thoreson, states that people are born in a neutral state. Environment, consisting of significant others and experience, shapes their behavior.

Three modes of learning are basic to behavioral counseling:[25]

1. Operant conditioning holds that if spontaneous behavior satisfies a need, it will occur with greater frequency. For example, a person who switches to a high-fiber diet and finds that constipation problems decrease will probably increase fiber in all meals.
2. Imitation does not involve teaching a new behavior; instead, the emphasis is on mimicking. For example, a hyperlipidemic client selects a low-cholesterol, low-fat snack after a spouse or friend has just ordered one in a restaurant.
3. Modeling extends the concept of imitation, which tends to be haphazard, by providing a planned demonstration. Modeling implies direct teaching of a certain behavior.[26] For example, an overweight client watches a videotape of someone who has lost a large amount of weight. The model's description or demonstration of successful weight loss behaviors helps the client begin a weight-loss program.

Behavioral counseling obviously varies from client to client, as each individual is responsible for shaping the environment to accommodate changes in behavior. Problem behaviors result from faulty learning, and the goal is to eliminate faulty learning and behavior and substitute more adaptive patterns of behavior.[27]

Gestalt Therapy

Gestalt counseling emphasizes confronting problems. Steps toward solving them involve experiencing them in the present rather than the past or the future. The major goal in Gestalt therapy is to make clients aware of all the experience they have disowned and recognize that individuals are self-regulating. Being aware of the hidden factors related to a problem is the key to finding an eventual solution.[28]

Using Gestalt therapy to help clients with dietary change involves asking them to recognize how many "disowned" factors can contribute to their dietary problems. Showing clients how to be responsible for regulating their behavior is a practical application of the Gestalt approach to counseling. The goal is for clients to take responsibility for making dietary changes.[29] For example, clients who continuously blame poor glucose control on parents who don't help them control foods or teachers who cause them to be under stress are disowning behaviors that they could control. Helping clients set reasonable behavioral goals can aid in solving the problem of disowning.

Family Therapy

In family therapy, behavior is examined as a system, and the family is considered a system of relationships that influence a client's behavior. The individual client is always seen in the context of relationships, with emphasis on understanding the total system in which the inappropriate behavior exists. The goal is to help individuals and families to change themselves and the systems within which they live.[30]

One of the major techniques used in family therapy is to involve the client's entire family in solving problems through open and closed questioning. Role playing may be used to illustrate both the negative aspects of "blaming" and the positive aspects, in which praising behavior change is emphasized.

Self-Management Approach

Researchers have found that behavioral approaches support short-term change[31] but usually fail to maintain change in the long run.[32,33] Leventhal proposed several reasons for this failure: behavioral techniques fail when contact with a health care professional is less frequent or absent, when initial symptoms of illness lessen, and when relapse into a previous behavior pattern does not provoke any symptoms.[34] Leventhal's theory of self-regulation is based on concepts from the behavioral approach and the health belief model,[35] self-efficacy,[36,37] and self-management.[38] The basic premise in self-regulation allows individuals to choose their own goals based on their perceptions of their illness and related challenges. Individuals seek, discover, and select coping behaviors and evaluate the outcome in emotional and cognitive terms. The nutrition counselor is a guiding expert who reinforces, supports, and encourages individuals as they select, evaluate, and adjust goals and strategies for behavior change.[39–42]

In the contemporary self-management approach,[43,44] nutrition counselors and clients are partners. Clients problem solve and use resources beyond those of the nutrition therapists. Clients develop skills and confidence (belief in personal efficacy) through guided mastery experiences, social modeling, social persuasion, and the reduction of adverse physiological reactions. Health care professionals and a social network encourage and cooperate with self-management practices.

The theories described above are only 6 of over 200 orientations to helping clients change their behavior. The communication and counseling skills presented in the next two chapters provide a format through which counselors can consider and use ideas based on these six theories. All theories are concerned with change—the generation of novel ways of thinking, being, deciding, and behaving. When a client who is trying to change a dietary behavior does so in a small way, the nutrition counselor has a beginning foundation with which to support further change. Integrating tenets of many theories into the treatment of a client's dietary problems is the goal. One theory may work best in promoting change at one stage in a client's treatment; another may work well at a different point. Chapter 3 discusses the client's readiness to change and provides ideas on ways to apply the theories described in this chapter.

IMPORTANCE OF NUTRITION COUNSELING IN MEDICAL NUTRITION THERAPY

Why is counseling important? Nutrition counseling provides a logical structure via strategies based on a variety of counseling theories for all dietary interviews. It sets the stage for optimum dietary adherence.

Dietary adherence, or how well clients follow practitioners' recommendations, should be the ultimate goal of all nutrition counseling sessions. Researchers have found that there are many deterrents to dietary adherence:

- the restrictiveness of the dietary pattern
- the required changes in lifestyle and behavior
- the fact that symptom relief may not be noticeable or may be temporary
- the interference of diet with family or personal habits
- other barriers:

1. cost
2. access to proper foods
3. effort necessary for food preparation[45]

Glanz has found that two positive counseling techniques appear to increase dietary adherence: (1) employing more strategies that influence client behavior and (2) involving clients more during the session.[46] She further specifies several strategies for maintaining dietary changes: (1) tailoring the dietary regimen and information about the regimen; (2) using social support inside and outside the health care setting; (3) providing skills and training in addition to information, such as assertiveness training skills and weighing and measuring skills; (4) ensuring effective client provider communication; and (5) paying attention to follow-up, monitoring, and reinforcement.[47]

Hosking lists conditions that increase dietary adherence in hypertensive clients on salt-restricted eating patterns:

- diet programs that are individualized, fully explained, and adapted to the client's preferences and lifestyle
- regular revisits to the same nutrition counselor
- involvement of the family
- reinforcement of the eating pattern from every member of the treatment team[48]

Several research studies have reported that adherence is better when the counselor is warm and empathetic and shows interest ("Call me if there is a problem") and demonstrates genuine concern ("I will call in a week").[49-59]

Counseling skills help eliminate the hit-or-miss philosophy that allows little assurance for success. This hit-or-miss philosophy tends to be inefficient, because the nutrition counselor must backtrack when strategies fail. To provide structure and organization, many counseling models resemble the systems approach described below.[60,61]

Systems Approach to Nutrition Counseling

Models provide a sequenced path for counselors to follow and list essential components in each step of the process. Figure 1–2 shows one model by which nutrition counselors can avoid missing a vital part of the process. In this model, the counselor wears many hats. The first is that of a diagnostician preparing for the interview by reviewing all available data in the medical record, diet records, diet recalls, diet histories, interviews with family members, and other sources.

The session begins with an explanation of the counseling relationship with enough detail that the client knows precisely what will take place. In this stage, the practitioner is a teacher informing the client of what the relationship is.

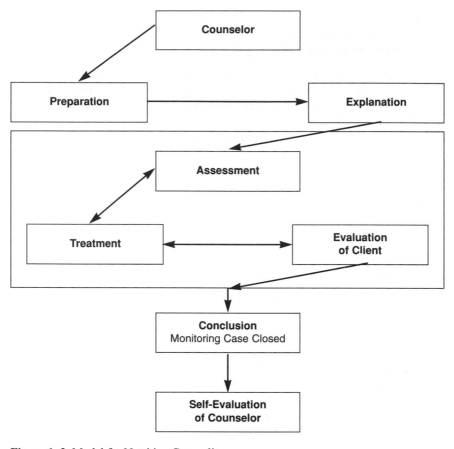

Figure 1–2 Model for Nutrition Counseling

During the assessment phase, once again in the role of diagnostician, the counselor evaluates the client's nutrition status and relates food intake data to behavioral indicators. The practitioner also must establish a safe, trusting, and caring environment, acting as empathizer. Mason et al. specify the categories of information necessary for assessment of clients' nutritional status:

- agricultural data
- socioeconomic data
- food consumption patterns
- dietary surveys
- special studies on foods

- vital and health statistics
- anthropometric studies
- clinical nutrition survey
- biochemical studies
- additional medical information[62]

As for the information necessary to assess behavior, Mason and colleagues designate several categories to analyze in determining baseline behaviors:

- general health practices
- health, attitudes, beliefs, and information
- physical activities
- educational achievements and language skills
- economic considerations
- environmental considerations
- social considerations[63]

In the treatment phase, the counselor's roles are those of expert and mutual problem solver, roles that usually can be combined only through diligent study and practice. Most novices at counseling tend to be either expert or empathizer. When the two roles are used in combination they can facilitate adherence to diet, but singly each can be detrimental to effective counseling.

Many practitioners are familiar with the all-knowing counselor who approaches clients with an air of authority. Clients are overwhelmed by these experts' self-confidence and taken in by the appearance of wisdom. However, when clients return home, they find it very difficult to follow the diet. They tend to forget much of what was said during the counseling session and are incapable of self-direction in adhering to the new regimen. The clients' solution in such a case is to continue with old eating habits.

On the other hand, counselors who are empathizers can become so involved with the client's problems that they lose sight of their other role of information disseminators. Counselors can run into conflicts when they see a client is in error but feel that revealing the mistake may damage the individual's pride and ability to follow the diet. "Eating cheesecake out a few times won't matter," the counselor says. To the client on a low-cholesterol diet, this may be a signal to go ahead and continue poor eating habits. Back at home, the client may comment to a family member, "The nutritionist said eating cheesecake in a restaurant just a few times wouldn't hurt. Three nights a week doesn't seem too often."

In evaluating clients, counselors once again become diagnosticians. If no solution to the problem has been reached, counseling reverts to the assessment or treatment phase. In some cases the clinicians may decide to refer a client to another practitioner more experienced with the problem.

In concluding the counseling session, the counselor should share a few words of wisdom, in which case the counselor becomes the expert again. Ending the program involves more than just closing the case. Monitoring the client's performance in the real world is important to continued dietary adherence. This means calling to check on progress and, with the individual's permission, checking with significant others to determine how they feel the client has progressed.

The last step involves self-evaluation of the counselor's performance. In this case, the counselor becomes the learner, building on past experience to improve present skills.

COUNSELING SKILLS

The basic steps just discussed are a part of counseling, but the complexities go beyond what Figure 1–2 indicates. Chapters 2 and 3 review these skills and ways to use them.

Communication Skills

Basic to all counseling is a knowledge of communication skills. Without these, treatment cannot and will not take place.

Counseling

Once clinicians have acquired this foundation, they then can learn various counseling skills to aid clients in achieving dietary goals. These skills involve assessment, treatment (including planning and implementation), and evaluation. Counseling skills integrate theories and make use of communication skills in assessing, treating, and evaluating the client's dietary problems.

Assessment

Nutrition counseling involves a process of targeting behaviors involving eating habits. Initially a careful assessment of current eating behaviors is important. Knowing what is eaten prior to making a change allows the individual to target specific foods and make substitutes.

Assessment involves more than asking clients, "Do you have a problem?" It is a carefully thought out plan to determine areas in which problems occur. Assessment in nutrition counseling includes ascertaining what clients are eating and why they make certain food selections.[64] The example that follows illustrates several potential responses to a weight-control client.

A client returns for a visit following the diet instruction and reports a problem: "I just haven't lost any weight on the diet you recommended." There are several counselor responses:

1. "Did you follow all of my advice?"
2. "Well, what have you been eating?"
3. "What is your typical day like?"

These three questions indicate various levels of communication skills. The first question is stated in a way that immediately places the client on the defensive. The client feels compelled to give a glowing picture or a multitude of excuses. The second question focuses only on eating behaviors, disregarding totally the surrounding circumstances that may have instigated the behavior. Depending on the tone of voice, it also may make the client feel compelled to reply with what the counselor wants to hear. The third question is stated sensitively and with a show of caring, characteristic of Rogerian style. It does not imply a reprimand, allows the client time to elaborate on what actually happened, and gives the counselor the information necessary to assess the situation. It sets the stage for the Rogerian style of learning.

For practicing nutrition counselors, the most frequent problem during an interview is a rush to give advice. It is important to stop and take time to assess the situation first. Only then provide advice, allowing the clients to assist by suggesting and describing how they expect to apply those recommendations in a true-to-life situation.

Treatment

Beyond understanding initial eating habits, counselors and their clients then make decisions about how to manage change. They determine which foods to modify or substitute to achieve a change in a targeted nutrient. Self-monitoring is crucial.[65,66]

In giving clients strategies to remedy nutrition problems or provide treatment, counselors once again must proceed slowly and involve the clients in planning and setting attainable goals. Counselors frequently decide before the interview how the problems should be solved and try to force clients into preformed molds. They do not give clients an opportunity to participate. In this phase, mutually decided goals will achieve the most success. **Counselors should use the following sequence of steps in setting goals:**

1. Identify nutrition goals.
   - Define desired nutrition behaviors (what to do).
   - Determine conditions or circumstances (where and when to do it).
   - Establish the extent or level (how much or how often to do it).

2. Identify nutrition subgoals (a subgoal for a long-term goal of eliminating snacks would be to eliminate the morning snack and determine a workable substitute behavior).

3. Establish client commitment, which includes identifying obstacles that might prevent goal attainment and listing resources needed for goal attainment.[67]

The strategy chosen to help implement these goals once again requires active listening to involve the clients in reaching solutions. Strategies are numerous and require knowledge and experience in counseling psychology. **Counselors should ask the following questions to help tailor strategies to each individual's situation:**

- Why is the client here?
- Is the problem the client describes all or only part of the problem? (Many nutrition counselors have thrown their hands up in despair, saying, "He just isn't motivated to follow this diet." In such a case, the real problem may hinge on emotional stress that must be treated before nutrition counseling can take place. The client might be referred to a psychologist or other professional for help before or concurrent with the nutrition counseling session.)
- What are the problematic nutrition behaviors and related concerns?
- Can I describe the conditions contributing to poor nutrition adherence?
- Am I aware of the present severity and intensity of the nutrition problem?[68]

For some clients, the problem may be lack of sufficient information to follow the desired regimen. For example, a person with renal disease who follows a low-protein eating pattern routinely has elevated urine urea nitrogen levels inconsistent with diet records that show excellent compliance. After requesting that the cook in her favorite restaurant slice one ounce of chicken off the actual portion of "Chicken Oscar" (her favorite entree), she is surprised: one ounce is much smaller than she guessed. For weeks, her concept of one ounce of meat has been much greater than the actual amount. Providing enough information for the client to follow a new eating pattern is the first step.

The second step may involve solving a problem of a different nature—forgetting. For example, a guest at a party realizes that he has no idea what ingredients are in the main dish. If before going to the party he has placed a cue on the refrigerator, "Call hostess to check on what is being served for the party tomorrow," the client can avoid a potentially awkward situation.

The third step in treating dietary problems is much more difficult. It involves diagnosing a problem involving lack of commitment to a dietary regimen. The term "lack of commitment" is not meant to reflect badly on the client but to diagnose accurately poor dietary adherence. For example, a person with diabetes may decide, "I just want to be free from dietary worries for a while. Life is so complicated. I want to forget my diet and splurge." The counselor cannot say, "Fine, don't worry about it for a week," but the counselor can say, "What can we do to streamline your dietary efforts? Let us begin by identifying when diet is most frequently a problem." Identification may require the client to keep a diary of thoughts before and following meals that could include all thoughts about food. For example, "I ate that chocolate cake even though I knew it would be too high in carbohydrate after that huge dinner." If a pattern of negative thoughts seems to occur frequently at dinner time, the client needs strategies to help make that meal a more positive experience.[69–71] By identifying a major problem time, the client may be able to work out menus in advance, elicit help from family in meal preparation on specified nights, rely on precalculated exchanges for each meal, build in time to relax before each meal, and work on more positive self-thoughts. By using the client's suggestions and combining ideas, the counselor and client can find a solution to the lack of commitment.

Evaluation

The last phase, evaluation, provides a reassessment of progress for both clients and counselors. Much of the questioning used during the assessment phase can be reused here, focusing on the desired objective and whether it was met. The counselor should monitor the client for a time in the real world, asking permission to check with significant others as to whether they feel the person is doing well.

Counselor self-evaluation frequently does not take place because of time constraints. It can be very important to review what went on in an interview and then to determine what made it a success and what might have improved its efficacy or quality.

COUNSELING SPECTRUM

Nutrition counselors assume a variety of roles. During the sessions some role changes take place automatically; others require a great deal of practice and effort. The role of the counselor falls on a spectrum such as that in Figure 1–3,

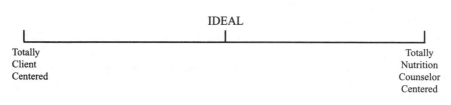

IDEAL

Totally
Client
Centered

Totally
Nutrition
Counselor
Centered

Figure 1–3 The Nutrition Counseling Spectrum

including some of the positions on both ends. When counseling is totally dominated by client requests and tangential topics, little behavior change will take place. A session totally dominated by a counselor who provides only information without listening to client concerns can be equally unproductive. The ideal is a mix of client and counselor interaction.

NOTES

1. M. Mason et al., *The Dynamics of Clinical Dietetics,* 2nd ed. (New York: John Wiley & Sons, 1982), 49.

2. Mason, *The Dynamics,* 45.

3. L. Snetselaar et al., "Reduction of Dietary Protein and Phosphorus in the Modification of Diet in Renal Disease Feasibility Study," *Journal of the American Dietetic Association* 94 (1994): 986–990.

4. S. Klahr et al., "The Effects of Dietary Protein Restriction and Blood Pressure Control on the Progression of Chronic Renal Disease," *New England Journal of Medicine* 330 (1994): 877–884.

5. J. Trager, *Food Book* (New York: Grossman Publishers, 1970), 262–263.

6. T. Jefferson to Dr. Vine Utley, 21 March 1819, The Thomas Jefferson Memorial Foundation, Monticello, Charlottesville, VA.

7. M.A. Ohlson, "The Philosophy of Dietary Counseling," *Journal of the American Dietetic Association* 63 (1973): 13.

8. L.S. Selling and M.S.S. Ferraro, *The Psychology of Diet and Nutrition* (New York: W.W. Norton & Co., 1945), 164–166.

9. A.E. Ivey et al., *Counseling and Psychotherapy, Integrating Skills Theory and Practice,* 2nd ed. (Englewood Cliffs, NJ: Prentice-Hall, 1987), xiv.

10. Ohlson, "Philosophy of Dietary Counseling," 13.

11. Selling and Ferraro, *Psychology of Diet and Nutrition,* 164–166.

12. Ivey et al., *Counseling and Psychotherapy,* xiv.

13. B. Stefflre and K.B. Matheny, *The Function of Counseling Theory* (Boston: Houghton Mifflin, 1968), 11.

14. M. Lorr, "Client Perception of Therapeutic Relation," *Journal of Counseling and Clinical Psychology* 29 (1965): 148.

15. S.K. Gerber, *Responsive Therapy: A Systematic Approach to Counseling Skills* (New York: Human Science Press, Inc., 1986), 30.

16. Stefflre and Matheny, *The Function of Counseling Theory,* 11.

17. Gerber, *Responsive Therapy,* 30–31.

18. Stefflre and Matheny, *The Function of Counseling Theory,* 11.

19. Stefflre and Matheny, *The Function of Counseling Theory,* 11.

20. C.R. Rogers, *Client-Centered Therapy* (Boston: Houghton Mifflin, 1951), 487.

21. J.J. Pietrofesa et al., *Counseling: Therapy Research and Practice* (Chicago: Rand McNally College Publishing Co., 1978), 71–72.

22. Ivey et al., *Counseling and Psychotherapy,* 429.

23. A. Ellis, *Reason and Emotion in Psychotherapy* (New York: Lyle Stuart, 1962), 49.

24. Ellis, *Reason and Emotion in Psychotherapy,* 28.

25. Pietrofesa et al., *Counseling: Therapy Research and Practice,* 77.

26. J.T. Spence et al., *Behavioral Approaches to Therapy* (Morristown, NJ: General Learning Press, 1976), 5.

27. Ivey et al., *Counseling and Psychotherapy,* 427.

28. Pietrofesa et al., *Counseling: Therapy Research and Practice,* 80–84.

29. Ivey et al., *Counseling and Psychotherapy,* 430.

30. M. Bowen, *Family Therapy in Clinical Practice* (New York: Aronson, 1978), 102–104.

31. J.M. Dunbar et al., "Behavioral Strategies for Improving Compliance," in *Compliance in Health Care,* ed. R.S. Haynes et al. (Baltimore, MD: The Johns Hopkins University Press, 1979), 174–190.

32. H. Leventhal and L. Cameron, "Behavioral Theories and the Problem of Compliance," *Patient Education and Counseling* 10 (1987): 117–138.

33. R.R. Wing, "Behavioral Treatment of Severe Obesity," *American Journal of Clinical Nutrition* 55 (1992):545S–551S.

34. H. Leventhal et al., "A Self-Regulation Perspective," in *Handbook of Behavioral Medicine,* ed. W.D. Gentry (New York: Guilford Press, 1984), 369–436.

35. N.K. Janz and M.H. Becker, "The Health Belief Model: A Decade Later," *Health Education Quarterly* 11 (1984): 1–47.

36. A. Bandura, "Self-Efficacy: Toward a Unifying Theory of Behavioral Change," *Psychological Review* 84 (1977): 191–215.

37. A. Bandura, "Self-Efficacy Mechanism in Physiological Activation and Health-Promoting Behavior," in *Neurobiology of Learning, Emotion and Affect,* ed. J. Madden (New York: Raven Press, 1991), 229–270.

38. D.L. Tobin et al., "Self-Management and Social Learning Theory," in *Self-Management of Chronic Disease: Handbook of Clinical Interventions and Research,* ed. K.A. Holroyd and T.L. Greer (Orlando, FL: Academic Press, 1986), 29–55.

39. J.A. Trostle, "Medical Compliance as an Ideology," *Social Science and Medicine* 27 (1988): 1299–1308.

40. D.J. Steele et al., "The Activated Patient; Dogma, Dream, or Desideratum? Beyond Advocacy: A Review of the Active Patient Concept," *Patient Education and Counseling* 10 (1987): 3–23.

41. G.C. Stone, "Patient Compliance and the Role of the Expert," *Journal of Social Issues* 35 (1979): 34–59.

42. T.S. Szasz and M.H. Hollender, "A Contribution to the Philosophy of Medicine: The Basic Models of the Doctor-Patient Relationship," in *Encounters Between Patients and Doctors,* ed. J.D. Stockle (Boston: Massachusetts Institute of Technology Press, 1987), 165–177.

43. H. Holman and K. Lorig, "Perceived Self-Efficacy in Self-Management of Chronic Disease," in *Self-Efficacy: Thought Control of Action,* ed. R. Schwarzer (Washington, DC: Hemisphere Publishing Company, 1992), 305–323.

44. K. Lorig et al., "The Beneficial Outcomes of the Arthritis Self-Mangement Course Are Not Adequately Explained by Behavior Change," *Arthritis and Rheumatism* 32 (1989): 91–95.

45. K. Glanz, "Nutrition Education for Risk Factor Reduction and Patient Education: A Review," *Preventive Medicine* 14 (1985): 721.

46. K. Glanz, "Dietitians' Effectiveness and Patient Compliance with Dietary Regimens," *Journal of the American Dietetic Association* 75 (1979): 631.

47. Glanz, "Nutrition Education," 745.

48. M. Hosking, "Eating Out: Salt and Hypertension," *Medical Journal of Australia* 2 (1979): 352.

49. M.H. Becker and L.A. Maiman, "Strategies for Enhancing Patient Compliance," *Journal of Community Health* 6 (1980): 113–135.

50. Z. Ben-Sira, "Affective and Instrumental Components in Physician-Patient Relationship: An Additional Dimension of Interaction Theory," *Journal of Health and Social Behavior* 21 (1980): 170–180.

51. R.B. Posner, "Physician-Patient Communication," *American Journal of Medicine* 77 (1984): 59–64.

52. M.R. Dimatteo and D.D. DiNicola, *Achieving Patient Compliance: The Psychology of the Medical Practitioner's Role* (New York: Pergamon Press, 1982), 78.

53. M.M. Kayvenhoven et al., "Written Simulation of Patient-Doctor Encounters," *Family Practice* 1 (1983): 25–29.

54. D.C. Turk et al., *Pain and Behavioral Medicine: A Cognitive-Behavioral Perspective* (New York: Guilford Press, 1983), 182–183.

55. M. Stewart, "Patient Characteristics Which Are Related to the Doctor-Patient Interaction," *Family Practice* 1 (1983): 30–36.

56. C.L. Peck and N.J. King, "Compliance and the Doctor-Patient Relationship," *Drugs* 30 (1985): 78–84.

57. G.V. Glass and R.M. Kliegl, "An Apology for Research Integration in the Study of Psychotherapy," *Journal of Counseling and Clinical Psychology* 51 (1984): 28–41.

58. S.B. Baker et al., "Measured Effects of Primary Prevention Strategies," *Personnel and Guidance Journal* 62 (1984): 459–464.

59. J.T. Beck and S.R. Strong, "Stimulating Therapeutic Change with Interpretations," *Journal of Counseling Psychology* 29 (1982): 551–559.

60. Glanz, "Dietitians' Effectiveness and Patient Compliance," 631.

61. N.R. Stewart et al., *Systematic Counseling* (Englewood Cliffs, NJ: Prentice-Hall, 1978), 54.

62. Mason et al., *Dynamics of Clinical Dietetics,* 108–109.

63. Mason et al., *Dynamics of Clinical Dietetics,* 124–126.

64. Mason et al., *Dynamics of Clinical Dietetics,* 110, 121.

65. D.E. Smith and R.R. Wing, "Diminished Weight Loss and Behavioral Compliance During Repeated Diets in Obese Patients with Type II Diabetes," *Health Psychology* 10 (1991): 378–383.

66. W.A. Sperduto et al., "The Effect of Target Behavior Monitoring on Weight Loss and Completion Rate in a Behavior Modification Program for Weight Reduction," *Addictive Behaviors* 11 (1986): 337–340.

67. M.L. Russell, *Behavioral Counseling in Medicine* (New York: Oxford University Press, 1986), 79, 116, 127.

68. W.H. Cormier and L.S. Cormier, *Interviewing Strategies for Helpers, Fundamental Skills and Cognitive Behavioral Intervention,* 2nd ed. (Monterey, CA: Brooks/Cole Publishing, 1985), 220–221.

69. Cormier and Cormier, *Interviewing Strategies for Helpers,* 296.

70. M.J. Mahoney and K. Mahoney, *Permanent Weight Control, A Solution to the Dieter's Dilemma* (New York: W.W. Norton & Company, 1976), 46–48.

71. M.J. Mahoney, *Strategies for Solving Personal Problems* (New York: W.W. Norton & Company, 1979), 85–101.

CHAPTER 2

Communication Skills

CHAPTER OBJECTIVES

1. List three characteristics necessary to perform optimum nutrition counseling.
2. Define the following three forms of nonverbal behavior: (a) kinesics, (b) paralinguistics, and (c) proxemics.
3. Apply appropriate responses to given client nonverbal behaviors.
4. Apply appropriate listening responses to given client statements.
5. Apply appropriate action responses to given client statements.
6. Apply appropriate sharing responses to given client statements.
7. Apply appropriate teaching responses to given client statements.

EFFECTIVE COUNSELOR-CLIENT RELATIONSHIPS

Communication skills form the foundation for nutrition counseling (Figure 2–1). To learn these skills, practitioners start not by examining their clientele but by looking at themselves. What characteristics should an effective nutrition counselor possess?

Personal Characteristics of Counselors

Ivey describes counseling as a process of facilitating another person's growth.[1] The way counselors respond to others can greatly influence how clients think and act in the future. The mere act of encouraging clients to talk as opposed to ignoring what they say may influence their lives greatly.

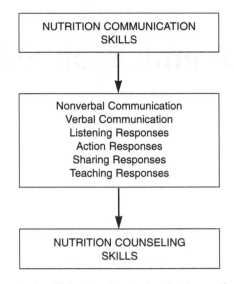

Figure 2–1 Communication Skills As a Foundation for Counseling

According to Russell, a good rapport between the nutrition counselor and client is essential to behavior change.[2] From the moment of initial contact, the nutrition counselor strives to develop an open, positive relationship in which the client senses the counselor's acceptance and understanding. To change their behavior, clients must feel comfortable freely relating intimate details of lifestyle to the counselor.

Cormier et al. suggest a variety of personal characteristics necessary to be an effective counselor.[3] Practitioners recognize intuitively that being understanding, conveying respect, and being themselves help create and maintain a more positively channeled session. The way they view themselves and their priorities, values, and expectations can alter the process positively or negatively.

Nelson-Jones describes some characteristics that helpers bring to a nutrition interview. Helpers come with motives, a learning history, thinking skills, capacity to feel, sense of worth, fears and anxieties, sexuality, gender role identity and expectations, values, ethics, culture and cross-cultural skills, race and racial attitudes and skills, and social class.[4]

Cormier and Cormier focus on three problems with self-image that can result in negative consequences during an interview: competence, power, and intimacy.[5] Counselors' attitudes can involve the concept of competence. Feelings of incompetence can lead to avoidance of controversial issues in counseling sessions. Nutrition counselors may be afraid to say that there are no direct or absolute answers to clients' questions. Counselors or clients may regard a truthful answer, such as "The evidence is not in at this time," as a sign of incompetence—the very trait the practitioners hope to avoid. Closely tied to feelings of incompetence are those of inadequacy, fear of failure, and fear of success. Counselors with these feelings unconsciously try to keep their negative self-images alive by using several behaviors. They may avoid positive interactions by negating positive feedback and making self-deprecating or apologetic comments. For example, an obese client who has lost weight says, "I really think you're a terrific counselor." A fearful counselor will reply, "Oh, no, I haven't done that much" instead of simply thanking the client for the compliment, "Thank you. Keep in mind you have done all of the work."

The second potential self-image problem, power, can make counselors feel both omnipotent and fearful of losing control or being weak or unresourceful. In the authoritarian role, counselors try to persuade clients to obey suggestions without question; practitioners dominate the content and direction of the interview, thinking, "I am in charge." If clients resist or do not respond, the outcome for counselors is resentment and anger. The weak and unresourceful counselor may occupy a subordinate role, complaining, "If you would just do as I say." On the other hand, the powerful practitioner tends to be dictatorial and overly silent; rarely participates in the interview; and, because of this aloof attitude, often loses credibility.

The third potential self-image problem focuses on feelings about intimacy. These can involve two extremes, affection and rejection. Counselors who are fearful of rejection try to elicit only positive feelings from clients, avoiding confrontation at all costs and ignoring negative cues. This type of counselor may even get involved in doing clients favors. Counselors who try to do everything for their clients may be eliminating independent problem solving. Practitioners at the opposite end of the spectrum try to ignore positive client feelings. They tend to act overly gruff and distant to avoid the closeness they fear. This type of counselor always tries to maintain the authoritarian role of "expert" to maintain distance. (Appendix A presents a counselor self-image checklist.)

Counselors As Growth Facilitators

One of the most crucial of all traits in nutrition counseling is the ability to facilitate growth—the art of helping clients achieve their goals and function on their own.

Ivey identifies four participants in an interview: the nutrition counselor and his or her cultural and historical background, and the client and his or her cultural and historical background.[6] For example, touching that is appropriate in many South American cultures represents an invasion of privacy among many North Americans. Concreteness is valued highly in North American culture but may be irrelevant to Asians, who communicate ideas more subtly. Facilitative counselors understand that the mode of being in the world differs among cultures.

As counselors see the world through their clients' eyes, they facilitate growth and provide concrete and specific strategies for behavior change. (See the segment on strategies in Chapter 3.)

Facilitative Levels

Researchers have delineated growth facilitative levels that counselors assume at various points in acquiring nutrition communication skills.[7] The levels below illustrate a gradual progression in the counselors' ability to respond appropriately to clients' problems.

- *Level 1:* The response shows no understanding and no direction in relation to the client's position. When the client brings up a crucial personal topic, the counselor starts talking about his or her own personal problems.
- *Level 2:* The response shows no understanding but some direction. The counselor presents only general advice: when the client expresses difficulty with a weight-loss strategy, the response is, "Well, don't worry about it."
- *Level 3:* The response shows understanding but no direction. The counselor might say, "You feel afraid because you're not sure how to avoid food offers from friends."
- *Level 4:* The response shows understanding and some direction. The counselor reacts to the client's deficits and provides details related to the problems: saying, "You feel afraid because you can't say 'no' and you want to avoid eating high-calorie foods."
- *Level 5:* The response shows understanding and specific direction. It contains the deficit, the goal, and one explicit step for overcoming the problem and reaching the objective: "You feel afraid because you can't say 'no' and you want to avoid eating high-calorie foods. How would you feel about exploring positive ways to say 'no'?

There are no perfect "super counselors" who have all the characteristics to make all sessions successful. Even positive characteristics may not always enhance the interview. Beyond personal characteristics that affect the sessions are the skills that require practice. When these skills are mastered, counseling takes on the characteristics necessary to achieve behavior change.

NONVERBAL COMMUNICATION

Client Nonverbal Behavior

Clients' nonverbal behavior can affect the direction of the interview. Effective counselors can identify nonverbal cues as signals for unspoken feelings.[8]

Cormier and Cormier describe three forms of client nonverbal behavior: kinesics, paralinguistics, and proxemics. Kinesics includes a variety of physical behaviors (e.g., facial expressions, body language). Paralinguistics refers to how the client's message is delivered (e.g., tone of voice). Proxemics involves environmental and personal space.[9] Appendix 2–A presents possible meanings associated with each behavior for each region of the body and a general category of autonomic responses. The table is designed to increase awareness of different behaviors; it is not intended to make all nutrition counselors experts on all client feelings. The effect or meaning of each nonverbal behavior varies from person to person and culture to culture.

Ivey contrasts nonverbal attending patterns in European-North American, middle-class culture with patterns of other cultures.[10] European-North American, middle-class cultures consider direct eye contact as a sign of interest. However, even in that culture, people often maintain more eye contact while listening and less while talking. When clients are uncomfortable about a topic, they may avoid eye contact. Some African Americans in the United States may have reverse patterns; they may look more when talking and slightly less when listening. Among some American Indian groups, eye contact by the young is a sign of disrespect. Some cultural groups (American Indian, Inuit, or Aboriginal Australian groups) avoid eye contact when talking about serious subjects.

Passons describes several ways of responding to nonverbal client behaviors "involving congruence, mixed messages, silence, changing cues, and refocusing for direction."[11] Nutrition counselors can use these suggestions to decide on a reply to client statements about dietary adherence.

- *Congruence.* Are the clients' nonverbal messages congruent with the verbal ones? An example might be the individual with diabetes who comes for the first follow-up interview. With furrowed brow, the client sends this confused message to the counselor: "How do I fill in this record? I have forgotten your directions." The counselor can make a mental note of the congruence in behaviors or ask the client to explain the meaning of the nonverbal conduct: "I noticed that your brow was furrowed. What does that mean?" The response could provide specific information on why the record was not completed. Was it too difficult? Did measuring the foods interfere with meal preparation for the family? Was the counselor's description of the information needed on the record unclear?
- *Mixed messages.* Is there a mixed message or discrepancy between the verbal and nonverbal messages? For example, a client comes in after having followed a no-added-salt eating pattern for several weeks and states, "It's going really [pause] well. I've had [pause] very few problems," while looking down and leaning away. The nutrition counselor can deal with these discrepancies

in one of three ways: (1) simply to take mental note; (2) to describe the discrepancy to the client, for example, "You say the diet is really going well and that there are few problems but you were looking down and really spoke with a lot of hesitation"; (3) to reply, "I noticed you looked away and paused as you said that. What does that mean?"

- *Silence.* Are there nonverbal behaviors with silence? Silence does not mean that nothing is happening. It can have different meanings from one culture to another. In some cultures silence denotes respect. Sue points out that for the Chinese and Japanese, silence means a desire to resume speaking after making a point. Once again the nutrition counselor can mentally note the silence, describe it to the client, or ask the client to explain it.[12]

- *Changing cues.* Is it necessary to distract or interrupt clients by focusing on nonverbal behavior? It may be needed to change the flow of the interview because continuation of the topic may be unproductive. If clients are pouring out a lot of information or rambling, a change in the direction of the interview may be useful. In such instances, nutrition counselors can distract clients from the verbal content by refocusing on nonverbal behavior. For example, for unproductive content in a client's messages, a counselor might say, "Our conversation so far has been dealing with your inability to cope with your spouse's unsupportive comments about your low-protein eating pattern. Are you aware that you have been gripping the sides of your chair with your hands while you speak?" Nutrition counselors must decide very carefully whether such distractions can be destructive or productive to the interview. If the change in flow makes the client feel unable to continue to air feelings, the distraction could be detrimental. Experienced counselors probably will find that their own intuition helps in knowing when to interrupt.

- *Refocusing for redirection.* Are there pronounced changes in the client's nonverbal behavior? Initially the client may sit with arms crossed, then become more relaxed, with arms unfolded and hands gesturing. Once again, counselors can respond either overtly or covertly. A nutrition counselor might respond to a seemingly more relaxed client by saying, "You seem more relaxed now. Do you feel less tense?"

Counselor Nonverbal Communication

The counselor's nonverbal communication can have a great impact on the relationship. Based on analogue research, Cormier and Cormier report that the nonverbal counselor behaviors that seem to be most important include expressions in the eyes and face, head nodding and smiles, body orientation and posture, some vocal cues, and physical distance between practitioners and clients.[13] Counselors can determine whether they are demonstrating desirable behaviors by asking someone to observe their nonverbal behaviors. Appendix B is a checklist that a third-party observer can mark while evaluating the counselor's nonverbal behavior. One word of caution: counselors should not try to apply these behaviors to themselves in a rigid way. Inflexible conformity can increase their tension in an interview, and clients will sense their nonverbal expression of that tension.

VERBAL COMMUNICATION

The counselor's knowledge and command of verbal skills can play an important part in directing the interview.

Conversational Style

Beginning counselors tend to fall into a kind of conversational mode that is very comfortable for them. Such a style is typical of a friendly chat with a neighbor. As a part of this conversation, they are under extreme pressure to provide an immediate solution for the client's problem.

Certain aspects of conversational style interfere with the objectives of counseling:[14]

- *Cocktail party "small talk":* Responding to a client at the beginning of an interview with, "Did you see the diet recipes in today's paper?"
- *Expressions of blame, criticism, or judgment: Client:* "The diet has gone badly this week." *Nutrition Counselor:* "I can certainly see that from this weight graph."
- *Expressions of advice offered in a preaching or self-righteous tone:* "You should really learn to have more self-control with this diet," or "You really ought to lose 20 pounds."
- *Expressions of sympathy in a patronizing tone:* "I really feel sorry for you. You seem to get absolutely no support from your family in following this diet," or "Now that you've told me your problems with weight loss, I'm sure I can make you feel better."
- *Threats or arguing:* "You'd better follow the low-protein eating pattern for your own good," or "I think your constant rejection of my suggestions is uncalled for."
- *Rigidity or inflexibility:* "There is only one right way to approach a low-cholesterol, fat-controlled eating pattern," or "Your suggestions won't work with a low-sodium diet."
- *Overanalyzing, overinterpreting, or intellectualizing:* "I think you find being overweight enjoyable, or you would follow the diet."

- *Several questions at once:* "How do you feel about following a low-cholesterol diet? Does it fit into your family life? If 'no,' why isn't it working out? Could you tell me?"
- *Extensive self-disclosure, sharing the counselor's own problems:* "I've been thinking a lot about my weight loss attempts as you were talking. I, too, have had several problems. For instance . . . ."

Each of these examples illustrates the importance of using appropriate communication skills during a session.

Counselor-Client Focus Identification

Once nutrition counselors have altered their conversational style appropriately, there are several specific ways they can learn to provide direction and focus for an interview. **Ivey delineates seven categories of subject focus:**

1. *Focus on the client:* "Laura, you sound upset. Could you tell me more about your feelings as you work to get your blood glucose levels in the 70–100 mg/dL range?"
2. *Focus on the main theme or problem:* "You had a terrible argument with your husband and then had a hypoglycemic reaction (encourager for discussion). Could you tell me about your symptoms before having a hypoglycemic reaction? (open question). Focusing on the person could lead the client to talk more about personal issues, whereas focusing on the main theme or problem encourages discussion of what happened and the facts of the situation. In both cases, listening skills combine with focusing to lead the client in very different directions. Which of the two alternatives is best? Both may be useful in obtaining a complete summary of the situation; at the same time, either could be overused.
3. *Focus on others:* This might include the husband or other people.
4. *Focus on family:* Many times client issues will relate to their families.
5. *Focus on mutual issues or group:* This focus involves the nutrition counselor and client relationship or the entire family.
6. *Focus on the nutrition counselor:* This focus includes self-disclosure or an "I" statement.
7. *Focus on cultural/environmental/contextual issues:* These are broader issues often not readily apparent, such as racial or sexual issues, family values, or economic trends. Example focus topics include issues of cultural identity, experiences of racism, sexism, or social class. Many clients also represent cultures of cancer survivors, people coping with other illnesses, or those suffering joblessness in a slow economy. People who experience issues such as these may manifest depression or other types of personal distress.[15]

In the North American culture, we are accustomed to making "I" statements and focusing on what an individual can do to help himself or herself. Counselors have to realize that this may clash with the world views of many minority people whose traditions focus on family. It may be hard for them to sever themselves from others in their family and just think of themselves. Their sense of self is often collective in nature, and their being may be authenticated mainly in terms of others. A balanced focus is needed between individual, family, and cultural expectations.

Lavelle suggests three areas of focus:[16]

1. affective focus
2. behavioral focus
3. cognitive focus

The verb "to feel" is used frequently when counselors want to focus affectively ("You are feeling very frustrated by your desire to follow the diet and your family's uncooperativeness."). Behavioral-focused sentences usually contain verbs such as "to do," "to act," or "to behave" ("What are you doing about this?"). A cognitive focus is revealed by such verbs as "to think" or "to tell oneself" ("What are you telling yourself when you eat the entire pie?").

The verb can be in the past, present, or future tense, which determines the time focus of the sentence. Too much focus on the past or future may indicate an avoidance of the present. An example might be this description of weight loss by one client. "My first husband was always supportive. My second husband wants me to be small but he always tempts me with high-calorie snacks. Still, he always talks about the future when I will be thin." This client is dwelling on both the past and the future but does not seem to recognize the importance of present goal setting.

The following examples show how verbal focusing might be used in response to a client who says: *"I'm having a conflict about wanting to lose weight but have no one at home who supports me when we eat out"*:

- *Client-Cognitive-Present Focus:* "You find yourself thinking about wanting to lose weight but also wanting to eat out with the family." In this response, the client-subject focus is reflected in "You find yourself," the cognitive focus by "thinking about," and the present time focus by the present tense of the verb "find."
- *Client-Affective-Present Focus:* "You're feeling concerned about wanting to lose weight and also wanting to eat out with your family."
- *Group-Behavioral-Future Focus:* "Perhaps this is an area we will explore together and see what you can do."
- *Problem-Cognitive-Present Focus:* "Losing weight is not always easy. When I think about it, there are lots of obstacles to try to overcome."

- *Cultural/Environmental-Cognitive/Behavioral-Past Focus:* "This is a conflict many weight-loss clients have faced because of the ideas our culture has given us about what people should eat in social situations."

LISTENING RESPONSES

Listening responses are the first step in forming a repertoire of communication skills involving clarifying, paraphrasing, reflecting, and summarizing.[17]

Clarifying

Clarification is posing a question, often after an ambiguous client message. Clarification may be used to make the previous message explicit and to confirm the accuracy of the counselor's perceptions of it. An example of incorrect use of clarification is:

> *Client:* "I wish I didn't have to fill in those diet records. They seem so silly to me."
> *Counselor:* "So, are you saying you don't like my diet aids?"
> *Client:* "I like all of them and the record has been useful, but I just don't feel as though it is helping me at this point."

In the next example, a statement of clarification establishes exactly what was said without relying on assumptions and inferences that are not confirmed or explored:

> *Client:* "I wish I didn't have to fill in those diet records. They seem so silly to me."
> *Counselor:* "Are you saying that you don't see any purpose to filling in the diet record?"
> *Client:* "No, I really don't. I just don't think I need them at this point."

Paraphrasing

Paraphrasing is restating or rephrasing the client's message in the counselor's own words. For example, the client says: "I don't mind eating low-protein foods at home, but my job requires that I travel one week of every month. It is impossible to follow the diet when eating in restaurants!" **In paraphrasing, counselors can:**

- Restate the message to themselves.
- Identify the content part of the message ("I don't mind eating low-protein foods at home," "My job requires one week of travel a month," "It is impossible to follow the diet when eating in restaurants").
- Translate the message into their own words. ("You can follow the diet at home but have problems following it in restaurants").

Reflecting

Reflection of feelings is used to rephrase the affective part of the message. This form of listening response has three purposes: (1) to encourage expression of more feelings, (2) to help clients experience feelings more intensely so they can become aware of unresolved problems, and (3) to help clients become more aware of feelings that dominate them.

For example, a client comments: *"I feel so depressed. Sometimes trying to match the foods I'm eating to insulin dosages seems useless."* In reply, counselors can:

- Restate the client's message to themselves.
- Identify the affective part of the message ("I feel so depressed").
- Translate the clients' affective words into their own words. ("You sometimes feel frustrated with following the eating pattern for your diabetes").

One word of caution: a reflection is more than just beginning a statement with the words "You feel . . . ." It is a reflecting back of the emotional part of the message with appropriate affect words. (Commonly used affect words are listed in Table 2–1.)

Summarizing

The fourth listening response, summarization, requires extending the paraphrase and reflection responses. It is a rather complex skill that includes paying

Table 2–1 Commonly Used Affect Words

Happiness	Sadness	Fear	Uncertainty	Anger
Happy	Discouraged	Scared	Puzzled	Upset
Pleased	Disappointed	Anxious	Confused	Frustrated
Satisfied	Hurt	Frightened	Unsure	Bothered
Glad	Despairing	Defensive	Uncertain	Annoyed
Optimistic	Depressed	Threatened	Skeptical	Irritated
Good	Disillusioned	Afraid	Doubtful	Resentful
Relaxed	Dismayed	Tense	Undecided	Mad
Content	Pessimistic	Nervous	Bewildered	Outraged
Cheerful	Miserable	Uptight	Mistrustful	Hassled
Thrilled	Unhappy	Uneasy	Insecure	Offended
Delighted	Hopeless	Worried	Bothered	Angry
Excited	Lonely	Panicked	Disoriented	Furious

Source: From *Interviewing Strategies for Helpers: Fundamental Skills and Cognitive Behavioral Interventions* by W.H. Cormier and L.S. Cormier. Copyright © 1991, 1985, and 1975 by Brooks/Cole Publishing Company, Pacific Grove, California 93950, a division of International Thomson Publishing Inc. By permission of the publisher.

attention to both content and feelings. It also includes elements of purpose, timing, and effect of the statements (process). Brammer recommends the following guidelines for summarization:

- Attend to major topics and emotions apparent as the client speaks.
- Summarize key ideas into broad statements.
- Do not add new ideas.
- Decide whether it is wise for you as a counselor to summarize or ask the client to summarize the broad themes, agreements, or plans.

To make this decision, counselors should review the purpose of the summarization:

- Was it to encourage the client at the beginning of the interview?
- Was it to bring scattered thoughts and feelings into focus?
- Was it to close the discussion on the major theme of the interview?
- Was it to check your understanding of the interview's progress?
- Was it to encourage the client to explore the basic theme of the interview more carefully?
- Was it to end the relationship with a progress summary?
- Was it to reassure the client that the interview was progressing well?[18]

Many summarization responses include references to both cognitive and affective messages:

> *Client:* "I want to follow the diet we discussed, but so many things pull me toward food—parties, friends, my family, etc. Above all this, though, I know I want to see my blood cholesterol come down."
>
> *Counselor:* "You feel torn. You want to reduce your blood cholesterol level, but sometimes you feel reluctant to avoid all of the people and things pulling you toward food" (summarization of emotion) or "You know that you do want to reduce your blood cholesterol level" (summarization of contents).

ACTION RESPONSES

The previous listening responses deal primarily with the client's message from the client's point of view. For nutrition counseling to progress, the process must move beyond the client's point of view to use of responses based on counselor-generated data and perceptions. These are counselor directed and are labeled *active responses*. They involve a combination of counselor perceptions and hypotheses, and client messages and behaviors.[19]

The purpose of active responses is to help clients recognize the need for change and positive action in solving nutrition problems. Active replies include probing, attributing, confronting, and interpreting responses.[20]

Probing

In nutrition counseling, an important part of gathering information on clients' eating patterns involves the art of probing. Probing can involve both open and closed questions.[21] Initially, it should be aimed at eliciting the most information possible. The clients should feel free to respond at length on any problem that may limit adherence to the eating pattern. The most direct way to probe is to ask open-ended questions that begin with "what," "when," "how," "where," "could," "why," or "who." Such questions require more than just "yes" or "no" responses. **Probing has a variety of purposes, including the following:**

- to begin an interview
- to encourage client elaboration or to obtain information
- to elicit specific examples of clients' nutrition-related behaviors, feelings, or thoughts
- to develop client commitment to communicate by inviting the client to talk and by providing guidance toward a focused interaction[22]

The first word of certain open questions can determine client responses. *What* questions most often lead to facts. "What happened?" "What are you going to do?" *How* questions often lead to a discussion about processes or sequences or to feelings. "How could that be explained?" "How do you feel about that?" *Why* questions most often lead to a discussion of reasons. "Why did you allow that to happen?" "Why do you think that is so?" *Could* questions are considered maximally open and contain some of the advantages of closed questions in that the client is free to say "No, I don't want to talk about . . . ." Could questions reflect less control and command than others. "Could you tell me more about your situation?" "Could you give me a specific example?" "Could you tell me what you'd like to talk about today?"[23]

Once the clients have provided adequate information for assessment of the nutrition problem, counselors can help focus attention on central issues by using closed questions.[24] When the clients then have a focus on which to concentrate, open invitations to talk may be used again. In becoming skilled interviewers, counselors learn to use a balance of open and closed questions. Various types of interviews use different proportions of open and closed questions.

An example of the use of open-ended probes follows:

> *Client* (a 25-year-old male who is trying to follow a 20 percent fat eating pattern): "I really have problems getting my wife to cook low-fat

meals. She says she wants to cook the way her mother taught her. I feel really frustrated about everything."

Counselor: "What else do you think or feel frustrated about?" "How long have you been feeling this way?" "When are some specific times you feel frustrated?" "Who are you with when you feel frustrated?" "What do you do when you feel frustrated?"

Counselors should keep in mind that extensive self-disclosure requests can be damaging to clients. Janis reports that seeking high self-disclosure or asking clients about material they would not usually share with other family members or friends has a detrimental effect on adherence to diet.[25] Asking the client personal questions about current and past sorrows, sex life, guilt feelings, secret longings, and similar private events can result in the client's becoming demoralized despite the counselor's positive comments and acceptance. In contrast, moderate levels of questions about feelings that focus on strengths as well as weaknesses enhance dietary adherence.[26]

After the client has discussed at length several specific frustrating instances, **the counselor can focus the interview with closed probes such as:**

- "Is your wife aware that you feel frustrated in these situations?"
- "Have you spoken to your wife about these frustrating instances?"
- "Can you speak with your wife about these problem situations?"
- "Do you see any solutions to this particular frustration?"

Attributing

Attributing responses point to the client's current potential for being successful in a designated activity. This response has several purposes:

- to encourage the client who lacks initiative or self-confidence to do something
- to expand the client's awareness of personal strength
- to point out a potentially helpful client action[27]

In deciding whether to use this response, counselors focus on inferring how the client will react. Will the attributing response "reinforce the client's action-seeking behavior or the client's feelings of inadequacy?"[28] This response is facilitative only when there is a basis for recognizing the client's ability to pursue a desired action. It is not simply a pep talk to smooth over or discount true feelings of discouragement. Feelings should be reflected and clarified first. Finally, the attributing response should be used when the client is ready for action but seems hesitant to initiate a step without some encouragement. **An example of an attributing response is as follows:**

Client (a 30-year-old woman who has tried repeatedly to lose weight): "I'm really discouraged with trying to lose weight at this point. I feel like I can't do anything right. Not only has it affected me personally but now it is affecting my family. I just don't feel I can do anything right."
Counselor: "Although you feel discouraged with weight loss right now, you still have those personal qualities you had when you lost weight before."

Confronting

Ivey describes confrontation as a complex of skills resulting in a client's examination of core issues. It may be contained in a paraphrase ("You want to see good blood sugars, but you hate watching the amount of foods you eat at parties"), a reflection of feeling ("On the one hand you are angry about having a disease that forces you to watch what you eat, but on the other hand you are grateful that following an eating pattern can improve your blood sugars"), or any other skills. When client discrepancies, mixed messages, and conflicts are confronted skillfully and nonjudgmentally, clients are encouraged to talk in more detail and resolve problems.[29]

A confronting response can be a descriptive statement of the client's mixed messages or an identification of an alternate view or perception of something the individual distorts. There are two intended purposes behind a confronting response: to identify the client's mixed or distorted messages and to explore other ways of perceiving the client's self or situation.[30]

Confronting responses can have very powerful effects. Counselors should keep several basic rules in mind before using them:

- Make the confronting response a description instead of a judgment or evaluation of the client's message or behavior.
- Cite specific examples of the behavior rather than making vague inferences.
- Prior to confronting the client, build rapport and trust.
- Offer the confrontation when the client is most likely to accept it.
- Do not overload the client with confrontations that make heavy demands in a short time.[31]

The timing of a confronting response is important. A confrontation should always take place at a time when clients do not feel threatened, not when it is totally unexpected. Adequate time for talking and listening should be provided in the interview.

Counselors' feelings also are important. Johnson clearly emphasizes confronting clients only if the practitioners are genuinely interested in improving the relationship,[32] never with the idea of punishing or criticizing clients. Before confronting, counselors should try to list their reasons for wanting to challenge discrepancies, distortions, or unproductive behaviors. Exhibit 2–1 describes eight components of effective confrontation by counselors.[33]

Clients' reactions to a confrontation vary. Ivey describes five types of reactions.

1. *Denial.* The client may deny that an incongruity or mixed message exists or fail to hear that it is there. ("I'm not angry about having to change my fat intake. I do feel deprived, but definitely not angry.")
2. *Partial examination.* The individual may work on a part of the discrepancy but fail to consider the other dimensions of the mixed message. ("Yes, I feel deprived. Perhaps I should be angry, but I can't really feel it.")
3. *Acceptance and recognition, but no change.* The client may engage the confrontation fairly completely, but make no resolution. Much of counseling operates at this level or at level 2. Until the client can examine incongruity, immobility, and mixed messages accurately, developmental change will be difficult. ("I guess I do have mixed feelings about it. I certainly miss eating spontaneously. It makes me angry and I ask why I have to deal with this at a time when I want to do whatever I feel like doing.")
4. *Generation of a new solution.* The client moves beyond recognition of the incongruity and puts things together in a new and productive way. ("Yes, you've got it. I've been avoiding my deep feelings of anger, and I think it's getting in my way. If I'm going to move on, I'll have to allow myself to admit that I am angry.")
5. *Development of new, larger, and more inclusive constructs, patterns, or behaviors—transcendence.* A confrontation is most successful when the client recognizes the discrepancy, works on it, and generates new thought patterns or behaviors to cope with and perhaps resolve the incongruity. ("I like the plan we've worked out. You've helped me see that mixed feelings and thoughts are part of every change situation.")[34]

If clients seem confused about the meaning of the confrontation, the counselors may not have been specific or concise enough; or confessed lack of understanding may be a way of avoiding the impact of the confrontation.

Sometimes clients may seem to accept the confrontation. If they show a sincere desire to change behavior, their acceptance probably is genuine. However, they may agree verbally with the counselors but, instead of pursuing the confrontation, may do so only to entice practitioners not to discuss the topic in the future.

There is no defined way to deal with negative reactions to a confrontation, but the components of effective confrontation (Exhibit 2–1) can be used to repeat the relationship statement or describe the counselor's own feelings and perceptions. The sequence might go like this:

Exhibit 2–1 Components of Effective Confrontation

1. *Personal statements:* These opening statements usually begin with the pronoun "I." Included in this statement are expressions of feelings, attitudes, or opinions. Examples are:
   "I need to talk to you."
   "There is something I've been hearing over and over in our conversation that I would like to speak to you about."
   "I have been confused during this session by something you've been saying."

2. *Relationship statements:* Define your relationship with the other person. An example is:
   "Lately we've been trying to work together to come up with some possible solutions to your binge eating."

3. *Description of behavior:* A description of a specific behavior would include specific time and place of occurrence. An example is:
   "From your description, binge eating occurs on weekends during parties."

4. *Descriptions of your feelings and interpretations of the client's situation:* An example: "I am confused when you say that you want to stop eating at parties but you feel compelled to continue because of social pressure. There seem to be two messages here."

5. *Understanding response:* This to be sure that what you have said is what the client has understood.
   Counselor: "Do you see what I mean?" "Is this the way you see things?"
   Client: "Yes."

6. *Perception check:* This is stated as a question to the client to double-check thoughts and feelings at this point.
   Counselor: "How do you feel about what I am saying?"
   Client: "I can see that I seem to be giving a mixed message. I want to lose weight but there are always obstacles when I go to parties. Friends always ask me to eat; I feel compelled to say 'Yes'."

7. *Interpretive response:* This is a paraphrase of what the client said in 5 and 6. An example is:
   "From what you have said, you seem to feel this same confusion. You want to lose weight but there is always someone pushing you to eat to be sociable."

8. *Constructive feedback:* This component of confrontation calls for working together for a solution. Alternatives are presented and weighed. The counselor, at this point, should allow the client to make suggestions on how to solve the problem. Examples are:
   "Can you think of a solution?"
   "This might be one solution. What else can we come up with?"
   "I'd like to talk about it again after we've thought about it for a while."

Source: From David W. Johnson, *Reaching Out: Interpersonal Effectiveness and Self-Actualization.* Copyright © 1972 by Allyn and Bacon. Adapted with permission.

Counselor: "Both of our goals are to help eliminate binge eating at parties." (relationship statement)

Client: "Actually I'm not sure I can ever achieve that, even though I do want to lose weight." (mixed message)

Counselor: "You say you want to lose weight but one of the major causes is too difficult to overcome." (description of counselor feelings and perceptions)

Client: "No, I guess you just don't understand. You've never been in my shoes." (discredit the counselor)

Counselor: "Because I've never been in your shoes doesn't mean we can't work on a solution together. I have had experience with many cases like yours. You seem to exhibit many qualities that show me that you can handle this problem." (attributing statement) "You are open about the difficulties you face and can describe specific instances where problems occur." (attributing statement) "Let's look at those specifics and try to come up with some solutions." (constructive feedback)

Ivey indicates that an overly confronting, charismatic counselor can prevent client growth.[35] In a confrontation, the counselor tries to point out discrepancies in attitudes, thoughts, or behaviors. Clients who come to nutrition counselors for help invariably give double messages: "I want to follow this diet, but I don't want to change my life to do it." Because almost all clients either overtly or covertly make this statement, confrontation becomes an important skill for nutrition counselors in facilitating behavior change.

Confrontation must be used with great sensitivity to individual and cultural differences. Within the United States and Canada, there are a variety of cultures and peoples who may object to strong confrontations. In regard to Native American, Canadian Inuit, and traditional Latina/Latino people, confrontational statements may not be helpful, particularly in the early stages of the helping process. Moreover, any individual who is particularly sensitive may prefer softer, more indirect confrontations.

Keeping caution in mind, any time the counselor can encourage clients to confront themselves and think about situations in new ways, the counselor can greatly facilitate growth. Some clients respond best to direct, assertive confrontations. Again, flexibility and the counselor's ability to respond to the unique person is essential.

Interpreting

An interpreting response is an active reply that gives a possible explanation of or association among various client behaviors. **It has three intended purposes:**

1. to identify the relationship between the client's behavior and nonverbal messages
2. to examine the client's behavior using a variety of views or different explanations
3. to help the client gain self-understanding as a basis for behavior change or action

There are several specific ground rules for interpreting responses.[36] Counselors must be careful about timing, and clients should demonstrate some degree of readiness for self-exploration or self-examination before an interpreting response is used. This response is best given at the beginning or middle phase of an interview so both the counselor and client have sufficient time to work through the client's reaction. It is important for the counselor's interpretation to be based on the client's actual message. Practitioners must eliminate their own biases and values and offer the interpretive response tentatively, using such words as, "I wonder if," "It's possible that," "Perhaps," or "Maybe." Finally, counselors ask clients whether the message is accurate.

Brammer offers these guidelines for counselors in interpreting responses:

- Look for the client's basic message.
- Paraphrase the message to the client.
- Add your own understanding of what the message means (motive, defense, needs, style, etc.).
- Keep the language simple and the level close to the client's message.
- Indicate that you are offering tentative ideas.
- Elicit the client's reactions to your interpretations.[37]

Ivey describes the interpreting response as a part of the essence of what the clients have said (emotionally and intellectually) and as a summary that adds other relevant data.[38] An interpreting response provides the client with a new way to view the situation. Such a change in view may result in changes in thoughts and behaviors.

The following is an interpreting response:

> *Client* (an overweight middle-aged man): "I'm really discouraged with this dieting. I am at the point where I feel like I can't win. I've been to doctors and weight-loss groups. I've taken diet pills. It's at the point where I can't think straight at work because my thoughts are always on dieting. I feel very depressed."
>
> *Counselor:* "I wonder if you're allowing your preoccupation with weight loss to interfere with your ability to cope?" (This interpreting response makes an association between the client's desire to lose weight and resulting feelings and behavior.)

Or: "Is it possible that you're trying to find an easy, magic way to lose weight when that solution may not exist?" (This interpreting response offers a possible explanation of the client's weight-loss behaviors.)

The interpreting response can be a powerful influencer for clients who are locked into feelings of failure. It is a core skill that is vital to encouraging behavior change.

SHARING RESPONSES

The sharing responses involve counselor self-expression and content that refers to the practitioner, the client, or the emotions of either one. Counselors can use two sharing responses: self-disclosure and immediacy.

Self-Disclosure

Self-disclosure is a response in which counselors verbally share information about themselves. Cormier and Cormier describe four purposes:

1. to provide an open, facilitative counseling atmosphere
2. to increase the client's perceived similarity between self and the counselor to reduce the distance resulting from role differences
3. to provide a model to assist in increasing the client's disclosure level
4. to influence the client's perceived or actual behavioral changes[39]

There are several basic ideas to keep in mind before using self-disclosure. First, self-disclosure is a controversial communication skill. Cormier, Cormier, and Weisser caution that if the counselor's beliefs differ significantly from the client's on a given issue, it is probably better for the counselor to remain silent.[40]

Ivey states that extensive self-disclosures take the focus away from the client and should be avoided but that moderate levels of self-disclosure help show clients how they come across to others. For example, "Oh, I really have trouble resisting desserts, too. It's tough isn't it? But I figure it's worth it to resist them and work toward a normal weight."[41]

Moderate levels of self-disclosure help establish a basis for similarity and enhance interpersonal influence. Counselors who rarely self-disclose may add to the distance between themselves and their clients. Self-disclosing statements should be similar in content and mood to the clients' message. Self-disclosure can be demographic, personal, positive, or negative.

In demographic disclosures, counselors talk about nonintimate events. For example:

"I have had some failures in low-cholesterol meal preparation, also."
"I have not always used good self-control skills in following a balanced diet."

In personal disclosures, counselors reveal private personal events. For example:

"Well, I don't always feel loving toward my husband (wife), especially when he (she) is unsupportive of my efforts in meal preparation."

"I think it is very natural to want to please close friends. There are times when I've accepted food at parties when I really didn't want it, but I cared so much about the person offering it that I couldn't say 'No.'"

In positive self-disclosure, counselors reveal positive strengths, coping skills, or positive successful experiences. For example:

"I'm really a task-oriented person. When I decide what must be done, I work until the task is completed."

"It's important to be as open with my husband (wife) as possible. When he (she) upsets me, I try to tell him (her) honestly exactly how I feel."

In negative self-disclosure, counselors provide information about personal limitations or difficult experiences. For example:

"I also have trouble expressing opinions, I guess I am wishy-washy some of the time."

"Sometimes I'm also afraid to tell my husband (wife) how I really feel. Then my frustration builds to a climax and I just explode."

Ivey lists three key dimensions of self-disclosure:

1. *Personal pronouns.* A counselor self-disclosure inevitably involves "I" statements or self-reference using the pronouns *I, me,* and *my.*
2. *Verb for content or feeling or both.* "I think . . . ," "I feel . . . ," and "I have experienced . . . " all indicate some action on the part of the counselor.
3. *Object coupled with adverb and adjective descriptors.* "I feel happy about your being able to assert yourself more directly in restaurants." "My experience with asserting myself in restaurants was similar to yours."[42]

Two examples of self-disclosure can apply to the same situation: the client is feeling like a failure because no one supports weight loss. The counselor responds:

"I, too, have felt down about myself at times."

"I can remember feeling depressed when everyone seemed to take lightly something that was important to me, like eating a favorite dish at my favorite restaurant."

Immediacy

The second sharing response, immediacy, involves the counselor's reflections on a present aspect of a thought or feeling about self, clients, or a significant relationship issue. The verbal expression of immediacy may include the listening responses of reflection and summation, the active responses of confrontation and interpretation, or the sharing response of self-disclosure. **Examples of the three categories of immediacy are:**

1. *Counselor immediacy:* The counselor reveals personal thoughts of immediacy at the moment they occur: "It's good to see you again;" or "I'm sorry I didn't follow that. I seem to have trouble focusing today. Let's go over that again."
2. *Client immediacy:* The counselor states something about the client's behavior or feeling as it occurs in the interview: "You seem uncomfortable now;" or "You're really smiling now. You must be very pleased."
3. *Relationship immediacy:* The counselor reveals personal feelings or thoughts about experiencing the relationship: "I'm glad that you are able to share those feelings you have about following the diet with me;" or "It makes me feel good that we've been able to resolve some of the problems with your diet."

Immediacy has two purposes: (1) it can bring expressed feelings or unresolved relationship issues into the open for discussion, and (2) it can provide immediate feedback about the counselor's and client's feelings and aspects of the relationship as they occur in the session. When making an immediacy response, counselors should (1) describe what they see as it happens, (2) reflect the "here and now" of the experience, and (3) reserve this response for initiating exploration of the most significant or most influential feelings or issues.

TEACHING RESPONSES

Much of nutrition counselors' work involves teaching clients how to change eating behaviors. Change means clients learn new ways to deal with themselves, others, or environmental situations. Counselors may teach new eating behaviors, new awareness or new perceptions of past and present behaviors, or how clients can teach themselves. Three verbal responses associated with teaching and learning can give structure to what ordinarily might be haphazard teaching: instructions, verbal setting operations, and information giving.[43]

Instructions

Instructions involve one or more statements in which the counselors tell clients what changes in current intake are necessary to achieve new eating behaviors, how new eating behaviors might occur, and what the allowable limits are. When using instruction responses, counselors instruct, direct, or cue the clients to do something. Instructions may deal with what should happen within or outside the interview and can be both informing and influential. Instructions have two main purposes: (1) to influence or give cues to help clients respond in a certain way, and (2) to provide information necessary to acquire, strengthen, or eliminate a response.

After giving instructions, counselors should ascertain whether the clients really understand the directions. Clients are asked to repeat what was said to help the counselors know whether they communicated the message accurately. The counselors then ask clients to use the instructions.

Instructions can be worded in many ways. "You should do something" is likely to put a client on the defensive. It is too demanding. More useful words are "I'd like you to," "I'd appreciate it," or "I think it would help if." Clients are more likely to follow instructions that are linked to positive or rewarding consequences.

Verbal Setting Operation

The second teaching response, the verbal setting operation, attempts to predispose someone to view a situation or an event in a certain way before it takes place. This response includes a statement describing a treatment and the potential value of counseling and/or treatment for clients. The purposes of verbal setting operations are to motivate clients to understand the purpose of and to use counseling and/or treatment.

Goldstein suggests that some initial counseling structure may prevent negative feelings in clients that result from lack of information about what to expect.[44] Initial structuring should focus upon and clarify counselor and client role expectations. This type of structuring should be detailed, deliberate, and repeated.

The following are examples of verbal setting operations:

- *To provide an overview of nutrition counseling,* the counselor says: "I believe it would be helpful if I first talked about what nutrition involves. We will spend some time talking together to find out first the kinds of nutrition concerns you have and what you want to do about them. Then we will work as a team to identify solutions for each concern. Sometimes I may ask you to do some things on your own outside the session."
- *To discuss the purpose of nutrition counseling,* the counselor says: "These sessions may help you change eating behaviors to achieve weight loss. The action plans you'll carry out, with my assistance, can help you learn to eat wisely in situations that may be of concern to you."
- *To check the client's understanding of nutrition counseling,* the counselor asks: "How does this fit with your expectations?"

Information Giving

Much of the nutrition counselor's responsibility involves the third teaching response, information giving. Below are specific guidelines to follow when giving information:

- Identify information presently available to client.
- Evaluate client's present information. Is it valid? Are databases sufficient? Insufficient?

The following guidelines can be used in determining what information to give:

- Identify the kind of information useful to the client.
- Identify possible reliable sources of information.
- Identify any preferred sequencing of information (i.e., option A before option B).

The following guidelines indicate how to deliver information:

- Limit the amount of information given at one time.
- Ask for and discuss client's feelings and biases about information.
- Know when to stop giving information so action is not avoided.
- Wait for the client's cue of readiness for additional information after providing a large group of facts.
- Present all relevant facts; don't protect client from negative information.
- Be specific, clear, detailed, concrete, and simple in communicating and giving instructions.
- Organize the material. Information given in the first third of communication is remembered longer. The first instruction given is usually remembered the longest.
- Provide advanced organizers (For example, "First, we will look at your current eating habits. Second, you will describe the changes you might make in the types of foods you currently eat.").
- Repeat important information.
- Use concrete illustrations, anecdotes, and self-disclosure to heighten the personal relevance of the material.
- Use oral and written material together. Supplement with slides, audiotapes, videotapes, films, anatomical models, diagrams, charts, and other aids.
- Check the client's comprehension, asking for a restatement of key features of a message.
- Involve significant others.[45-52]

Table 2–2 presents examples of information giving both inside and outside a nutrition counseling session.

Table 2–2 Aspects of Information Giving

Counselor's Instructions	In the Interview	Outside the Interview
What to do	"Please repeat what I have asked you to do in responding to your husband's (wife's) nonsupportiveness toward your diet. I want to be sure I am communicating the request accurately."	"Please keep a record of your thoughts before your conversations with your husband (wife)."
How to do	"When you say this, pretend that I am your husband (wife). Look at me and maintain eye contact while you say it."	"Write your thoughts down on a note card and bring them in next week."
Allowable limits	"Say it in a strong, firm voice. Don't speak in a soft, weak voice. Look at me while you say it."	"Remember to record these thoughts before, not after, you speak."

CHOOSING THE APPROPRIATE RESPONSE

One of the most important processes in counseling involves deciding when to use the responses just described. Steps toward determining appropriate responses include: (1) identification of the purposes of the interview and of the counselor responses and (2) assessment of the effects of the selected replies and strategies on client answers and outcomes. When one response or strategy does not achieve its intended purpose, the counselor can use discrimination to identify and select another that is more likely to achieve the desired results or focus.

Cormier and Cormier describe three parts of an interview that can be used in determining which responses or strategies to select:

1. Counselor identifies purposes of the interview and responses.
2. Counselor selects and implements the response.
3. Counselor determines if resulting client verbal and nonverbal responses achieve the purpose or distract from the purpose.[53]

These authors also describe a step-by-step process for counselors in conducting an effective interview:

1. Define the purpose of the interview.
2. Define the purpose of your initial response.

3. Make your initial response.
4. Identify client verbal and nonverbal responses.
5. Label those client responses as goal related or distracting.
6. Set a plan for the next response.[54]

The nutrition counselor's first step is to listen carefully to each of the client's statements. The counselor must think about whether each statement is related to or distracts from the purpose of the interview. Having made this determination, the counselor can select and use responses he or she believes will achieve the objective. If client responses are goal related, practitioners may decide that their own replies and comments are on target; however, if they note several statements that are distracting, it may be necessary to analyze what they have been saying.

For example, one of the major goals of a counseling session may be to identify steps to help change eating behaviors in an overweight adult male. The counselor has suggested cutting down on midmorning snacking by switching from high-calorie snack foods that are low in nutrients to low-calorie, high-nutrient foods. The client indicates that this change will not work for him. After determining that this is a distracting client response, the practitioner will need to formulate and use an alternate response, perhaps a new action step. Regardless of what that next response is, the important point is that the counselor can identify a purpose or direction, assess whether the client's answers are related to that goal, and select alternative replies with a rationale in mind. Counselors should make these assessments cognitively. This step-by-step procedure should be used in thinking through an interview.

What follows is an example of how those steps might apply in a nutrition counseling session, in which the purpose of the interview is to listen to the client (a 26-year-old woman) describe factors contributing to her inability to lose weight over the past two years.

> *Counselor:* "According to your chart, Dr. B. sent you to see me again today. He writes here that you've been trying to lose weight and need some help in determining what factors have contributed to the lack of weight loss. Is that correct?" (The purpose of the initial response is to double-check the client's rationale for attending the interview.)
>
> *Client* (fidgeting): "Well, that's true. Sometimes I think that all I have to do is to look at food and I gain weight."
>
> (Counselor thinks: The client admits that she has a weight problem (indirectly). She seems to be discounting the contributing factors (distracting response). In frustration, she tries to absolve herself from blame by attributing her problem to some unknown phenomenon that makes her gain weight at the very sight of food. For my next response I will check her thoughts as to her control over the weight gain.)

Counselor: "From what you have said you seem to think that your weight gain is out of your control. How well does that describe what you are thinking?"

Client: "Well, sometimes I feel that way but I suppose I do have some control."

(Counselor thinks: Okay, the client is now admitting to having some control. I will focus next on areas where she may feel she has some control.)

Counselor: "What are some areas related to your weight gain that you do feel you can control?"

Client: "Well, I guess I could just stop buying groceries."

(Counselor thinks: She either did not understand my question or she is feeling defensive about having to discuss situations where she might have control but doesn't exercise the option. My next response will focus on the idea of shopping and I will give her some examples using a self-disclosing response.)

Counselor: "Well, sometimes when I go shopping and I'm very hungry, I tend to buy more food and high-calorie snacks."

Client (voice pitch goes up, tone gets louder): "How would you know what it's like to go shopping and want foods you shouldn't have? You're not overweight."

(Counselor thinks: My example seemed to make the client avoid the issue of contributing factors even more. She seems to have built up a great deal of frustration. Perhaps exploring her feelings about grocery buying might give me some clues. I will respond to her question and then direct the focus to her concern about buying groceries.)

Counselor: "I really can't know what it's like to be in your shoes. I can only express a situation similar to yours that I have been in. I guess buying groceries is a very important concern for you because it is tied so closely to your desire to lose weight. What feelings do you have while you're shopping?"

Client (loud voice): "I feel like a child in a candy store. Here is everything I love, everything that gives me pleasure, but I am forbidden to touch any of it. Then my kids and my husband are saying, 'Oh, go on honey (or mom) buy it; we love it. We shouldn't have to suffer just because you don't have any willpower.'"

(Counselor thinks: That's the most verbal she has been. It's the first indication that she is willing to explore the situation. It seems that one of the factors contributing to her lack of ability to lose weight is her nonsupportive husband and children. I might check this theory out further.)

Counselor: "Are you saying that your family really doesn't give you a lot of support in losing weight?"

Client: "Yes. Being overweight is bad enough but, when your own family gives you no support, losing weight is almost impossible."

(Counselor thinks: The client seems to feel very strongly about this lack of family support. I will try to get at how this affects the way she feels in specific situations where nonsupport is apparent.)

Counselor: "Having your family respond negatively when you try to buy low-calorie foods and avoid high-calorie snacks seems to make you feel very frustrated. You would like them to praise your efforts. I guess having your family reject your efforts at weight loss may affect the way you see yourself, too."

Client (avoids eye contact): "What do you mean?"

(Counselor thinks: From the lack of eye contact and the client's verbal message, I believe either my response was unclear or she isn't ready to look at her self-image yet. I will approach this indirectly by asking her to describe some situations in which she has felt frustrated by lack of support from her family.)

Counselor: "Well, I'm not sure. Maybe you could tell me exactly what happens in a situation where your family is nonsupportive."

At this point the interview enters the area where additional counseling skills are necessary. Chapter 3 discusses those skills and how they can help nutrition counselors in formulating plans and applying strategies during interviews.

NOTES

1. A.E. Ivey, *Intentional Interviewing and Counseling: Facilitating Client Development in a Multicultural Society,* 3rd ed. (Pacific Grove, CA: Brooks/Cole Publishing, 1994), 9.

2. M.L. Russell, *Behavioral Counseling in Medicine: Strategies for Modifying At-Risk Behavior* (New York: Oxford University Press, 1986), 37.

3. W.H. Cormier et al., *Interviewing and Helping Skills for Health Professionals* (Belmont, CA: Wadsworth Health Sciences Division, 1984), 41–42.

4. R. Nelson-Jones, *Lifeskills Helping: Helping Others Through a Systematic People Centered Approach* (Pacific Grove, CA: Brooks/Cole Publishing, 1993), 67.

5. W H. Cormier and L.S. Cormier, *Interviewing Strategies for Helpers: Fundamental Skills and Cognitive Behavioral Interventions,* 2nd ed. (Monterey, CA: Brooks/Cole Publishing, 1985), 13–14.

6. Ivey, *Intentional Interviewing and Counseling,* 11–12.

7. R.R. Carkhuff and R.M. Pierce, *The Art of Helping: Trainer's Guide* (Amherst, MA: Human Resources Development Press, 1975), 178–182.

8. G. Egan, *The Skilled Helper: A Problem Management Approach to Helping* (Pacific Grove, CA: Brooks/Cole Publishing, 1994), 93.

9. Cormier and Cormier, *Interviewing Strategies for Helpers: Fundamental Skills and Cognitive Behavioral Interventions,* 67–78.

10. Ivey, *Intentional Interviewing and Counseling,* 29.

11. W.R. Passons, *Gestalt Approaches in Counseling* (New York: Rinehart and Winston, 1975), 103–105.

12. D.W. Sue, "Culture Specific Strategies in Counseling: A Conceptual Framework," *Professional Psychology: Research and Practice* 21, no. 6 (1990): 426.

13. Cormier and Cormier, *Interviewing Strategies for Helpers: Fundamental Skills and Cognitive Behavioral Interventions,* 81–83.

14. W.H. Cormier and L.S. Cormier, *Interviewing Strategies for Helpers: A Guide to Assessment, Treatment and Evaluation* (Monterey, CA: Brooks/Cole Publishing, 1979), 50.

15. Ivey, *Intentional Interviewing and Counseling,* 216.

16. J.J. Lavelle, "Comparing the Effects of an Affective and a Behavioral Counselor Style on Client Interview Behavior," *Journal of Counseling Psychology* 24 (1977): 174.

17. L.M. Brammer, *Helping Relationship Process and Skills* (Englewood Cliffs, NJ: Prentice-Hall, 1985), 26–34.

18. Brammer, *Helping Relationship Process and Skills,* 26–34.

19. Cormier and Cormier, *Interviewing Strategies for Helpers: Fundamental Skills and Cognitive Behavioral Interventions,* 113.

20. Cormier and Cormier, *Interviewing Strategies for Helpers: A Guide to Assessment, Treatment and Evaluation,* 79.

21. Ivey, *Intentional Interviewing and Counseling,* 49.

22. Cormier and Cormier, *Interviewing Strategies for Helpers: Fundamental Skills and Cognitive Behavioral Interventions,* 115.

23. Ivey, *Intentional Interviewing and Counseling,* 56.

24. Ivey, *Intentional Interviewing and Counseling,* 56.

25. I.L. Janis, "Improving Adherence to Medical Recommendations: Prescriptive Hypotheses Derived from Recent Research in Social Psychology," in *Handbook of Psychology and Health, Vol. 4, Social Psychology of Aspects of Health,* ed. A. Baum et al. (Hillsdale, NJ: Erlbaum, 1984), 113–148.

26. M.R. DiMatteo and C.C. DiNicola, *Achieving Patient Compliance: The Psychology of the Medical Practitioner's Role* (New York: Pergamon Press, 1982), 107.

27. Cormier and Cormier, *Interviewing Strategies for Helpers: A Guide to Assessment, Treatment and Evaluation,* 80.

28. Cormier and Cormier, *Interviewing Strategies for Helpers: A Guide to Assessment, Treatment and Evaluation,* 81.

29. Ivey, *Intentional Interviewing and Counseling,* 190.

30. Cormier and Cormier, *Interviewing Strategies for Helpers: Fundamental Skills and Cognitive Behavioral Interventions,* 118.

31. Cormier and Cormier, *Interviewing Strategies for Helpers: Fundamental Skills and Cognitive Behavioral Interventions,* 120–121.

32. D.W. Johnson, *Reaching Out: Interpersonal Effectiveness and Self-Actualization* (Englewood Cliffs, NJ: Prentice-Hall, 1972), 159–172.

33. Johnson, *Reaching Out: Interpersonal Effectiveness and Self-Actualization,* 165.

34. Ivey, *Intentional Interviewing and Counseling*, 201.

35. Ivey, *Intentional Interviewing and Counseling*, 95.

36. Cormier and Cormier, *Interviewing Strategies for Helpers: Fundamental Skills and Cognitive Behavioral Interventions*, 127.

37. Brammer, *Helping Relationship, Process and Skills*, 94–95.

38. Ivey, *Intentional Interviewing and Counseling*, 287–291.

39. Cormier and Cormier, *Interviewing Strategies for Helpers: Fundamental Skills and Cognitive Behavioral Interventions,* 29.

40. Cormier et al., *Helping Skills for Health Professionals*, 41.

41. Ivey, *Intentional Interviewing and Counseling*, 280–281.

42. Ivey, *Intentional Interviewing and Counseling,* 280.

43. Cormier and Cormier, *Interviewing Strategies for Helpers: A Guide to Assessment, Treatment and Evaluation*, 101.

44. A.P. Goldstein, "Relationship-Enhancement Methods," in *Helping People Change,* ed. F.H. Kanfer. (New York: Pergamon Press, 1975), 18.

45. J. Warpeha and J. Harris, "Combining Traditional and Nontraditional Approaches to Nutrition Counseling," *Journal of the American Dietetic Association* 93 (1993): 797.

46. T.T. Baldwin and G.A. Falciglia, "Application of Cognitive Behavioral Theories to Dietary Change in Clients," *Journal of the American Dietetic Association* 95 (1995): 1315–1316.

47. J.M. Johnson et al., "Comparison of Group Diet Instruction to a Self-Directed Education Program for Cholesterol Reduction," *Journal of the American Dietetic Association* 26 (1994): 140–145.

48. J. Dunbar, "Adhering to Medical Advice: A Review," *International Journal of Mental Health* 9 (1980): 70–87.

49. S.A. Eraker et al., "Understanding and Improving Patient Compliance," *Annals of Internal Medicine* 100 (1984): 258–268.

50. H. Leventhal et al., "Compliance: A Self-Regualtion Perspective," in *Handbook of Behavioral Medicine,* ed. W.D. Gentry (New York: Guilford Press, 1984), 377.

51. P. Ley, "Giving Information to Patients," *Social Psychology and Behavioral Medicine* (New York: Wiley, 1982): 339–373.

52. D.C. Turk et al., "Chronic Pain," in *Self-Management of Chronic Disease: Handbook of Clinical Interventions and Research*, ed. K.A. Holroyd and T.L. Creer (Orlando, FL: Academic Press, 1986), 446.

53. Cormier and Cormier, *Interviewing Strategies for Helpers: A Guide to Assessment, Treatment and Evaluation*, 117.

54. Cormier and Cormier, *Interviewing Strategies for Helpers: A Guide to Assessment, Treatment and Evaluation,* 118–124.

Appendix 2–A Client Nonverbal Behavior Checklist

Nonverbal Dimensions

Behaviors	Description of Counselor-Client Interaction	Possible Effect or Meanings
KINESICS		
Eyes		
Direct eye contact	Client has just shared concern with counselor. Counselor responds; client maintains eye contact.	Readiness or willingness for interpersonal communication or exchange; attentiveness
Lack of sustained eye contact	Each time counselor brings up the topic of client's family, client looks away.	Withdrawal or avoidance of interpersonal exchange; or respect or deference
	Client demonstrates intermittent breaks in eye contact while conversing with counselor.	Respect or deference
	Client mentions sexual concerns, then abruptly looks away. When counselor initiates this topic, client looks away again.	Withdrawal from topic of conversation; discomfort or embarrassment; or preoccupation
Lowering eyes—looking down or away	Client talks at some length about alternatives to present job situation. Pauses briefly and looks down. Then resumes speaking and eye contact with counselor.	Preoccupation

continues

Source: From *Interviewing Strategies for Helpers: Fundamental Skills and Cognitive Behavioral Interventions* by W.H. Cormier and L.S. Cormier. Copyright © 1991, 1985, and 1975 Brooks/Cole Publishing Company, Pacific Grove, California 93950, a division of International Thomson Publishing Inc. By permission of the publisher.

Appendix 2–A continued

Behaviors	Description of Counselor-Client Interaction	Possible Effect or Meanings
Eyes (cont'd)		
Staring or fixating on person or object	Counselor has just asked client to consider consequences of a certain decision. Client is silent and gazes at a picture on the wall.	Preoccupation; possibly rigidness or uptightness; pondering; difficulty in finding an answer
Darting eyes or blinking rapidly—rapid eye movements; twitching brow	Client indicates desire to discuss a topic yet is hesitant. As counselor probes, client's eyes move around the room rapidly.	Excitation or anxiety; or wearing contact lenses
Squinting or furrow on brow	Client has just asked counselor for advice. Counselor explains role and client squints, and furrows appear in client's brow.	Thought or perplexity; or avoidance of person or topic
	Counselor suggests possible things for client to explore in difficulties with parents. Client doesn't respond verbally; furrow in brow appears.	Avoidance of person or topic
Moisture or tears	Client has just reported recent death of father; tears well up in client's eyes.	Sadness; frustration; sensitive area of concern
	Client reports real progress during past week in marital communication; eyes get moist.	Happiness

continues

Appendix 2–A continued

Behaviors	Description of Counselor-Client Interaction	Possible Effect or Meanings
Eyes (cont'd)		
Eye shifts	Counselor has just asked client to remember significant events in week; client pauses and looks away; then responds and looks back.	Processing or recalling material; or keen interest; satisfaction
Pupil dilation	Client discusses spouse's sudden disinterest and pupils dilate.	Alarm; or keen interest
	Client leans forward while counselor talks and pupils dilate.	Keen interest; satisfaction
Mouth		
Smiles	Counselor has just asked client to report positive events of the week. Client smiles, then recounts some of these instances.	Positive thought, feeling, or action in content of conversation; or greeting
	Client responds with a smile to counselor's verbal greeting at beginning of interview.	Greeting
Tight lips (pursed together)	Client has just described efforts at sticking to a difficult living arrangement. Pauses and purses lips together.	Stress or determination; anger or hostility
	Client has just expressed irritation at counselor's lateness. Client sits with lips pursed together while counselor explains the reasons.	Anger or hostility

continues

Appendix 2–A continued

Behaviors	Description of Counselor-Client Interaction	Possible Effect or Meanings
Mouth (cont'd)		
Lower lip quivers or biting of lip	Client starts to describe her recent experience of being laughed at by colleagues at work because she is trying hard to follow her new eating pattern. As client continues to talk, her lower lip quivers; occasionally she bites her lip.	Anxiety, sadness, or fear
	Client discusses loss of parental support after a recent divorce. The problems associated with this home situation make following a new eating pattern difficult. Client bites her lip after discussing this.	Sadness
Open mouth without speaking	Counselor has just expressed feelings about a block in the relationship. Client's mouth drops open; client says was not aware of it.	Surprise; or suppression of yawn—fatigue
	It has been a long session. As counselor talks, client's mouth parts slightly.	Suppression of yawn—fatigue

continues

Appendix 2–A continued

Behaviors	Description of Counselor-Client Interaction	Possible Effect or Meanings
Facial Expressions		
Eye contact with smiles	Client talks very easily and smoothly, occasionally smiling; maintains eye contact for most of session.	Happiness or comfortableness
Eyes strained; furrow on brow; mouth tight	Client has just reported strained situation with a spouse who dislikes her efforts to cut down on fat intake. Client then sits with lips pursed together and frowns.	Anger; or concern; sadness
Eyes rigid, mouth rigid (unanimated)	Client states: "I have nothing to say"; there is no evident expression or alertness on client's face.	Preoccupation; anxiety; fear
Head		
Nodding head up and down	Client has just expressed concern over own health status and what the new eating pattern will do to improve health; counselor reflects client's feelings. Client nods head and says "That's right."	Confirmation; agreement; or listening, attending
	Client nods head during counselor explanation.	Listening; attending
Shaking head from left to right	Counselor has just suggested that client's continual lateness to sessions may be an issue that needs to be discussed. Client responds with "No," and shakes head from left to right.	Disagreement; or disapproval

continues

Appendix 2–A continued

Behaviors	Description of Counselor-Client Interaction	Possible Effect or Meanings
Head (cont'd)		
Hanging head down, jaw down toward chest	Counselor initiates topic of termination. Client lowers head toward chest, then says, "I am not ready to stop the counseling sessions."	Sadness; concern
Shoulders		
Shrugging	Client reports that spouse just walked out with no explanation. Client shrugs shoulders while describing this.	Uncertainty; or ambivalence
Leaning forward	Client has been sitting back in the chair. Counselor discloses something personal; client leans forward and asks counselor a question about the experience.	Eagerness; attentiveness; openness to communication
Slouched, stooped, rounded, or turned away from person	Client reports feeling inadequate and defeated because of snacking; slouches in chair after saying this.	Sadness or ambivalence; or lack of receptivity to interpersonal exchange
	Client reports difficulty in talking. As counselor pursues this, client slouches in chair and turns shoulders away from counselor.	Lack of receptivity to interpersonal exchange

continues

Appendix 2–A continued

Behaviors	Description of Counselor-Client Interaction	Possible Effect or Meanings
Arms and Hands		
Arms folded across chest	Counselor has just initiated conversation. Client doesn't respond verbally; sits back in chair with arms crossed against chest.	Avoidance of interpersonal exchange; or dislike
Trembling and fidgety hands	Client expresses fear of weight gain; hands tremble while talking about this.	Anxiety or anger
	In a loud voice, client expresses resentment; client's hands shake while talking.	Anger
Fist clenching of objects or holding hands tightly	Client has just come in for initial interview. Says that he or she feels uncomfortable; hands are closed together tightly.	Anxiety or anger
	Client expresses hostility toward husband; clenches fists while talking.	Anger
Arms unfolded—arms and hands gesturing in conversation	Counselor has just asked a question; client replies and gestures during reply.	Accenting or emphasizing point in conversation; or openness to interpersonal exchange
	Counselor initiates new topic. Client readily responds; arms are unfolded at this time.	Openness to interpersonal exchange

continues

Appendix 2–A continued

Behaviors	Description of Counselor-Client Interaction	Possible Effect or Meanings
Arms and Hands (cont'd)		
Rarely gesturing, hands and arms stiff	Client arrives for initial session. Responds to counselor's questions with short answers. Arms are kept down at side.	Tension or anger
	Client has been referred; sits with arms down at sides while explaining reasons for referral and irritation at being here.	Anger
Legs and Feet		
Legs and feet appear comfortable and relaxed	Client's legs and feet are relaxed without excessive movement while client freely discusses personal concerns.	Openness to interpersonal exchange; relaxation
Crossing and uncrossing legs repeatedly	Client is talking rapidly in bursts about problems; continually crosses and uncrosses legs while doing so.	Anxiety; depression
Foot-tapping	Client is tapping feet during a lengthy counselor summary; client interrupts counselor to make a point.	Anxiety; impatience—wanting to make a point
Legs and feet appear stiff and controlled	Client is open and relaxed while talking about job. When counselor introduces topic of marriage, client's legs become more rigid.	Uptightness or anxiety; closed to extensive interpersonal exchange

continues

Appendix 2–A continued

Behaviors	Description of Counselor-Client Interaction	Possible Effect or Meanings
Total Body		
Facing other person squarely or leaning forward	Client shares a concern and faces counselor directly while talking; continues to face counselor while counselor responds.	Openness to interpersonal communication and exchange
Turning of body orientation at an angle, not directly facing person, or slouching in seat	Client indicates some difficulty in "getting in to" interview. Counselor probes for reasons; client turns body away.	Less openness to interpersonal exchange
Rocking back and forth in chair or squirming in seat	Client indicates a lot of nervousness about an approaching conflict situation. Client rocks as this is discussed.	Concern; worry; anxiety
Stiff—sitting erect and rigidly on edge of chair	Client indicates some uncertainty about direction of interview; sits very stiff and erect.	Tension; anxiety; concern

PARALINGUISTICS

Voice Level and Pitch		
Whispering or inaudibility	Client has been silent for a long time. Counselor probes; client responds, but in a barely audible voice.	Difficulty in disclosing
Pitch changes	Client is speaking at a moderate voice level while discussing job. Then client begins to talk about unsupportive friends at work and voice pitch rises considerably.	Topics of conversation have different emotional meanings

continues

Appendix 2–A continued

Behaviors	Description of Counselor-Client Interaction	Possible Effect or Meanings
Fluency in Speech		
Stuttering, hesitations, speech errors	Client is talking rapidly about feeling uptight in certain social situations; client stutters and makes some speech errors while doing so.	Sensitivity about topic in conversation; or anxiety and discomfort
Whining or lisp	Client is complaining about having a hard time losing weight; voice goes up like a whine.	Dependency or emotional emphasis
Rate of speech slow, rapid, or jerky	Client begins interview talking slowly about a bad weekend. As topic shifts to client's feelings about self, client talks more rapidly.	Sensitivity to topics of conversation; or topics have different emotional meanings
Silence	Client comes in and counselor invites client to talk; client remains silent.	Reluctance to talk; or preoccupation
	Counselor has just asked client a question. Client pauses and thinks over a response.	Preoccupation; or desire to continue speaking after making a point; thinking about how to respond
	A Chinese client talks about own family. Pauses; then resumes conversation to talk more about same subject.	Desire to continue speaking after making point

continues

Appendix 2–A continued

Behaviors	Description of Counselor-Client Interaction	Possible Effect or Meanings
Autonomic Responses		
Clammy hands, shallow breathing, sweating, pupil dilation, paleness, blushing, rashes on neck ˙	Client discusses the exciting prospect of having two desirable job offers. Breathing becomes faster and client's pupils dilate.	Arousal—positive (excitement, interest) or negative (anxiety, embarrassment)
	Client starts to discuss binge eating; breathing becomes shallow and red splotches appear on neck.	Anxiety, embarrassment
PROXEMICS		
Distance		
Moves away	Counselor has just confronted client; client moves back before responding verbally.	Signal that space has been invaded; increased arousal, discomfort
Moves closer	Midway through session, client moves chair toward helper.	Seeking closer interaction, more intimacy
Position in Room		
Sits behind or next to an object in the room, such as table or desk	A new client comes in and sits in a chair that is distant from counselor.	Seeking protection or more space
Sits near counselor without any intervening objects	A client who has been in to see counselor before sits in chair closest to counselor.	Expression of adequate comfort level

CHAPTER 3

Counseling Skills To Facilitate Self-Management

CHAPTER OBJECTIVES

1. List the stages through which clients pass in the course of changing a behavior.

2. Describe each stage.

3. Apply the skills described in assessing the readiness-to-change stages.

4. Apply the adherence thermometer and the motivation, confidence, and readiness-to-change thermometer to a variety of nutrition situations where adherence may be a problem.

5. Apply eight motivational strategies to nutrition-related adherence problems.

6. Apply the stages of change to goal setting by asking appropriate questions.

This chapter describes ways in which nutrition counselors motivate people to change. The secret to change lies in self-management. Emphasis is on client responsibility for behavior and for dealing with and planning the future. The nutrition counselor sets up an environment that is a transient support system that prepares the client to handle social and personal demands more effectively. The nutrition counselor's role is one of providing the most favorable conditions for change.[1]

THE STAGES OF CHANGE

Communication skills discussed in Chapter 2 provide a basis for facilitating a state of readiness or eagerness to change. Prochaska and DiClemente describe a model of how change occurs.[2] They describe a series of six stages through which people pass in the course of changing a behavior:

1. precontemplation
2. contemplation
3. determination
4. action
5. maintenance
6. relapse

Miller and Rollnick illustrate the Prochaska-DiClemente model with a wheel of change shown in Figure 3–1.[3]

The wheel indicates that it is normal for everyone involved in changing eating habits to go around the process several times before achieving stable changes. In research with smokers, Prochaska and DiClemente found that smokers ordinarily went around the wheel between three and seven times (with an average of four) before finally quitting completely. This wheel recognizes relapses in changing behaviors as a normal stage in change. Knowing this, the self-managing client avoids feeling disheartened when relapse occurs. By distinguishing different stages of readiness for change, the nutrition counselor approaches clients differently,

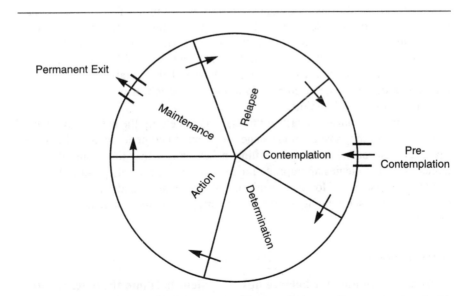

Figure 3–1 Prochaska and DiClemente's Six Stages of Change. *Source:* Reprinted with permission from W.R. Miller and S. Rollnick, *Motivational Interviewing: Preparing People To Change Addictive Behavior*, p. 15, © 1991, The Guilford Press.

depending on where they are in the process of change.[4] Each stage requires a different skill. Problems of clients being unmotivated or resistant occur when a nutrition counselor uses inappropriate strategies for a client's current stage of change.

Precontemplation

As illustrated in Figure 3–1, the entry point to the process of change is the precontemplation stage. This is the point at which the client has not even contemplated having a problem or needing to make a change. Words like, "I'm not interested in what I eat," may be common. A person in the precontemplative stage needs information and feedback to raise his or her awareness of the problem and possibility of change. Nutrition advice for eating changes is counterproductive at this point.[5]

Contemplation

Once some awareness of the problem arises, the person enters a period of ambivalence: the contemplation stage. The contemplator considers change and rejects it. As nutrition counselors listen to the contemplator, they hear reasons for concern and justifications for unconcern. This is a normal and characteristic stage of change, although sometimes its manifestations are misattributed to pathological personality traits or defense mechanisms. The contemplator seesaws between reasons to change and reasons to stay the same. *A person who falls into this stage may say the following:* "I really do eat low-fat foods most of the time. Probably I do eat out too often, but my friends and my husband always talk me into going to high-fat restaurants. But at home I do a really good job. It is just that lately we seem to eat out all of the time."

The nutrition counselor's task at this stage is to help tip the balance in favor of change. This is the most common stage for clients to come to the nutrition counselor for assistance in changing eating behaviors. A nutrition counselor who launches into strategies appropriate for the action stage at this point is likely to engender resistance. However, working on advantages and disadvantages to continuing or discontinuing a nutrition therapy may help the client see changes differently.

Determination

From time to time the balance tips. The client falls into the determination stage. *At this stage, the client may say the following:* "I've got to start eating more low-fat dairy products! This is serious! Something has to change. What can I do? How can I change?"

The determination stage is like a window of opportunity that opens for a brief period of time. If during this time the person enters into action, the change process continues. If not, the person slips back into contemplation. The nutrition counselor's task when a client is in the determination stage is not one of motivating but rather matching. At this point, the client needs help in finding a change strategy or a goal that is acceptable, accessible, appropriate, and effective.

Action

The action stage is what is most often termed counseling. The client engages in actions that bring about change. The goal during this stage is to produce a change in the problem area.

Maintenance

Making a change does not guarantee maintenance of that change. Obviously, human experience includes good intentions and initial changes, followed by minor ("slips") or major ("relapses") steps backward. During the maintenance stage, the challenge is to sustain the change accomplished by previous action and to prevent relapse.[6] Maintaining a change may require a different set of skills and strategies from those needed to accomplish the change in the first place. Reducing dietary fat may be an initial step, followed by the challenge of maintaining reduced fat intake.

Relapse

Finally, if relapse occurs, the individual's task is to start around the wheel again rather than becoming stuck in this stage. Slips and relapses are normal, expected occurrences as a person seeks to change any long-standing pattern of behavior. The nutrition counselor's task here is to help the client avoid discouragement and demoralization, continue contemplating change, renew determination, and resume action and maintenance efforts.

ASSESSMENT OF THE CLIENT'S READINESS FOR CHANGE

Assessing which stage a person is in is a very important part of the process of counseling. The adherence thermometer in Figure 3–2 provides a way of helping clients work through the process of identifying which stage they are currently in or whether relapse is occurring.

When the nutrition counselor is assessing where the clients fit into the model, it is important to ask, *"How ready are they?"* **Giving advice is not appropriate at this point. Avoid lists of dos and don'ts.** It is important to use

ALWAYS

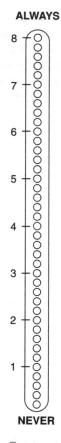

NEVER

Figure 3–2 Adherence Thermometer. Courtesy of Kaiser Permanente, Portland, Oregon.

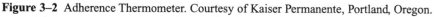

the listening skills discussed in Chapter 2 to hear where clients feel they are in the process of change. This is when open-ended questions can help to explore current eating behavior and progress. "Tell me more about _____." "Tell me more about 'sometimes.' At what times do you follow your low-fat eating pattern, and at what times don't you?" "How are you feeling about limiting the fat in foods you choose?" "The last time we met, you were working on _____. How is that going?" As clients speak, use positive responses to affirm, compliment, and reinforce.

At this point, it is appropriate to provide objective feedback about dietary intake. Show clients feedback forms indicating changes in lipids or saturated fat or blood glucose levels. Compare client results with normative data or other interpretative information. After giving feedback, ask about the client's overall response, "What do you make of all this information?"

Determine the client's readiness to change by showing the readiness-to-change thermometer (Figure 3–3). Ask the question, "How interested are you in making changes to eat foods lower in saturated fat and cholesterol?" This thermometer provides the clues to where a client is in readiness to change. Each point on the thermometer includes a different stage in change. "Not interested in changing what I eat" falls into the precontemplative stage. "Thinking about it in the next month" is suggestive of the contemplation phase. "Thinking about it in the next week" implies determination. "Already starting to do it" shows the action stage. The final stage of maintenance involves already "doing it."

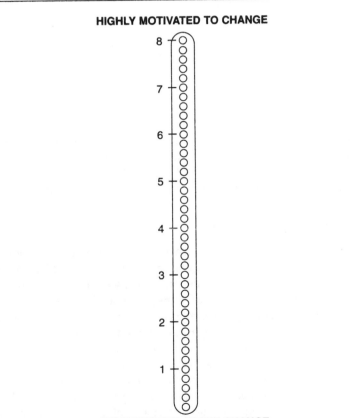

Figure 3–3 Motivation, Confidence, and Readiness-To-Change Thermometer. Courtesy of Kaiser Permanente, Portland, Oregon.

MOTIVATIONAL STRATEGIES

Keeping in mind the stages of change, the nutrition counselor might ask this question, "What strategies can a counselor use to enhance motivation for change?" Researchers have found that there are identifiable factors that motivate people to change. Miller provides a detailed review of this extensive literature.[7] From that research, **eight general motivational strategies can be identified:**

1. giving advice
2. identifying and removing barriers
3. providing choices
4. decreasing desirability of a present behavior
5. practicing empathy
6. providing feedback
7. clarifying goals
8. active helping

Giving Advice

Advice alone is not likely to be sufficient to induce change in a majority of individuals, but the motivating influence of clear and compassionate advice is valuable. Brief and systematic advice from a physician can increase the likelihood that medical patients will stop smoking or change their alcohol use.[8–12] Miller and Rollnick propose elements of effective advice.[13] Advice should clearly identify the problem or risk area, explain why change is important, and advocate specific change.

Identifying and Removing Barriers

A second effective motivation approach involves identifying and removing significant barriers to change efforts. A contemplator may be willing to consider entering treatment, but also may be inhibited or discouraged from doing so by specific practical barriers, such as cost, transportation, child care, shyness, waiting time, or safety concerns. These barriers may interfere not only with treatment entry, but with change efforts more generally. Once the nutrition counselor identifies barriers, the task is to assist the client in practical problem solving.

Sisson and Mallams provide a good example of the power of simple strategies for overcoming barriers.[14] Their goal was to increase attendance at initial Alcoholics Anonymous (AA) meetings. The counselor gave one group the usual encouragement: an explanation of the importance of attendance, a schedule of available meeting times and places, and exhortation to attend. A second group, chosen at random, received systematic help in overcoming barriers to attendance. While the client was in the office, the counselor placed a prearranged telephone call to an AA member. Acting as a buddy, the AA member then spoke to the client, offering to provide transportation and to accompany the client to the first meeting. They agreed on a meeting time, and the member attained the client's telephone number in order to place a reminder call on the evening before the agreed-upon meeting. Marked results occurred. Every client in the latter group attended AA; in the former (encouragement) group, not a single client made it to the first AA meeting.

Some barriers are very tangible, such as cost or transportation. Other factors are less tangible but also significant: delays, comfort, a sense of belonging, cultural appropriateness. Long delays in a waiting room or assignment to a waiting list can discourage participation. It may be better to offer clients an effective brief intervention than place them on a waiting list for treatment.[15–17] Child care during treatment is an access issue for many women. Transportation and safety may be special concerns for the elderly. Language and cultural sensitivity are issues in counseling people from different racial and cultural backgrounds.

Some barriers to change are more attitudinal than overt. A person may fear that changing will result in adverse consequences[18] or cut off important sources of positive reinforcement. An individual's circle of friends or cultural context may encourage the perception that the "problem" behaviors are really quite normal and acceptable, and that no change is needed. Removal of these barriers to change may require more cognitive and informational strategies that require the client to think about alternatives.

Providing Choices

The effective nutrition counselor provides choices. Offering clients choices among alternative approaches may decrease resistance and dropout rates and may improve compliance and outcomes.[19–22] Similarly, acknowledging freedom of choice with regard to treatment goals may enhance client motivation.

Decreasing Desirability of a Present Behavior

Decreasing the desirability of a present behavior is important in the contemplation stage. At this point, the client is weighing the benefits and costs of change against the merits of continuing as before. Motivation strategies for the contemplation stage involve removing weights from the status quo side of the balance, and increasing weights on the change side of the scales. An important task for the nutrition counselor is to identify the client's positive incentives for continuing his or her present behavior. How and why is this behavior desirable to the client? Clear positive incentives allow the nutrition counselor to seek effective approaches for decreasing, undermining, or counterbalancing them. Change in affective or value dimensions of desirability alter behavior.[23,24] Relationships and environment, along with individual desire, work to change behavior.

Practicing Empathy

Practicing empathy toward all clients favors motivation for change. Experimental and correlational studies show that an empathic counseling style results in low levels of client resistance and greater long-term behavior change.[25,26]

As discussed in Chapter 2, empathy is not an ability to identify with a person's experiences. It is a learnable skill for understanding another's meaning through the use of reflective listening, whether or not the listener has actually had similar experiences. Although a nutrition counselor skilled in empathic listening can make it look easy and natural, this is a demanding counseling style. It requires sharp attention to each new client statement, and a continual generation of hypotheses as to the underlying meaning. Nutrition counselors reflect back to the client their best guesses as to meaning, often adding to the client's content. The client responds, and the whole process starts over again. Reflective listening is easy to copy or do poorly, but quite challenging to do well. It is a key element to behavior change.

Providing Feedback

Providing clients with feedback on changes in dietary intake is valuable to future change. If the clients do not know where they are, it is difficult to plan how to get somewhere else. People sometimes fail to change because they do not receive sufficient feedback about their current situation. Clear knowledge of the present situation is a crucial element of motivation for change. Checkups that provide information about how a behavior is harmful yield long-term changes.[27,28] Self-monitoring dietary behaviors can be very helpful to clients on a daily basis as they change behaviors.[29–32]

In the world of nutrition, feedback is often overemphasized. It is important, but feedback alone cannot achieve change. Compare feedback with standards. It is this process of self-evaluation—comparing perceived status with personal standards—that influences whether change will occur.[33]

Clarifying Goals

Helping clients set clear goals facilitates change.[34] Clients must see goals as realistic and attainable, or they will expend little effort to reach the goal, even if they acknowledge it as important.[35] Goals are of little use if clients lack feedback about the present situation. Motivation for change occurs when goals and feedback work together.

Goal setting involves asking the right questions to elicit in which stage the client falls. An initial stage of goal setting (which corresponds with the precontemplation or contemplation stage of change) may involve unreadiness or ambivalence. The goal for the nutrition counselor is to build motivation and help tip the client's decisional balance in favor of change. **Important questions to ask include the following:**

- What do you think about eating food high in saturated fat and cholesterol? Any dislikes?
- What are some of the good reasons for not making changes in your eating habits?
- Are there any reasons why you might want to make a change in your eating habits?
- Ideally, how would you like to be eating?
- What do you think might happen if you keep eating like this the rest of your life?

In this stage, it is important to address the client's ambivalence. Explore reasons for ambivalence without controlling or passing value judgments on responses to the above questions. Use of confrontation skills described in Chapter 2 may be important now if clients are in precontemplative stages. In the contemplation stage, assessing thoughts and feelings about self and the problem is important.

The second stage of goal setting (which corresponds with the determination stage of change) involves a serious consideration of making changes in eating habits. The nutrition counselor's goal is to strengthen commitment to change by eliciting from the client reasonable goals and strategies for change. The following questions would be helpful in this stage:

- What are your reasons for wanting to eat foods lower in saturated fat and cholesterol?
- What has helped you eat foods low in saturated fat and cholesterol in the past?
- What do you think needs to change?
- What are your ideas for making a change in your eating?

In this stage, the window is open for action. The questions above provide ways to let the client know that there are ways to approach the action stage.

The third stage of goal setting corresponds with the action/maintenance stage of change. In this stage, the goal of the nutrition counselor is to help the client take additional steps to change and deal with backward slips. At this point, the following questions are helpful:

- What do you like about low-fat eating?
- What are you doing that is working?
- How would you change what you are now doing?
- Is there anything else you see as a challenge?

In this action/maintenance stage, client and nutrition counselor negotiate a plan. The questions above provide ideas that tell the nutrition counselor what the client wants to do. The goal is to balance the differences between what the nutrition counselor wants and what the client wants to do.

It is important to follow up on whether goals are being met. The time of contact should be shortly after the client tries the goal. If the client is not able to meet the goal, the goal is faulty. Recycling (revising goals) is a positive step and not a sign of failure. Help the client set contingency plans. If plan X does not work, use plan Y.

Active Helping

At the end of a session, keep directions clear. Always be sure to leave clients with a sense of hope, not shame. Exhibit 3–1 provides the client with a few clear positive steps toward dealing with backward slips.

Exhibit 3–1 Dealing with Backward Slips

1. **Stay calm and listen to any negative thoughts and turn them into positive thoughts.**
   a. Listen to your thoughts.
   b. Decide if your thoughts help or hurt your progress.
      i. What messages are you giving yourself?
      ii. Are they positive and helpful, or negative and limiting?
   c. Stop your negative thoughts.
   d. Reword your negative thoughts to make them into positive messages.
      i.   Think about the successful changes you've already made.
      ii. Be specific.
      iii. Use the present tense.
      iv. Forget what *should* be.
   e. Replace the negative thought with the positive message.
   f. Repeat your positive message to yourself, as often as possible.
2. **Learn from your slip.**
   a. What type of high-risk situation triggered your slip?
   b. What went wrong in your high-risk situation?
   c. What strategies have you successfully used before to prevent a slip in this type of situation?
3. **Make a plan to get back on track.**
   a. What two steps can you take today to get yourself back on track?
   b. How can you reward yourself when you get back on track?

CONCLUSION

Each of the chapters that follow on eating pattern change related to chronic disease states provides information on how to move clients to appropriate stages on the wheel of change (Figure 3–1). To make these moves, knowledge about risk factors (the behaviors or conditions that place one at risk) and the ways in which risk factors can be reduced is necessary.[36]

Chapters 4 through 9 give ideas for tools that provide knowledge. Beyond knowledge, clients need skills that can first be modeled by the nutrition counselor and then practiced by the client.[37] Finally, clients must be confident that they are capable of changing their behavior.[38]

To move within the wheel of change a variety of behavior skills are necessary. The interventions needed to move a client toward the desired behavior vary by stage.[39-41] To move from **precontemplation to contemplation,** a knowledge of past performance is necessary. A graph of dietary intake is suggested in many of the following chapters. Encouragement and reevaluation of the positive new information can then begin to have the desired effect.

Moving from **contemplation to preparation** requires practicing new behaviors. Writing a menu is suggested in the chapters that follow. Once again, giving feedback on change in diet over time is very important. To move from the **preparation stage to the action stage** requires several different behavioral techniques. Cueing devices are described in the following chapters (e.g., a reminder on the refrigerator). This is the point at which social support is very important. Setting specific goals or designing contracts are important behavioral devices in this change step. Learning how to cope with problems and acquiring social and self-reinforcement is important in this move.

To move from **action to maintenance** is a process of refining. Seeing a setback as an example of how to cope is important in this stage of change. The nutrition counselor bolsters the ability to handle change by referring to times when change *was* achieved. At this point the nutrition counselor encourages people to feel good about themselves as they progress toward a goal and have positive thoughts.

In summary, the behavior change wheel includes numerous behavioral strategies. As change occurs, the strategies used may change also.

NOTES

1. H. Kanfer and L. Gaelic-Buys, "Self-Management Methods," in *Helping People Change: A Textbook of Methods,* ed H. Kanfer and P.J. Goldstein (New York: Pergamon Press, 1991), 306.

2. J. Prochaska and C. DiClemente, "Transtheoretical Therapy: Toward a More Integrative Model of Change," *Psychotherapy: Theory, Research and Practice* 19 (1982): 276–288.

3. W.R. Miller and S. Rollnick, *Motivational Interviewing: Preparing People To Change Addictive Behavior* (New York: Guilford Press, 1991), 14.

4. R. Davidson et al., eds., *Counseling Problem Drinkers* (London: Tavistock/Routledge Publishers, Inc., 1991).

5. S. Rollnick and I. MacEwan, "Alcohol Counselling in Context," in *Counseling Problem Drinkers*, ed. R. Davidson et al. (London: Tavistock/Routledge Publishers, Inc., 1991), 97–114.

6. G.A. Marlatt and J.R. Gordan, eds., *Relapse Prevention: Maintenance Strategies in the Treatment of Addictive Behaviors* (New York: Guilford Press, 1985).

7. W.R. Miller, "Motivation for Treatment: A Review with Special Emphasis on Alcoholism," *Psychological Bulletin* 98 (1985): 84–107.

8. J. Chick et al., "Counselling Problem Drinkers in Medical Wards: A Controlled Study," *British Medical Journal* 290 (1985): 965–967.

9. G.A. Elvy et al., "Attempted Referral and Intervention for Problem Drinking in the General Hospital," *British Journal of Addiction* 83 (1988): 83–89.

10. H. Kristenson et al., "Identification and Intervention of Heavy Drinking in Middle Aged Men: Results and Follow-Up of 24–60 Months of Long-Term Study with Randomized Controls," *Alcoholism: Clinical and Experimental Research* 7 (1983): 203–209.

11. M.A.H. Russell et al., "Effect of General Practitioner's Advice Against Smoking," *British Medical Journal* 297 (1988): 663–668.

12. P. Wallace et al., "Randomized Controlled Trial of General Practitioner Intervention in Patients with Excessive Alcohol Consumption," *British Medical Journal* 297 (1988): 663–668.

13. Miller and Rollnick, *Motivational Interviewing,* 20, 21, 203–208.

14. R.W. Sisson and J.H. Mallams, "The Use of Systematic Encouragement and Community Access Procedures To Increase Attendance at Alcoholics Anonymous and Al-Anon Meetings," *American Journal of Drug and Alcohol Abuse* 8 (1981): 371–376.

15. K.B. Harris and W.R. Miller, "Behavioral Self-Control Training for Problem Drinkers: Mechanisms of Efficacy," *Psychology of Addictive Behaviors* 4 (1990): 82–90.

16. M. Sanchez-Craig, "Brief Didactic Treatment for Alcohol and Drug-Related Problems: An Approach Based on Client Choice," *British Journal of Addiction* 85 (1990): 169–177.

17. M.M. Schmidt and W.R. Miller, "Amount of Therapist Contact and Outcome in a Multidimensional Depression Treatment Program," *Acta Psychitrica Scandinavica* 67 (1983): 319–332.

18. S.M. Hall, "The Abstinence Phobia," in *Behavioral Analysis and Treatment of Substance Abuse*, ed. N.A. Krasnegor (Rockville, MD: National Institute on Drug Abuse, 1979): 55–67.

19. R.M. Costello, "Alcoholism Treatment and Evaluation: In Search of Methods," *International Journal of Addictions* 10 (1975): 251–275.

20. B. Kissin et al., "Selective Factors in Treatment Choices and Outcomes in Alcoholics," in *Recent Advances in Studies of Alcoholism*, ed. N.K. Mello and J.H. Mendelson (Washington, DC: U.S. Government Printing Office, 1971): 781–802.

21. M.W. Parker et al., "Patient Autonomy in Alcohol Rehabilitation: I. Literature Review," *International Journal of the Addictions* 14 (1979): 1015–1022.

22. Sanchez-Craig, "Brief Didactic Treatment for Alcohol and Drug-Related Problems."

23. H. Leventhal, "Fear Appeals and Persuasion: The Differentiation of a Motivation Construct," *American Journal of Public Health* 61 (1971): 1208–1224.

24. D. Premack, "Mechanisms of Self-Control," in *Learning Mechanisms in Smoking*, ed. W.A. Hunt (Chicago: Aldine, 1970): 107–123.

25. G.R. Patterson and M.S. Forgatch, "Therapist Behavior as a Determinant for Client Noncompliance: A Paradox for the Behavior Modifier," *Journal of Consulting and Clinical Psychology* 53 (1985): 846–851.

26. W.R. Miller and R.G. Sovereign, "The Check-Up: A Model for Early Intervention in Addictive Behaviors," in *Addictive Behaviors: Prevention and Early Intervention*, ed. T. Loberg et al. (Amsterdam: Swets and Zeitlinger, 1989): 219–231.

27. H. Kristenson, et al., "Identification and Intervention of Heavy Drinking in Middle-Aged Men: Results and Follow-Up of 24–60 Months of Long-Term Study with Randomized Controls," *Alcoholism: Clinical and Experimental Research* 7 (1983): 203–209.

28. Miller and Sovereign, "The Check-Up."

29. R.R. Wing, "Behavioral Treatment of Severe Obesity," *American Journal of Clinical Nutrition* 55 (1992): 5455–5515.

30. D.E. Smith and R.R. Wing, "Diminished Weight Loss and Behavioral Compliance during Repeated Diets in Obese Patients with Type II Diabetes," *Health Psychology* 10 (1991): 378–383.

31. W.A. Sperduto et al., "The Effect of Target Behavior Monitoring on Weight Loss and Completion Rate in a Behavior Modification Program for Weight Reduction," *Addictive Behaviors* 11 (1986): 337–340.

32. R.C. Baker and D.S. Kirschenbaum, "Self-Monitoring May Be Necessary for Successful Weight Control," *Behavior Therapy* 24 (1993): 395–408.

33. F.H. Kanfer and L. Gaelick, "Self-Management Methods," in *Helping People Change*, 3rd ed., ed. F.H. Kanfer and A.P. Goldstein (Elmsford, NY: Pergamon Press, 1986): 283–345.

34. E.A. Locke et al., "Goal Setting and Task Performance: 1969–1980," *Psychological Bulletin* 90 (1981): 125–152.

35. A. Bandura, "Self-Efficacy Mechanism in Human Agency," *American Psychologist* 37 (1982): 122–147.

36. E.W. Maibach and D. Cotton, "Moving people to behavior change," in *Designing Health Messages,* eds. E.W. Maibach and L. Parrott (Thousand Oaks, CA: Sage Publications, Inc., 1995): 44.

37. A. Bandura, "Self-efficacy mechanism in physiological activation and health-promoting behavior," in *Neurobiology of Learning, Emotion and Affect* (New York, NY: Raven Press, 1991), 46.

38. R. Wood and A. Bandura, "Social cognitive theory of organizational management," *Academy of Management Review,* 14 (1989): 361–384.

39. N.D. Weinstein, "The precaution adoption process," *Health Psychology,* 7 (1988): 355–386.

40. J. Prochaska, et al., "In search of how people change: Application to addictive behaviors," *American Psychologist,* 47 (1992): 1102–1114.

41. T. Baranowski, "Beliefs as motivational influences at stages in behavior change," *International Journal of Community Health Education,* 13 (1992): 3–29.

PART II

Application of Interviewing and Counseling Skills

Part II discusses problems in eating behaviors that are associated with certain prescribed dietary patterns involving modifications in calories, fat, cholesterol, carbohydrates, protein, and sodium. Each chapter begins with a review of research on the association between nutrients and the disease, followed by a discussion of research on compliance with an eating pattern in which specified nutrients are restricted. Suggestions follow for assessing individual behaviors that are inappropriate to the prescribed eating pattern. Treatment of such behaviors is then analyzed in terms of strategies to combat lack of knowledge, forgetfulness, and lack of commitment.

Strategies to deal with clients' lack of knowledge are both informational and behavioral. Informational strategies focus on imparting facts about the regimen. Behavioral strategies include many ways to change behavior by identifying information in terms of the antecedents and consequences of target behaviors without necessarily intervening directly with respect to nutrition or health knowledge and attitudes. Suggestions for modifying these antecedents and consequences are proposed as steps toward behavior change. Strategies to solve problems of forgetfulness include behavioral techniques such as cueing.

Clients who seem to be less committed to dietary change may benefit from strategies designed to intervene directly to change their attitudes. These strategies focus on persuasion through engaging relevant motivations or increasing clients' readiness to change by affecting their attitudes. Behavioral strategies are frequently coupled with these motivational strategies to increase commitment to a modified eating pattern. A summary of Chapter 3 is included in Figure II–1. It includes concepts related to motivational interviewing. This outline will help counselors when dealing with problem motivation behaviors. The counselor must individualize these strategies for each client, because some may be inappropriate for some individuals. Discussion of suggested assessment and treatment strategies for specific dietary patterns are important if this book is used as a classroom text, because there are many ways to solve each nutrition-related problem.

Chapters 4 through 9 provide examples of three types of adherence tools: (1) *monitoring devices* that help determine how well clients are adhering to their

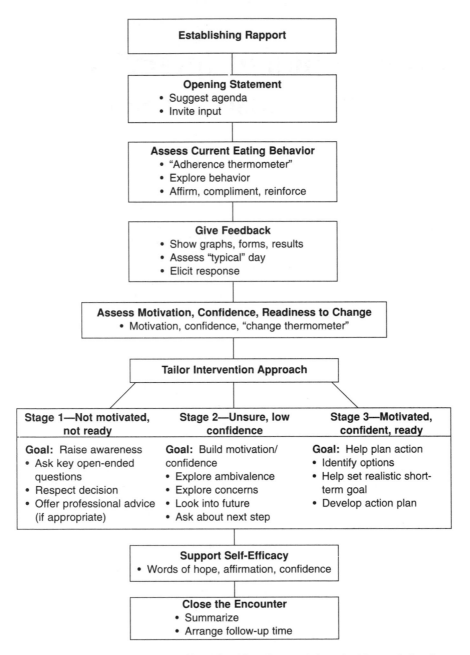

Figure II–1 Motivational Intervention Algorithm. *Source:* Adapted with permission from S. Rollnick and W. Miller, "What Is Motivational Interviewing?" *Behavioral Cognitive Psychotherapy,* Vol. 23, pp. 325–334, © 1995, Wisepress Ltd.

dietary patterns, (2) *informational devices* that supplement the basic dietary instruction, and (3) *cueing devices.* Each tool:

- has a goal or an objective
- gains the client's attention
- is concise and to the point
- allows for individual differences in eating habits

Health professionals who do not have formal training in dietetics should work closely with a registered dietitian in recommending changes for modified regimens. For example, the modified eating pattern for clients with renal insufficiency (Chapter 7) includes changes in many nutrients. Registered dietitians trained in the field should be consulted.

Exhibits II–1 and II–2 are qualitative and quantitative evaluations of communication skills styles to use during practice sessions in which peers or clients evaluate the counselor's progress with counseling skills. They can also be used to check that counselors have acquired basic skills before beginning Part II of this book.

The qualitative scoring (Exhibit II–1) involves a subjective judgment by a rater or by the client (or both) about aspects of the counselor's style. After observing

---

Exhibit II–1 Qualitative Rating of Counselor's Helping Style

	Rarely	*Occasionally*	*Undecided*	*Often*	*Almost Always*
1. Did the nutrition counselor appear to be comfortable with the client and with the subject areas discussed?					
2. Did the counselor avoid imposing values on the client?					
3. Did the counselor remain objective?					
4. Did the counselor focus on the client, not just on the procedure of providing a diet instruction?					
5. Were the counselor's skills spontaneous and non-mechanical?					
6. How would you describe the likelihood of the client's returning to this nutrition counselor again?					
Comments from Rater or Client					

Source: From *Interviewing Strategies for Helpers: Fundamental Skills and Cognitive Behavioral Interviews* by W.H. Cormier and L.S. Cormier. Copyright © 1991, 1985, and 1975 by Wadsworth Inc. Adapted by permission of Brooks/Cole Publishing Company, Pacific Grove, California 93950, a division of International Thomson Publishing Inc. By permission of the publisher.

Exhibit II–2 Quantitative Rating of Counselors

Nutrition Counselor Statement No.	Verbal Responses — Listening				Verbal Responses — Action				Sharing		Teaching			Nonverbal — Eyes		Face		Body						Paralinguistics	
	Clarification	Paraphrase	Reflection of Feeling	Summarization	Probe	Ability Potential	Confrontation	Interpretation	Self-Disclosure	Immediacy	Instructions	Verbal Setting Operation	Information Giving	Initiates Eye Contact	Breaks Eye Contact	Head Nods	Smiles	Body Facing Client	Body Turned Away	Body Leaning Forward	Body Leaning Backward	Body Relaxed	Body Tense	Completed Sentences	Broken Sentences, Speech Errors
1																									
2																									
3																									
4																									
5																									
6																									
7																									
8																									
9																									
10																									
Total																									

Source: From *Interviewing Strategies for Helpers: Fundamental Skills and Cognitive Behavioral Interviews* by W.H. Cormier and L.S. Cormier. Copyright © 1991, 1985, and 1975 Wadsworth Inc. Adapted by permission of Brooks/Cole Publishing Company, Pacific Grove, California 93950, a division of International Thomson Publishing Inc. By permission of the publisher.

the interview for each of the six items, the rater or client checks the box for items that represent the appropriate judgment about the counselor for most of the interview. Comments can be added at the bottom of the rating sheets.

The quantitative scoring (Exhibit II–2) involves counting certain of the counselor's verbal and nonverbal responses. For each statement by the counselor, the client or rater indicates the type of verbal and nonverbal response. At the end of the interview, the responses associated with each category are tallied.

The following chapters give examples of nutrition as a means of preventing disease and/or its complications, and ways to use counseling skills to promote adherence to new eating patterns. Each new eating pattern focuses on disease prevention and long-term maintenance as opposed to brief therapeutic symptom management.

CHAPTER 4

Nutrition Counseling in Treatment of Obesity

CHAPTER OBJECTIVES

1. Identify common inappropriate behaviors associated with weight gain or overeating.

2. Identify steps in assessing individual eating behaviors.

3. Identify strategies to treat inappropriate eating behaviors contributing to weight gain.

4. Generate appropriate strategies to counsel overweight clients to control eating patterns.

5. Recommend certain dietary adherence tools for weight-loss clients.

THEORIES AND FACTS ABOUT NUTRITION AND OBESITY

Obesity is one of the most common medical disorders in the United States. At least 26 percent of adult Americans are significantly overweight,[1,2] and the prevalence of obesity reaches 50 percent in women in minority populations (American Indian, African American, and Hispanic).[3,4]

Epidemiology studies show a clear excess mortality associated with obesity and increased risk for diabetes, heart disease, stroke, hypertension, gallstones, and certain types of cancer.[5] Assessment of the obese client requires both clinical and laboratory techniques. The major diseases associated with obesity (coronary heart disease, diabetes, and high blood pressure) and their nutritional associations are discussed in Chapters 5, 6, and 8.

Identification, Measurement, and Classification of Obesity

Obesity is an excessive amount of body weight for a given stature. It is also defined as an excessive amount of total body fat (adipose tissue) relative to the amount of lean body tissue. Regional adiposity is the accumulation of an excessive amount of fat tissue in a particular area of the body, such as in the abdominal area or the hips and thighs. Researchers also use statistical definitions of *overweight* or *obesity*, based on body dimensions and connect these with risk for adverse health outcomes.[6]

Relative weight uses the ratio of actual weight to some standard of desirable weight. The most widely used standards are the Metropolitan Life Insurance Tables (Table 4–1). A second relative weight standard is the 85th percentile of weight for height for a given age group, using the 85th percentile of 20- to 29-year-olds as the standard for comparison. Weight and height can also be related by other ratios such as weight divided by height and height divided by the cube root of weight (ponderal index).

Several laboratory-based methods provide estimates of body fat. Body density derived from underwater weighting and converted to a proportion of fat in the body is considered the gold standard procedure. The method assumes that a two-compartment model of body composition is adequate for the purpose of obtaining a valid measure of body fat content. This is a reasonable assumption, provided that the density of fat-free tissue does not vary widely. Unfortunately, it does fluctuate with disease (e.g., osteoporosis), growth, aging, exercise, and malnutrition. Erroneous estimates of body fat content occur under a variety of circumstances, although the magnitude of the errors in terms of percentage of body fat is relatively small.

Nutrition counselors also use other methods to estimate body fat content that do not require the density of fat-free tissues to be constant from person to person. Most notable is the dual emission X-ray absorptiometry (DEXA). It exposes the body to a very small dose of radiation and is thought to provide an accurate measure of total body fat content. Several other techniques of estimating total body fat are used in laboratories. They include isotopic dilution to assess body water, body potassium content to assess skeletal muscle mass, computed tomography (CT) scanning and magnetic resonance imaging (MRI) to assess body fat at a large number of sites or over the whole body. All these methods are expensive; require elaborate instrumentations; and, in some instances, provide data that are difficult to anlayze. These methods are confined to the laboratory and are used almost exclusively for research purposes.

Simple approaches to estimate body fat content include body mass index (BMI)—the prediction of body fat from simple anthropometric measurements (see Appendix C) such as skinfolds and circumferences—and, more recently, bioelec-

Table 4-1 Weights Associated with Lowest Mortality for Men and Women, 1983

Height (with Shoes)	Weight (in Indoor Clothing), lb		
	Small Frame	Medium Frame	Large Frame
Men[a]			
5'2"	128–134	131–141	138–150
5'3"	130–136	133–143	140–153
5'4"	132–138	135–145	142–156
5'5"	134–140	137–148	144–160
5'6"	136–142	139–151	146–164
5'7"	138–145	142–154	149–168
5'8"	140–148	145–157	152–172
5'9"	142–151	148–160	155–176
5'10"	144–154	151–163	158–180
5'11"	146–157	154–166	161–184
6'0"	149–160	157–170	164–188
6'1"	152–164	160–174	168–192
6'2"	155–168	164–178	172–197
6'3"	158–172	167–182	176–202
6'4"	162–176	171–187	181–207
Women[b]			
4'10"	102–111	109–121	118–131
4'11"	103–113	111–123	120–134
5'0"	104–115	113–126	122–137
5'1"	106–118	115–129	125–140
5'2"	108–121	118–132	128–143
5'3"	111–124	121–135	131–147
5'4"	114–127	124–138	132–151
5'5"	117–130	127–141	137–155
5'6"	120–133	130–144	140–159
5'7"	123–136	133–147	143–163
5'8"	126–139	136–150	146–167
5'9"	129–142	139–153	149–170
5'10"	132–145	142–156	152–173
5'11"	135–148	145–159	155–176
6'0"	138–151	148–162	158–179

[a]Weights at ages 25–59 based on lowest mortality. Weight in pounds according to frame (in indoor clothing weighing 5 lb, shoes with 1" heels).

[b]Weights at ages 25–59 based on lowest mortality. Weight in pounds according to frame (in indoor clothing weighing 3 lb, shoes with 1" heels).

Courtesy of Metropolitan Life Insurance Company.

tric impedance analysis (BIA). The BMI (kg/m^2), typically used in large-scale population studies, is a valid marker of body mass for height but is only a moderately valid surrogate for measuring body fat content. Fatness can be measured by a number of techniques, but in epidemiologic studies it is usually measured by the skinfold thickness. When the BMI is above 30 kg/m^2, skinfold measurements for the top 5 to 10 percent of the population and BMI are almost superimposable. BIA has considerable merit, but more research is needed on its limitations and on the conditions under which it is best used. In general, these methods provide estimates of mean total body fat for a group of patients, but are not accurate for an individual.

There are a variety of clinical and laboratory approaches available to measure body dimensions, estimate body tissue mass, and categorize individuals as overweight or obese. Weight and stature are the most widely used and readily available measures to indicate whether individuals are overweight or obese. Among the weight-for-stature indices available, various cutoff points for BMI (kg/m^2) are used to allocate persons to the overweight or obese categories. The World Health Organization has endorsed adapting the obesity grading system proposed by Garrow:[7] Grade 1 obesity, BMI 25.0 to 29.9; Grade 2, BMI 30.0 to 39.9; Grade 3, BMI greater than 40.[8] Other researchers have used slightly different BMI cutoff points depending upon their interpretation of the scientific literature.[9–12] Regardless of the specific cutoff points and the associated nomenclature used, health risk increases with increasing BMI greater than 25, especially when accompanied by comorbidities or complicating factors.[13]

Criteria for Defining *Overweight* in the United States

Statistical reports from the U.S. government as well as from academic researchers reporting in scientific and medical journals use a survey-based BMI definition of *overweight*. Height and weight distributions of adult participants in the Second National Health and Nutrition Examination Survey (NHANES II) of the National Center for Health Statistics provide data for this definition. The overweight category includes adults ages 20 years or older who have a BMI greater than 27.8 for males and greater than 27.3 for females. This is a statistical definition that corresponds to the 85th percentile of BMI for persons ages 20 to 29 years in the NHANES II.[14]

Researchers support the rationale for using persons ages 20 to 29 years as the reference population by the observation that increases in body weight with age result from fat accumulation.[15] Body fat normally increases in both sexes after puberty, as adolescents enter young adulthood. By age 18, body fat accounts for approximately 15 to 18 percent of body weight in males, and 20 to 25 percent of body weight in females. Body fat content greater than 20 percent of body weight in males and greater than 30 percent in females might represent an excess amount of body fat at 18 years of age. In subsequent decades of adult life, body fat increases to approximately 30 to 40 percent of body weight, although this is probably not biologically necessary or desirable.[16]

Fat Distribution

Excessive amounts of weight involve excess body fat content but may also be associated with a large skeletal and muscle mass. Excess fat occurs in variable patterns of distribution—upper body and lower body. In addition, some individuals have more fat than others in the abdominal visceral (intraabdominal) compartment. Normal weight and obese men have more visceral fat on the average than normal weight and obese women. In both genders, the amount of visceral fat is thought to increase naturally with age.

The various types of human obesities carry different levels of risk for heart disease, diabetes, and other common diseases. Researchers have found that upper body obesity and visceral obesity are the high-risk types of obesity.[17–20]

Calculating Body Mass Index and Waist-to-Hip Ratio

A body mass nomogram is illustrated in Exhibit 4–1. BMI is calculated by dividing weight in kilograms by height in meters squared (kg/m^2), and waist-to-hip ratio (W:H) is calculated by dividing the waist measure by the hip (buttocks) measure.

Recommended Energy and Nutrient Levels

Government authorities such as the U.S. Food and Nutrition Board's Committee on Recommended Dietary Allowances and the Canadian Ministry of Health and Welfare have published recommended energy intakes for various groups by age and sex.[21] The energy Recommended Dietary Allowance (RDA) meets the needs of an average person. (RDAs do not necessarily apply to individuals, but, because they are the sole reference for calorie needs, they will be used here to address the needs of an average person.) An energy deficit of 3,500 calories is necessary for the loss of a pound of body fat. This means that with a deficit of 500 calories per day, an individual will lose a pound of weight each week. Whitney and Hamilton found that the loss of more than two pounds of body fat a week rarely can be maintained; they cautioned that a diet supplying less than 1,200 calories per day can be made adequate in vitamins and minerals only with great difficulty.[22]

Nutrient levels are important in promoting adequate nutrition. For adults, the RDAs are 0.8 grams of protein per kilogram of body weight per day.[23] For a 70-kilogram man, that would be 56 grams of protein per day, and for a 55-kilogram woman, 44 grams.

There is a considerable difference of opinion as to whether carbohydrates or fats should be reduced in an energy-restricted diet. Significant weight reductions

Exhibit 4–1 Body Mass Nomogram

To use this nomograph, place a straightedge across the scales for weight and height. The body mass index (BMI) is the number in the middle scale where the straightedge crosses it.

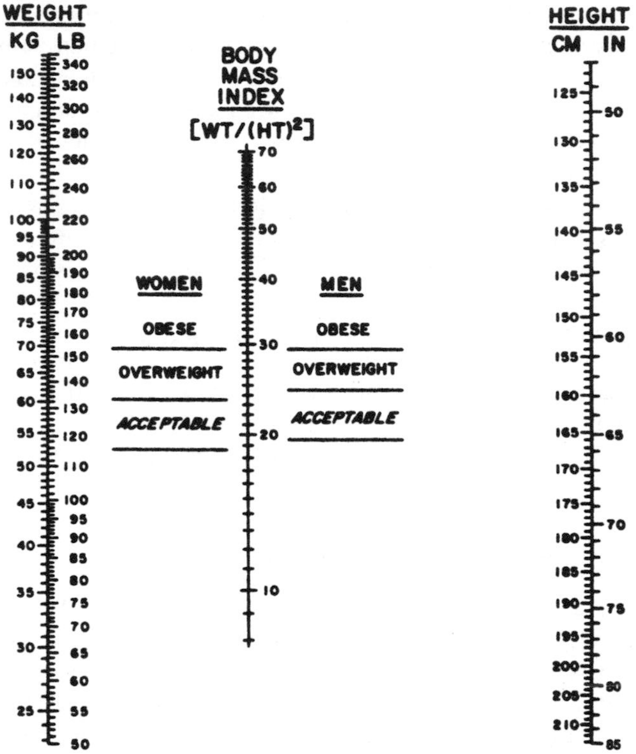

Source: Copyright © George A. Bray, 1978. Used with permission.

Use of BMI to Guide Therapeutic Intervention

BMI

≤23   Normal

>23 to <27   Intervention in the presence of ↑ serum cholesterol or family history of heart disease, diabetes, or hypertension

≥27   Intervention even in the absence of other risk factors

Source: Data from Burton BT, Foster WR, Hirsch J, Van Itallie TB. Health Implications of Obesity: An NIH Consensus Development Conference. *International Journal of Obesity.* 1985;9:155–169, MacMillan Press Ltd.

on carbohydrate-free diets probably result from loss of water bound to glycogen. Without carbohydrates in the diet, the body uses stored glycogen to maintain normal blood glucose levels. The water with its electrolytes that are bound to the glycogen is excreted by the kidneys.

An energy-restricted diet should provide vitamins and minerals at least equivalent to the RDAs. If calorie intake is very restricted, vitamin and mineral supplements may be needed.

The alcohol content of the diet should be assessed carefully at baseline, because clients tend to underestimate consumption. One gram of alcohol provides 7 calories. Beer and wine contain carbohydrates that also contribute calories. The calories from alcoholic beverages may be the difference between losing and gaining weight.

Water and other nonnutritive fluids are not restricted in an energy-restricted diet unless there are heart or kidney complications.

ADHERENCE WITH WEIGHT-LOSS PROGRAMS

Behavioral programs are among the most widely used approaches for weight loss. Weight loss during active treatment is of obvious importance, but the more crucial concern is whether obese persons can be helped to achieve long-term weight loss.[24] There is a body of data on follow-ups of one year and longer.[25–27] The results for the first year of follow-ups for behavioral treatment of obesity are encouraging. Wilson and Brownell found that weight losses at one year typically are similar to those following treatment and, sometimes, slightly better.[28] These findings for one year lend credence to the value of behavioral interventions. Consistent with one-year follow-up, weight maintenance at one and even two years posttreatment is promising.[29]

The medical team has many options available for weight-loss management. Before selecting a strategy, practitioners should analyze numerous methods. In weight-loss programs, unlike other areas of dietary change, practitioners have a great deal of research from which to draw conclusions. In the 1970s, much was written on treatments based on behavior modification and their effectiveness as compared with traditional dietary methods based on short-term evaluation.[30–32] Although weight losses resulting from behavior modification treatment strategies are statistically different from control group losses, these changes are small and not clinically significant, especially for grossly overweight persons.

Few long-term follow-up evaluations are available for dietary, medical, or behavior modification programs. However, 12-month and longer evaluations of behavior modification programs began to appear in the literature in the late 1970s. In a self-controlled behavioral program, Hall et al. found short-term weight losses that were not maintained over time.[33] Other studies have shown similar results.[34–36] Data from Stuart provide a single exception to these studies.[37] Using two key elements, individual behavior modification sessions coupled with booster sessions throughout the follow-up, Stuart found an average weight loss of 32 pounds for eight patients at 12 months.

Miller and Sims evaluated components of a weight-loss program to compare the successful client with the unsuccessful one.[38] Initially, stimulus control and contingency management (contracts) were found useful, but they were not significantly related to long-term success. This finding was corroborated in reports by Brownell and Stunkard[39] and by Wing,[40] suggesting that techniques necessary for weight maintenance may be quite different from those needed for short-term weight loss.

The majority of successful clients over a 12-month period used (1) cognitive restructuring techniques (positive self-thoughts), (2) exercise, (3) social skills (assertiveness skills), and (4) eating style changes.[41] Mahoney and Mahoney report that changes in perfectionistic standards, negative beliefs, and self-defeating private monologues are important to success in a 12-month weight-control program.[42]

Researchers have found that exercise is an ineffective method in losing significant weight.[43–47] In light of this finding, most recent weight-loss programs incorporate a multidisciplinary approach to weight control. The most successful programs utilize a combination of behavior change (exercise and nutrition behavior) and moderate to severe caloric restriction.[48,49]

Many studies have stressed the importance of social support in weight-loss maintenance. Mahoney and Mahoney reported a high correlation between weight loss and family support in a two-year follow-up study.[50] In a more controlled study, Brownell and coworkers evaluated the involvement of spouses in the weight loss program.[51] Subjects whose spouses were trained to be supportive showed three times the weight loss of clients whose spouses were not trained. Clients were also taught the interpersonal skills, such as assertiveness, that are necessary for requesting appropriate support from others.

Researchers' findings on eating style are contradictory.[52,53] Researchers have compared duration of eating, size of mouthfuls, time between bites, and chewing time of obese and nonobese individuals, but it is unclear whether these groups differ in these dimensions. Some researchers suggest that the "nonobese" eating style may be important in controlling food intake because it increases awareness of satiety cues and enhances feelings of self-efficacy and self-control.[54]

More research is needed in the form of controlled clinical trials (the Miller and Sims research was not in this category). Even though social skills training, exercise, and cognitive restructuring appear to influence long-term success, other forms of behavioral therapy should not be discounted. Indeed, combinations of behavioral techniques are provided below as examples of ways to deal with lack of commitment.

There are a variety of general techniques to facilitate weight loss. Honig and Blackburn review various psychological and nonpsychological strategies for treating overweight persons:[55]

- calorie counting
- behavior modification
- self-help groups, such as TOPS (Take Off Pounds Sensibly), Weight Watchers, and Overeaters Anonymous
- exercise programs
- gastric bypass surgery
- drugs to increase metabolic rate and suppress appetite
- popular "lose-pounds-quickly" diets

Van Itallie,[56] Shikora et al.,[57] and Staten[58] carefully review the problems associated with the last three methods listed.

INAPPROPRIATE EATING BEHAVIORS

The following thoughts are frequently associated with weight gain:

> *"I deserve it."*
> *"It's just no use. I have no willpower."*
> *"I'm bored."*
> *"I'm off that rotten diet now."*

Each of these thoughts can have a direct bearing on the individual's propensity to gain weight. Nutrition counselors must be aware of a variety of thought processes as well as overt eating behaviors. It is important to try to identify antecedents and consequences of inappropriate eating behaviors.

Many present or future clients begin thinking about weight loss in terms of going on and off diets: "I go on a diet to lose weight. Usually I can't stand the diet. I just wait until I lose 10 or 15 pounds and then go back to eating those really good foods I'm accustomed to." This syndrome frequently is associated with alternating increases and decreases in weight.

Nutrition counselors might consider trying to avoid the term *diet* in their instructions to describe a means toward weight loss. The rationale is that along with the word *diet,* the two negative words *going off* tend to follow. Many clients will suggest that food is a kind of reward: "When I finish the house work (or reach the 3 PM break at my job), I feel like I deserve a reward, so I just go to the refrigerator (or vending machines or cafeteria). Right there in front of me are all the rewards I need. I really deserve to eat in payment for my hard work."

Signals or cues to eat are everywhere. Counselors should study each client's environment and note specific cues that trigger inappropriate eating behaviors. At home, candy near the television set can trigger snacking responses that might not occur otherwise. TV commercials may provide a stimulus to go to the kitchen for potato chips, candy bars, beverages, etc.

Many clients admit that boredom can cause inappropriate eating behaviors: "I eat because there is nothing else to do." Counselors can suggest many substitutes for eating to eliminate boredom and possibly increase activity. In some cases, hobbies or chores (such as doing needlework or polishing shoes) can serve as substitutes for eating while watching TV.

Some inappropriate behaviors involve rapid eating. It appears that the client is saying, "How fast can I clear this plate?" Along with this behavior is the inability to listen when the body provides signals of fullness or satiety. Booth states that satiety may not originate solely from gastric motility and distention or a physiological state, and that the power of suggestion also may play a large role in providing signals of fullness.[59]

In the eating-chain syndrome as described by Ferguson, activities can be used to break up patterns that lead to inappropriate behaviors.[60] Ferguson says that eating occurs at one end of a chain of responses. If the nutrition counselor works backward from the terminal behavior of eating, events or cues in the environment that started the chain of events leading to it can be identified. Wardle focuses on cueing in research that has shown positive results in weight control.[61]

Much of what goes on in the client's head, such as negative thoughts, can trigger inappropriate eating behaviors. The client who is thinking, "I'm really a rotten person for eating that piece of candy. It's no use. I might as well eat until I'm stuffed," probably will overeat out of despair. Mahoney and Mahoney describe the reversal of this process as "cognitive ecology."[62] **By substituting positive thoughts for negative ones, clients can develop a built-in self-reward system.**[63,64]

In some cases, lack of exercise can be a problem. Some clients may complain, "I just don't feel like moving." Studies have shown that decreased caloric intake plus exercise can be beneficial.[65,66] In fact, more fat tissue is reduced (as opposed to muscle tissue) if exercise programs are included with lowered caloric intake.

In general, inappropriate eating behaviors and lack of exercise may contribute to weight gain. The first step in achieving weight loss is to identify accurately the inappropriate eating behaviors.

ASSESSMENT OF EATING BEHAVIORS

The nutrition counselor must assess clients' eating behaviors. The first step is to try to identify the general problem from the many that may surface in a general interview. In reality, overweight clients may not want to lose weight but appear at a counseling session because their spouse or doctor has sent them. In some cases the major problem may be psychological, and referral to a specialist in that field may be the best course of action.[67]

If referral does not seem necessary, the next step is data collection. Six factors related to weight gain should be emphasized:

1. eating patterns
2. food quantities
3. food quality
4. activity levels
5. food-related thoughts
6. food-related cues

Exhibit 4–2 presents instructions and a form to use in gathering information in each of these categories, and Exhibit 4–3 is a sample already filled out. Adherence Tool 4–1 is a questionnaire for clients to fill out, and a simplified monitoring device for use with goal attainment is provided in Adherence Tool 4–2. Brownell states that when assessing obese clients, it is important to cover the following categories:[68]

• physiology
• eating behaviors
• physical activity
• psychological and social adjustment

Physiological factors can include an assessment of cell size and number. In assessing physical status, several categories should be considered: endocrine, hypothalmic, cardiopulmonary, orthopedic, genetic, weight, and family history. Bray and Teague provide an algorithm for medical assessment and delineate the steps necessary in diagnosing medical problems of an obese client.[69-72]

In the physiological analysis, counselors also should be concerned about body fat, which can be assessed through a variety of tests. The one most commonly used is skinfold thickness, using a caliper. Body fat is an indicator of physical status. Appendix C provides information on physiological measures of nutritional status.

Assessing eating behaviors is very important to eventual treatment. The most frequently used assessment method is a diet record. This can provide details on food preferences, eating style, environmental cues to eating, and amounts eaten.

Physical activity is an important component in any weight-loss program. Nutrition counselors should check on the client's exercise during both working and nonworking hours. Equally important is psychological and social functioning. Psychological functioning can include positive and negative monologues as described earlier; social functioning deals with responses by spouse, children, coworkers, or friends to weight loss and eating behaviors.

Exhibit 4–2 Data Collection Chart

INSTRUCTIONS FOR FILLING OUT THE FOOD DIARY

Time: Starting time for a meal or snack

Minutes spent eating: Length of the eating episode in minutes

M/S: Meal or snack (Indicate type of eating by the appropriate letter)

H: Hunger on a scale of 0 to 3, with 0 = no hunger, 3 = extreme hunger

Body position: 1 = walking; 2 = standing; 3 = sitting; 4 = lying down

Activity while eating: Record any activity you carry out while eating, such as watching television, reading, functioning in a workplace, or sweeping the floor.

Location of eating: Record each place you eat, such as your car, workplace, kitchen table, living room couch, or bed.

Food type and quantity: Indicate the content of your meal or snack by kind of food and quantity. Choose units of measurement that you will be able to reproduce from week to week. Accuracy is not as important as consistency.

Eating with whom: Indicate with whom you are eating or whether you are eating that meal or snack alone.

Feelings before and during eating: Record your feelings or mood immediately before (B) or while (W) eating. Typical feelings are anger, boredom, confusion, depression, frustration, sadness, etc.

Minutes spent exercising today: Record the total number of minutes you spent exercising, followed by the type of exercise (walking, jogging, running, riding a bicycle or a horse, dancing, skiing, swimming, bowling, etc.).

FOOD DIARY

Day of Week _____   Name _____

Time	Minutes Spent Eating	M/S	H	Body Position	Activity While Eating	Location of Eating	Food Type and Quantity	Eating with Whom	Feeling Before (B) and While (W) Eating	Minutes Spent Exercising Today
6:00										
11:00										
4:00										

M = Meal; S = Snack

H: Degree of Hunger (0 = None; 3 = Maximum)

Body Position: 1 = Walking, 2 = Sitting, 3 = Standing, 4 = Lying Down

(B): Before   (W): While

Source: Adapted from *Habits Not Diets* by J.M. Ferguson, pp. 13–14, with permission of Bull Publishing Company, © 1976.

Exhibit 4–3 Example of a Completed Food Diary Form

SAMPLE

Day of Week ___Monday___   Name ___R.S.T.___

Time	Minutes Spent Eating	M/S	H	Body Position	Activity While Eating	Location of Eating	Food Type and Quantity	Eating with Whom	Feeling Before (B) and While (W) Eating	Minutes Spent Exercising Today
6:00										
7:20–30	10 min	M	0	3	Paper	Kitchen	8 oz. coffee, 1 cup cereal	Wife	Happy	40 minutes walking
8:15–20	5 min	S	0	2	Talking	Work	4 oz. whole milk 1 cake doughnut 8 oz. coffee	Friends	Tired (B)	
10:30–?	5 min	S	1	1	Walking	Hall	1 cake doughnut	Alone	Late (W)	
11:00										
12:30	1 min	S	2	2	Work	Desk	1–1.5 oz. Snicker	Alone	Late (W)	
3:30– 3:40	10 min	M	3	3	Reading	Restaurant	1–8 oz. Coke, 3 oz. chd. hamburger patty 1 hamburger bun	Alone	Tired (B)	
4:00										
5:30– 6:00	30 min	S	3	3	Paper, TV	L.R.	1 oz. Scotch 1/4 c. peanuts	Family	Tired (B)	
6:00– 7:00	1 hour	M	2	3	TV	D.R.	Beef TV dinner 1 c. ice cream	Family	Angry (B)	
9:00										
10:30– 10:45	15 min	S	0	2	TV	L.R.	1/2 c. ice cream	Wife	Bored (B)	

M/S: Meal or Snack
H: Degree of Hunger (0 = None, 3 = Maximum)
Body Position: 1 = Walking, 2 = Standing, 3 = Sitting, 4 = Lying Down
(B): Before   (W): While

Source: Adapted from *Habits Not Diets* by J.M. Ferguson, pp. 13–14, with permission of Bull Publishing Company, © 1976.

TREATMENT STRATEGIES

Treatment strategies for obesity include self-management, self-monitoring, stimulus-control methods, reinforcement techniques, and the readiness-to-change model. Current programs have incorporated cognitive restructuring approaches, exercise, and social support in the achievement of long-term weight loss. Brownell provides a detailed list of many specific techniques that may be of value in the treatment of obesity.[73] The treatment strategies described below deal with the following three problems: lack of knowledge, forgetfulness, and lack of commitment.

Strategies To Deal with Lack of Knowledge

At baseline, the client needs a clear understanding of information pertinent to weight gain. Adherence Tool 4–1 elicits information on current eating disorders. Baseline data should be compared with information collected during strategy implementation. Adherence Tool 4–3 provides suggestions on facilitating weight loss.

Strategies to combat inappropriate eating behaviors follow. One is substitution of non–food-related activities. With this method, it is necessary to work with the clients in developing a list of enjoyable activities, particularly those requiring substantial expenditure of energy. The information obtained in the Data Collection Chart (Exhibit 4–2) can suggest a starting point. It is preferable to select activities that fit into the clients' daily routine, based on their suggestions as to which ones

---

Exhibit 4–4 Activity Substitutes for Eating

Clients can resort to numerous activities as alternatives to overeating. They can:
- Rearrange furniture.
- Spend extra time with a friend.
- Play cards or a game with someone—chess, Monopoly, bridge, etc.
- Go to a movie, play, or concert.
- Do something for charity.
- Go to a museum.
- Take a quiet walk.
- Take a long, leisurely bubble bath.
- Balance their checkbook.
- Write a letter.
- Make a phone call to a friend or relative.
- Wash their hair.
- Start a garden.
- Do home repairs.
- Write a creative poem or story.
- Do some sewing or creative stitchery.
- Do a crossword puzzle.
- Go jogging.
- Play golf.
- Join a softball team.
- Jump rope.
- Take up weight lifting.
- Go hiking.
- Take up, or increase participation in, a sport.

would work best. This is a time when counselors' listening skills and encouragement for clients can generate solutions that will lead to optimum results. Instead of eating, clients can substitute other activities such as those in Exhibit 4–4.

Interposing time between eating episodes is a second method for diminishing the urge. This strategy may require the use of a cooking timer, alarm clock, etc. Clients are asked to delay a snack for a certain number of minutes. Gradually they will be able to increase the time between the urge to snack and the actual act of eating to 10 or 15 minutes. During this interlude, they should be encouraged to perform some other activity. Clients usually are amazed at how well this strategy curbs their appetites.

The third strategy is cue elimination. Exhibit 4–2 can help in determining which cues lead to improper eating. For example, by looking at a rough house plan and identifying where eating episodes are occurring, clients can set up roadblocks to those cues. Many clients will find their snacking locations show up in clusters around the television set, favorite chairs, or in the kitchen by the refrigerator or sink (or the cafeteria or vending machines at work). They may be shocked to find they eat in more places than they believed.

Ferguson has designed an exercise to help eliminate eating cues:[74]

1. Ask the clients to select a specific room in the house in which all eating should occur. This place should be regarded as relatively comfortable. They should be cautioned to avoid eating while working to break the chain of association between eating and other activities. The nutrition counselor could suggest that every designated eating place be special. For example, if clients must eat while working, if at all feasible a place mat and silverware should be set, with a real (not plastic) cup for coffee or tea. At home, candlelight, flowers, and attractive plates and silverware can make the designated place "special."
2. Ask the clients to change their usual eating place at the table. If, for example, it is the head, they should move to one side; if they usually sit at the side, change with someone on the other side. The rationale is to break long-standing cues at the table.
3. Ask the clients to separate eating from other activities—to avoid combining eating with telephone conversations, watching TV, reading, working, etc. The emphasis should be on food with others and on making eating enjoyable by focusing on the taste and texture of the ingredients.
4. Ask clients to remove food from all places (particularly visible ones) except appropriate storage areas in the kitchen and to keep stored food out of sight by placing it in cupboards, in opaque containers, or in the refrigerator.
5. Suggest that clients keep fresh fruits and vegetables for snacks in attractive containers.
6. Request that clients remove serving containers from the table during mealtimes.

Once nutrition counselors have helped clients eliminate cues, the strategy can turn to decreasing serving size slowly. The use of smaller plates and smaller portions will decrease total caloric consumption. Nouvelle cuisine, with its very small portions arranged artistically in the center of large plates, is an attractive alternative. The foods need not involve fancy French cooking; the regular menu can simply be restaged in a fancier setting at no additional cost.

Many of these strategies involve getting help from spouse, family, and/or friends. Clients should be told to explain the strategies to anyone seen regularly. Closest friends' understanding of the program rationale can provide moral support. Through teaching others, clients may grasp strategies more clearly. Appendixes D and E provide useful tools for recording eating behaviors.

Strategies To Deal with Forgetfulness

At social events, people may unknowingly forget to follow a diet. A note on the refrigerator can remind the client of an upcoming event, "Don't forget to plan for Jan's party." Planning may involve calling the hostess on the phone to obtain a list of party foods to be served. This same idea can help clients plan for problem times such as eating out, weddings, or anniversaries. The cues should be simple and visible, such as "Remember your restaurant engagement Friday at noon!" posted on the bathroom mirror.

Many problems occur when people act spontaneously and either unknowingly or by choice fall into old habits. By providing memory cues, planning ahead can give clients the time they need to avoid situations that lead to inappropriate eating behaviors.

Strategies To Deal with Lack of Commitment

When clients know what is causing inappropriate behaviors and have used memory joggers without success, they may be entering a phase in which altering their lifestyle to make changes in body size no longer seems important—the relapse phase. At this point, a review of the client's initial list of reasons for wanting to lose weight may be valuable in identifying why commitment is waning.

In a relapse stage, it is important to emphasize that slips are normal. They are expected whenever changes in long-standing behaviors occur. Slips can be positive because they provide lessons in dealing with problems associated with eating behavior changes. The nutrition counselor's goal is to help the client avoid discouragement and continue change in eating behaviors. Use the adherence thermometer (Figure 3–2) and the readiness-to-change thermometer (Figure 3–3). Discuss barriers to change and identify strategies to eliminate them.

One strategy involves exploring negative thoughts. In some cases negative thoughts result from repeated indiscretions. Positive thinking is a useful strategy to deal with negative thoughts. Appendix F gives examples of ways in which record-keeping can help uncover negative thoughts associated with inappropriate eating behaviors. Getting clients to see how often negative thoughts force excessive food consumption can be a first step to weight control. This change from negative to positive thinking is an activity in which clients are very much in charge. Counselors can provide examples of thoughts such as: "I'm such a failure. I can't do anything right. I might as well give up. Who cares if I stuff myself with this cake?"

This negative monologue can be transformed to more positive thinking: "I ate one piece of cake, and even though it is high in calories I can stop with that one piece. I'm really feeling good about being able to stop without going ahead and eating the entire cake." From that point on, the clients can formulate positive self-thoughts to replace their negative ones (see Appendix G).

For most people, increasing exercise in combination with decreasing calories is helpful. Exhibit 4–2 is used to determine baseline activity levels. Many of the suggestions listed as substitutes for eating in Exhibit 4–4 involve an increase in activity. Nutrition counselors should encourage clients to enroll in exercise programs but caution them to check with a physician first.

Client progress is evaluated by comparing current and past data, as in Exhibit 4–5. Graphs of weight loss over time associated with specific eating behaviors (i.e., fat intake) may provide valuable feedback. Tables or graphs also will show when successes occurred so that client can reflect on what specifically happened at those positive weight loss points. Clients can be asked to extend a strategy, possibly by increasing negative-to-positive thought transformations. If a strategy is not working, it should be revised. For example, if finding a designated eating place at work poses problems, the nutrition counselor may need to discuss other means of cue elimination (e.g., using a place mat, plate, and silverware). In some cases, a new strategy may be appropriate. If clients find it impossible to substitute noneating activities for routine snacking, it may be necessary first to work to eliminate negative monologues, and then to add other activities as monologues are transformed to a more positive mode.

Facilitating the desire for commitment may require more intensive counselor client interaction. This may involve periodic phone calls set up to assess compliance with behaviors identified in a contract such as the one shown in Exhibit 4–6.

Although individual counseling is important and is effective initially in tailoring the diet, group sessions can be very helpful in facilitating maintenance of a low-calorie eating pattern. Groups provide support, ideas, chastisement, and concern. They can be very potent factors in achieving behavior change. **The following are some basic group process guidelines:**

- Ask open questions to begin sessions and start conversations on successes or failures with weight loss.
- Use the group members as a source for problem-solving ideas.

Exhibit 4–5 Diet Maintenance Data Collection

Day of Week _____			Name _____	
Time	M/S	H	Food Type and Quantity	Minutes Spent Exercising and Type of Exercise
6:00 AM				
11:00 AM				
4:00 PM				
9:00 PM				

M/S: Meal or Snack
H: Degree of Hunger (0 = none; 3 = maximum)

Source: Adapted from *Habits Not Diets* by J.M. Ferguson, pp. 87, with permission of Bull Publishing Company, © 1976.

- Place yourself, the counselor, in the role of facilitator.
- Make eye contact with less verbal class members to draw them out.
- Use more positive group members to keep other members' negative thoughts at a minimum.
- Use basic interviewing and counseling skills.

The group process is more a matter of skill mastery than concept memorization. To gain skill in this area, counselors should request to observe a Weight Watchers meeting. Any group-process meeting that requires members' active participation is helpful.

CONCLUSION

In summary, nutrition counseling for weight loss requires a knowledge of cues that promote overeating, suggestions for planning ahead, and behavioral strategies to increase commitment to dietary change once readiness to change is determined.

Exhibit 4–6 Sample Contract

I will reward myself each day for avoiding a high-calorie snack from 8:00 AM to 12:00 noon. I will avoid those foods I frequently use:
- 3 doughnuts or
- 2 Hostess Twinkies or
- 24 chocolate drops

I will substitute instead one of the following low-calorie foods from home:
- 5 saltine crackers with reduced sugar fruit jam
- Sugar-free gum
- 5 pretzel sticks

If I accomplish this goal in three out of five working days, I will reward myself with one of the following:
- shopping spree
- visit to my best friend who lives 20 miles away
- a night out at the theater

If I do not achieve the above goal, I will receive no rewards.
Every Friday at 10:00 AM (nutrition counselor) will call to check on my progress.

Client_____

Friend or Spouse_____

Nutrition Counselor_____

Review of Chapter 4
(Answers in Appendix H)

1. In the following examples, identify the inappropriate eating behaviors associated with weight gain:

   "I have followed this diet so religiously, I'm really proud of myself. The agony of passing up cocktails and opting for the diet drink at a party, the embarrassment of refusing my friend's seven-layer torte, the pain of refusing the birthday cake my kids made especially for me, and on and on. Those days are behind me now. I lost 20 pounds and now I'm home free."

What syndrome is this sort of thinking leading to?_____

   "What is wrong with me? Don't I have any willpower? I look like a fat slob and yet I continue to eat. I'm just a hopeless case."

What syndrome does this sort of self-talk tell you as a counselor that the client is struggling with?

2. List three steps in assessing individual eating behaviors.

   a. _____

   b. _____

   c. _____

3. List six strategies that might be used to facilitate weight loss in the following two clients.

   Jan, a 30-year-old female, is nearly 20 pounds overweight. She is very upset over this and has tried many ways toward quick and easy weight control—diet pills, fasting, fad diets, etc. Jan has a family of four and works from 8 AM to 5 PM at a dress shop. She prepares breakfast for her family each morning, eats at a cafeteria for lunch, and fixes dinner for the family each evening. Her major problem, she indicates, is evening snacking.

   Dan, a 40-year-old male, is 30 pounds overweight. He frequently is depressed over his weight and has tried many lose-weight-quick treatments. All have failed. He lives alone and works nights on a line in a factory. He sleeps during the day and eats all of his meals away from home.

   a. _____

   b. _____

   c. _____

   d. _____

   e. _____

   f. _____

4. Describe one situation in which you would use one or more of those six strategies. Indicate your rationale.

   _____

   _____

   _____

   _____

NOTES

1. R. Sichieri et al., "Relative Weight Classifications in the Assessment of Underweight and Overweight in the United States," *International Journal of Obesity* 16 (1992): 303–312.

2. National Center for Health Statistics, M.F. Najjar and M. Rowland, "Anthropometric Reference Data and Prevalence of Overweight," *Vital Health Statistics* 11, no. 238 (1987): 238.

3. D.F. Williamson, et al., "The 10-Year Incidence of Obesity and Major Weight Gain in Black and White U.S. Women Aged 30–55 Years." *American Journal of Clinical Nutrition,* 53 (1987): 15155–15185.

4. D.F. Williamson et al., "The 10-Year Incidence of Overweight and Major Weight Gain in U.S. Adults," *Archives of Internal Medicine* 150 (1990): 665–672.

5. F.X. Pi-Sunyer, "Health Implications of Obesity," *American Journal of Clinical Nutrition* 53 (1991): 1595S–1603S.

6. S. Heshka et al., "Obesity: Clinical Evaluation of Body Composition and Energy Expenditure," in *Obesity Pathophysiology, Psychology and Treatment,* ed. G.L. Blackburn and B.S. Kanders (New York: Chapman and Hall, 1994), 39–56, 61–62.

7. J.S. Garrow, *Treat Obesity Seriously: A Clinical Manual* (London: Churchill Livingstone, 1981).

8. World Health Organization, *Report of a WHO Study Group: Diet, Nutrition, and the Prevention of Chronic Diseases,* WHO Technical Report, Series 797 (Geneva: 1990), 69–71.

9. G.A. Bray. "Obesity," in *Present Knowledge in Nutrition,* ed. M.L. Brown (Washington, DC: International Life Sciences Institute, 1990), 23–38.

10. T.B. Van Itallie, "Body Weight, Morbidity, and Longevity," in *Obesity,* ed. P. Bjorntorp (Philadelphia: J.B. Lippincott. Co., 1992), 361–369.

11. P.R. Thomas, *Weighing the Options, Criteria for Evaluating Weight-Management Programs* (Washington, DC: National Academy Press, 1995).

12. R.J. Kucsmarski, "Prevalence of Overweight and Weight Gain in the United States," *American Journal of Clinical Nutrition* 55 (1992): 495S–502S.

13. Bray, *Present Knowledge in Nutrition,* 23–38.

14. National Center for Health Statistics, 238.

15. T.B. Van Itallie, "Health Implications of Overweight and Obesity in the United States," *Annals of Internal Medicine* 103 (1985): 983–988.

16. Bray, *Present Knowledge in Nutrition,* 23–38.

17. A. H. Kissebah et al., "Health Risks of Obesity," *Medical Clinics of North America* 73 (1989): 111.

18. J. Vague, "Diabetogenic and Atherogenic Fat," in *Progress in Obesity Research,* ed. Y. Oomura et al. (London: John Libbey, 1991), 343–358.

19. R. E. Ostlund et al., "The Ratio of Waist to Hip Circumference, Plasma Insulin Level and Glucose Intolerance as Independent Predictors of the HDL2 Cholesterol Level in Older Adults," *New England Journal of Medicine* 322 (1990): 229.

20. P. Bjorntorp, "Criteria of Obesity," in *Progress in Obesity Research,* ed. Y. Oomura et al. (London: John Libbey, 1990), 655–658.

21. Food and Nutrition Board, *Recommended Dietary Allowances,* 10th ed. (Washington, DC: National Academy Press, 1989), 24–38.

22. E.N. Whitney and E.M.N. Hamilton, *Understanding Nutrition* (St. Paul, MN: West Publishing Co., 1981), 248.

23. Food and Nutrition Board, *Recommended Dietary Allowances,* 59.

24. K.D. Brownell and F.M. Kramer, "Behavioral Management of Obesity," in *Obesity Pathophysiology, Psychology and Treatment,* ed. G.L. Blackburn and B.S. Kanders (New York: Chapman and Hall, 1994), 231, 234.

25. K.D. Brownell and R.W. Jeffrey, "Improving Long-Term Weight Loss: Pushing the Limits of Treatment," *Behavior Therapy* 18 (1987): 353.

26. F.M. Kramer et al., "Long-Term Follow-Up of Behavioral Treatment for Obesity: Patterns of Weight Regain among Men and Women," *International Journal of Obesity* 13 (1989): 123–136.

27. T.A. Wadden et al., "Three-Year Follow-Up of the Treatment of Obesity by Very Low Calorie Diet, Behavior Therapy, and Their Combination," *Journal of Consulting and Clinical Psychology* 56 (1988): 925.

28. G.T. Wilson and K.D. Brownell, "Behavior Therapy for Obesity: An Evaluation of Treatment Outcome," *Advances in Behavior, Research and Therapy* 3 (1980): 49.

29. Brownell and Kramer, *Obesity Pathophysiology, Psychology and Treatment,* 236.

30. D.B. Jeffrey, "Prevalence of Overweight and Weight Loss Behavior in a Metropolitan Adult Population: The Minnesota Heart Survey Experience, *Addictive Behaviors* 1 (1975): 23–26.

31. G.R. Leon, "Current Directions in the Treatment of Obesity," *Psychological Bulletin* 83 (1976): 557–578.

32. A.J. Stunkard, "From Explanation to Action in Psychosomatic Medicine: The Case of Obesity," *Psychosomatic Medicine* 37 (1975): 195–236.

33. S.M. Hall et al., "Permanence of Two Self-Managed Treatments of Overweight in University and Community Populations," *Journal of Consulting Clinical Psychology* 42 (1974): 781–786.

34. W.M. Beneke and B.K. Paulsen, "Long Term Efficacy of a Behavior Modification Weight Loss Program: A Comparison of Two Follow-Up Maintenance Strategies," *Behavior Therapy* 10 (1978): 8–13.

35. R.R. Wing, "Behavioral Treatment of Severe Obesity," *American Journal of Clinical Nutrition 55* (1992): 545S–551S.

36. R.G. Kingsley and G.T. Wilson, "Behavior Therapy for Obesity: A Comparative Investigation of Long Term Efficacy," *Journal of Consulting and Clinical Psychology* 45 (1977): 288–298.

37. R.B. Stuart, "Behavior Control of Overeating," *Behaviour Research and Therapy* 5 (1967): 357–365.

38. P.M. Miller and K.L. Sims, "Evaluation and Component Analysis of a Comprehensive Weight Control Program," *International Journal of Obesity* 5 (1981): 57–65.

39. K.D. Brownell and A.J. Stunkard, "Behavior Therapy and Behavior Change: Uncertainties in Programs for Weight Control," *Behavior Research and Therapy* 16 (1978): 301.

40. R.R. Wing, "Behavioral Treatment of Severe Obesity," 545S–551S.

41. Miller and Sims, "Evaluation and Component Analysis of a Comprehensive Weight Control Program," 57–65.

42. M.J. Mahoney and K. Mahoney, "Treatment of Obesity: A Clinical Exploration," in *Obesity: Behavioral Approaches to Dietary Management,* ed. B.J. Williams et al. (New York: Brunner/ Mazel, 1976), 30–39.

43. J.H. Wilmore, "Body Composition in Sport and Exercise: Directions for Future Research," *Medicine and Science in Sports Exercise* 15 (1983): 21.

44. W.B. Zuti and L.A. Golding, "Comparing Diet and Exercise as Weight Reduction Tools," *Physical Sports Medicine* 4 (1976): 49.

45. G. Gwinup, "Weight Loss without Dietary Restriction: Efficacy of Different Forms of Aerobic Exercise," *American Journal of Sports Medicine* 15 (1987): 275.

46. G.A.L. Meijer, "Physical Activity: Implications for Human Energy Metabolism" (Ph.D. diss., University of Limburg at Maastricht, 1990).

47. J.O. Hill et al., "Effects of Exercise and Food Restriction on Body Composition and Metabolic Rate in Obese Women," *American Journal of Clinical Nutrition* 46 (1987): 622.

48. Council on Scientific Affairs, "Treatment of Obesity in Adults," *Journal of the American Dietetic Association* 260 (1988): 2547.

49. K.N. Pavlou et al., "Effects of Dieting and Exercise on Lean Body Mass, Oxygen Uptake, and Strength," *Medicine and Science in Sports Exercise* 17 (1985): 466.

50. Mahoney and Mahoney, "Treatment of Obesity," 30–39.

51. K.D. Brownell et al., "The Effect of Couples Training and Partner Cooperativeness in the Behavioral Treatment of Obesity," *Behaviour Research and Therapy* 16 (1978): 323–333.

52. M.J. Mahoney, "The Obese Eating Style: Bites, Beliefs and Behavior Modification," *Addictive Behaviors* 1 (1975): 47–53.

53. N. Adams et al., "The Eating Style of Obese and Non-Obese Women," *Behaviour Research and Therapy* 16 (1978): 225–232.

54. Beneke and Paulsen, "Long Term Efficacy," 8–13.

55. J.F. Honig and G.L. Blackburn, "The Problem of Obesity: An Overview," in *Obesity Pathophysiology, Psychology and Treatment,* ed. G.L. Blackburn and B.S. Kanders (New York: Chapman and Hall, 1994), 1–8.

56. T.B. Van Itallie, "Dietary Approaches to the Treatment of Obesity," in *Obesity,* ed. A.J. Stunkard (Philadelphia: W.B. Saunders Company, 1980), 249–261.

57. S.A. Shikora et al., "Surgical Treatment of Obesity," in *Obesity Pathophysiology, Psychology and Treatment,* ed. G.L. Blackburn and B.S. Kanders (New York: Chapman and Hall, 1994), 264–282.

58. M.A. Staten, "Pharmacologic Therapy for Obesity," in *Obesity Pathophysiology, Psychology and Treatment,* ed. G.L. Blackburn and B.S. Kanders (New York: Chapman and Hall, 1994), 283–299.

59. D.A. Booth, "Acquired Behavior Controlling Energy Input and Output," in *Obesity,* ed. A.J. Stunkard (Philadelphia: W.B. Saunders Company, 1980), 102.

60. J.M. Ferguson, *Habits Not Diets* (Palo Alto, CA: Bull Publishing Co., 1976), 65.

61. J. Wardle, "Conditioning Processes and Cue Exposure in the Modification of Excessive Eating," *Addictive Behaviors* 15 (1990): 387.

62. M.J. Mahoney and K. Mahoney, *Permanent Weight Control* (New York: W.W. Norton and Co., 1976), 46–68.

63. C.F. Telch et al., "Group Cognitive-Behavioral Treatment for the Nonpurging Bulimic: An Initial Evaluation," *Journal of Consulting Clinical Psychology* 58 (1990): 629.

64. M.R. Dimatteo and D.D. DeNicola, *Achieving Patient Compliance: The Psychology of the Medical Practitioner's Role* (New York: Pergamon Press, 1982), 236–237.

65. R. Woo et al., "Effect of Exercise on Spontaneous Caloric Intake," *American Journal of Clinical Nutrition* 36 (1982): 470–484.

66. J. O'Hill et al., "Effects of Exercise and Food Restriction on Body Composition," *American Journal of Clinical Nutrition* 46 (1987): 622–630.

67. M.L. Russell, *Behavioral Counseling in Medicine: Strategies for Modifying at Risk Behavior* (New York: Oxford University Press, 1986), 306–315.

68. K.D. Brownell, "Assessment of Eating Disorders," in *Assessment of Adult Disorders,* ed. D. Barlow (New York: Guilford Press, 1981), 366–374.

69. G.A. Bray and R.J. Teague, "An Algorithm for the Medical Evaluation of Obese Patients," in *Obesity,* ed. G.A. Bray (Philadelphia: W.B. Saunders Company, 1980), 240–248.

70. B.S. Kanders et al., "Obesity," in *Conns Current Therapy,* ed. R.E. Rakel (Philadelphia: W.B. Saunders Company, 1981), 524–531.

71. R.T. Frankel and M.Y. Yang, *Obesity and Weight Control: The Health Professional's Guide to Understanding and Treatment* (Gaithersburg, MD: Aspen Publishers, Inc., 1988).

72. F.X. Pi-Sunyer, "Obesity," in *Modern Nutrition in Health and Disease,* 7th ed., ed. M.E. Shils and V.R. Young (Philadelphia: Lea & Febiger, 1988), 795–816.

73. K.D. Brownell, *The LEARN Program for Weight Control* (Dallas, TX: American Health Publication Co., 1992).

74. Ferguson, *Habits,* 31–32.

Adherence Tool 4–1: Client Questionnaire for Low-Calorie Eating Patterns in Treating Obesity

The following questionnaire is a monitoring device that has been designed to efficiently collect patient information in clinical weight control programs. It has several functions.

Initially, it is a useful screening device or test of motivation. Individuals who will not take time to fill it out probably will not take time to participate fully in the behavioral weight-control program.

Second, the answers to these questions can be of great use to the therapist during the initial interviews and later during the weight-control sessions. The weight history allows the therapist to look systematically at the clients' own views of their weight problems, and at some of the environmental influences they feel are important to their weight problems. The history of past attempts to lose weight, the lengths of time they have stayed in weight-loss programs, and the reasons for past failure can all be useful. Also, clients' reports of mood changes during previous periods of weight loss can help you anticipate and deal with problems that might arise during treatment.

A brief medical history is included to give you a basis for referral. For example, if someone indicates he or she is a diabetic, and does not have a physician, you might suggest contacting a doctor before the weight-control program begins. Similarly, if someone indicates a history of heart disease, you may want to check with that person's physician before dealing with increased activity and exercise.

The questions about social and family history provide additional information that is of use medically (for example, the cause of parental death and the family weight history).

In most states the information contained in this questionnaire is confidential. Without *written* approval from the clients, this information cannot be divulged to interested individuals, physicians, insurance companies, or law enforcement agencies.

Adapted with permission from J.M. Ferguson, *Learning To Eat, Behavior Modification for Weight Control,* © 1975, Bull Publishing Company.

Name: _____ Sex: M F   Age: _____ Birthdate: _____

Address: _____ Home phone: _____

_____ Office phone: _____

WEIGHT HISTORY

1. Your present weight _____ Height _____
2. Describe your present weight (check one)

___ Very overweight   ___ About average

___ Slightly overweight

3. Are you dissatisfied with the way you look at this weight? (check one)

___ Completely satisfied   ___ Dissatisfied

___ Satisfied   ___ Very dissatisfied

___ Neutral

4. At what weight have you *felt* your best or do you think you would feel your best?_____

5. How much weight would you like to lose?_____

6. Do you feel your weight affects your daily activities?

___ No effect   ___ Often interferes

___ Some effect   ___ Extreme effect

7. Why do you want to lose weight at this time? _____

_____

8. What are the attitudes of the following people about your attempt(s) to lose weight?

	Negative (They disapprove or are resentful)	*Indifferent* (They don't care or don't help)	*Positive* (They encourage me and are understanding)
Husband			
Wife			
Children			
Parents			
Employer			
Friends			

continues

Adherence Tool 4–1   continued

9. Do these attitudes affect your weight loss or gain?   Yes   No

   If yes, please describe:_____

   _____

   _____

10. Indicate on the following table the periods in your life when you have been
    overweight. *Where appropriate,* list your maximum weight for each period
    and number of pounds you were overweight. Briefly describe any methods
    you used to lose weight in that five-year period (e.g., diet, shots, pills). Also
    list any significant life events you feel were related to either your weight gain
    or loss (e.g., college tests, marriage, pregnancies, illness).

Age	Maximum Weight	Pounds Overweight	Methods Used To Lose Weight	Significant Events Related to Weight Change
Birth				
0–5				
6–10				
11–15				
16–20				
21–25				
26–30				
31–35				
36–40				
41–45				
46–50				
51–55				

Age	Maximum Weight	Pounds Overweight	Methods Used To Lose Weight	Significant Events Related to Weight Change
56–60				
61–65				

11. How *physically* active are you? (check one)

___ Very active   ___ Inactive   ___ Average

___ Active   ___ Very inactive

12. What do you do for physical exercise and how often do you do it?

ACTIVITY (for example, swimming, jogging, dancing)	FREQUENCY (daily, weekly, monthly)

13. A number of different ways of losing weight are listed below. Please indicate which methods you have used by filling the appropriate blanks.

	Ages Used	Number of Times Used	Maximum Weight Lost	Comments (Length of Time Weight Loss Maintained; Successes; Difficulties)
TOPS (Take Off Pounds Sensibly)				
Weight Watchers				
Pills				
Supervised Diet				
Unsupervised Diet				
Starvation				
Behavior Modification				
Psychotherapy				
Hypnosis				
Other				

continues

Adherence Tool 4–1   continued

14. Which method did you use for the longest period of time? _____

_____

15. Have you had a major mood change during or after a significant weight loss? Indicate any mood changes on the following checklist.

	Not at All	A Little Bit	Moder- ately	Quite a Bit	Extremely
a. Depressed, sad, feeling down, unhappy, the blues	____	_____	_____	____	_____
b. Anxious, nervous, restless, or uptight all the time	____	_____	_____	____	_____
c. Physically weak	____	_____	_____	____	_____
d. Elated or happy	____	_____	_____	____	_____
e. Easily irritated, annoyed, or angry	____	_____	_____	____	_____
f. Fatigued, worn out, tired all the time	____	_____	_____	____	_____
g. A lack of self-confidence	____	_____	_____	____	_____

16. What usually goes wrong with your weight-loss programs? _____

_____

_____

MEDICAL HISTORY

17. When did you last have a complete physical examination? _____

18. Who is your current doctor? _____

19. What medical problems do you have at the present time? _____

_____

_____

20. What medications or drugs do you take regularly? _____

_____

_____

21. List any medications, drugs, or foods you are allergic to. _____

_____

_____

22. List any hospitalizations or operations. Indicate how old you were at each hospital admission.

      Age   Reason for hospitalizations

_____   _____

_____   _____

_____   _____

_____   _____

23. List any serious illnesses you have had that have not required hospitalization. Indicate how old you were during each illness.

      Age   Illness

_____   _____

_____   _____

_____   _____

_____   _____

24. Describe any of your medical problems that are complicated by excess weight.

_____

_____

_____

_____

_____

25. How much alcohol do you usually drink per week?_____

26. List any psychiatric contact, individual counseling, or marital counseling that you have had or are now having.

      Age   Reason for contact and type of therapy

_____   _____

_____   _____

_____   _____

_____   _____

continues

Adherence Tool 4–1   continued

SOCIAL HISTORY

27. Circle the last year of school attended:

    1 2 3 4 5 6 7 8   9 10 11 12   1 2 3 4   M.A.   Ph.D.

    Grade School   High School   College

    Other _____

28. Describe your present occupation _____

    _____

29. How long have you worked for your present employer? _____

30. Present marital status (check one):

    ____ Single

    ____ Married

    ____ Widowed

    ____ Divorced

    ____ Separated

    ____ Engaged

31. Answer the following questions for each marriage:

    Date of marriage   _____, _____ _____

    Date of termination   _____ _____ _____

    Reason (death, divorce, etc.) _____ _____ _____

    Number of children   _____ _____ _____

32. Spouse's Age _____ Weight _____ Height _____

33. Describe your spouse's occupation _____

34. Describe your spouse's weight (check one):

    ____ Very overweight

    ____ Slightly overweight

    ____ About average

    ____ Slightly underweight

    ____ Very underweight

35. List your children's ages, sex, heights, weights, and circle whether they are overweight, average, or underweight. Include any children from previous marriages, whether they are living with you or not.

Age	Sex	Weight	Height	Overweight			Underweight	
——	——	——	——	very	slightly	average	slightly	very
——	——	——	——	very	slightly	average	slightly	very
——	——	——	——	very	slightly	average	slightly	very
——	——	——	——	very	slightly	average	slightly	very
——	——	——	——	very	slightly	average	slightly	very

36. Who lives at home with you? _____

FAMILY HISTORY

37. Is your father living?   Yes   No   Father's age now, or age at and cause of death _____

_____

38. Is your mother living?   Yes   No   Mother's age now, or age at and cause of death _____

39. Describe your father's occupation _____

40. Describe your mother's occupation _____

41. Describe your father's weight while you were growing up (check one).

___ Very overweight

___ Slightly overweight

___ About average

___ Slightly underweight

___ Very underweight

42. Describe your mother's weight while you were growing up (check one).

___ Very overweight

___ Slightly overweight

___ About average

___ Slightly underweight

___ Very underweight

continues

Adherence Tool 4–1   continued

43. List your brothers' and sisters' ages, sex, present weights, heights, and circle
    whether they are overweight, average, or underweight.

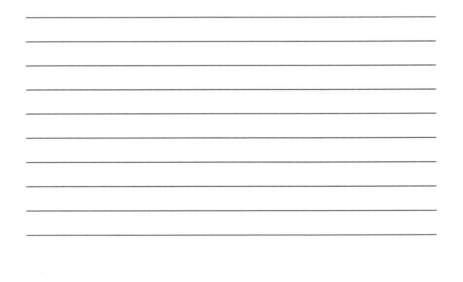

Age	Sex	Weight	Height		Overweight		Underweight	
⎯⎯	⎯⎯	⎯⎯⎯	⎯⎯⎯	very	slightly	average	slightly	very
⎯⎯	⎯⎯	⎯⎯⎯	⎯⎯⎯	very	slightly	average	slightly	very
⎯⎯	⎯⎯	⎯⎯⎯	⎯⎯⎯	very	slightly	average	slightly	very
⎯⎯	⎯⎯	⎯⎯⎯	⎯⎯⎯	very	slightly	average	slightly	very
⎯⎯	⎯⎯	⎯⎯⎯	⎯⎯⎯	very	slightly	average	slightly	very

44. Please add any additional information you feel may be relevant to your
    weight problem. This includes interactions with your family and friends that
    might sabotage a weight-loss program, and additional family or social history
    that you feel might help us understand your weight problem.

⎯⎯⎯⎯⎯⎯⎯⎯⎯⎯⎯⎯⎯⎯⎯⎯⎯⎯⎯⎯⎯⎯⎯⎯⎯⎯⎯⎯⎯⎯⎯⎯

⎯⎯⎯⎯⎯⎯⎯⎯⎯⎯⎯⎯⎯⎯⎯⎯⎯⎯⎯⎯⎯⎯⎯⎯⎯⎯⎯⎯⎯⎯⎯⎯

⎯⎯⎯⎯⎯⎯⎯⎯⎯⎯⎯⎯⎯⎯⎯⎯⎯⎯⎯⎯⎯⎯⎯⎯⎯⎯⎯⎯⎯⎯⎯⎯

⎯⎯⎯⎯⎯⎯⎯⎯⎯⎯⎯⎯⎯⎯⎯⎯⎯⎯⎯⎯⎯⎯⎯⎯⎯⎯⎯⎯⎯⎯⎯⎯

⎯⎯⎯⎯⎯⎯⎯⎯⎯⎯⎯⎯⎯⎯⎯⎯⎯⎯⎯⎯⎯⎯⎯⎯⎯⎯⎯⎯⎯⎯⎯⎯

⎯⎯⎯⎯⎯⎯⎯⎯⎯⎯⎯⎯⎯⎯⎯⎯⎯⎯⎯⎯⎯⎯⎯⎯⎯⎯⎯⎯⎯⎯⎯⎯

⎯⎯⎯⎯⎯⎯⎯⎯⎯⎯⎯⎯⎯⎯⎯⎯⎯⎯⎯⎯⎯⎯⎯⎯⎯⎯⎯⎯⎯⎯⎯⎯

⎯⎯⎯⎯⎯⎯⎯⎯⎯⎯⎯⎯⎯⎯⎯⎯⎯⎯⎯⎯⎯⎯⎯⎯⎯⎯⎯⎯⎯⎯⎯⎯

⎯⎯⎯⎯⎯⎯⎯⎯⎯⎯⎯⎯⎯⎯⎯⎯⎯⎯⎯⎯⎯⎯⎯⎯⎯⎯⎯⎯⎯⎯⎯⎯

⎯⎯⎯⎯⎯⎯⎯⎯⎯⎯⎯⎯⎯⎯⎯⎯⎯⎯⎯⎯⎯⎯⎯⎯⎯⎯⎯⎯⎯⎯⎯⎯

Adherence Tool 4–2:   Goal Attainment Chart (Monitoring Device)

Action Plan for Goal Attainment

Name:_____ Date: _____

1. Goal:_____

_____

_____

_____

2. Was goal achieved? _____

		Days						
Week	1	2	3	4	5	6	7
1							
2							
3							
4							

☆ = Yes, goal was achieved

○ = No, goal was not achieved

3. Significant events that helped or hindered goal attainment: _____

_____

_____

4. Rewards given for achieving goal: _____

_____

_____

_____

5. Comments/suggestions: _____

_____

6. Next contact date and time: _____

Adherence Tool 4–3: Don't Be Caught in the Trees (Informational and Cueing Device)

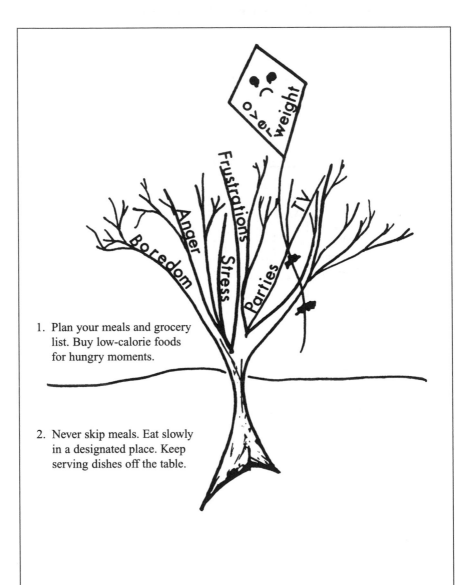

1. Plan your meals and grocery list. Buy low-calorie foods for hungry moments.

2. Never skip meals. Eat slowly in a designated place. Keep serving dishes off the table.

Adherence Tool 4–3 (continued)

3. Ask friends and family to help.

4. Leave a bit of everything on your plate. Eat from smaller plates.

5. Store food only in the kitchen.

6. When preparing foods, taste only once.

7. Let other people clean their own plates after eating.

CHAPTER 5

Nutrition Counseling in Prevention and Treatment of Coronary Heart Disease

---

CHAPTER OBJECTIVES

1. Identify common dietary misconceptions about fat- and cholesterol-modified patterns that lead to inappropriate eating behaviors.

2. Identify common dietary excesses that contribute to inappropriate eating behaviors associated with diets low in fat and cholesterol.

3. Identify specific nutrients that should be emphasized in assessing a baseline eating pattern before providing dietary instruction.

4. Identify strategies to treat inappropriate behaviors associated with fat- and cholesterol-modified eating patterns.

5. Generate strategies to deal with clients following low-fat and low-cholesterol eating patterns.

6. Recommend dietary adherence tools for clients on fat- and cholesterol-modified eating patterns.

CHOLESTEROL, FAT, AND CORONARY HEART DISEASE

Coronary heart disease (CHD) is the leading cause of death among adult Americans.[1] Based on this evidence, in 1993 the National Heart, Lung, and Blood Institute sponsored a Second Report of the Expert Panel on Detection, Evaluation, and Treatment of High Blood Cholesterol in Adults (Adult Treatment Panel II, or ATP II). The results of this group's deliberations were the National Cholesterol Education Program's (NCEP's) updated recommendations for cholesterol management.[2]

The NCEP report identifies low-density lipoproteins (LDL) as the primary target of cholesterol-lowering therapy. Dietary therapy remains the first line of treatment of high blood cholesterol, and drug therapy is reserved for patients who are considered to be at high risk for CHD. This report focuses on CHD risk status and serves as a guide to type and intensity of cholesterol-lowering therapy. High-density lipoprotein (HDL) is targeted as a negative CHD risk factor. The NCEP report emphasizes physical activity and weight loss as components of the dietary therapy of high blood cholesterol. The ATP II recommends that patients with high-risk LDL-cholesterol (>160 mg/dL), those with borderline-high-risk LDL-cholesterol (130–159 mg/dL) who have two or more risk factors, and those with CHD or other clinical atherosclerotic disease and an LDL-cholesterol >100 mg/dL should enter into a program of therapy. The first two groups qualify for primary prevention and the latter for secondary prevention. In primary prevention, most patients should receive dietary therapy and should increase physical activity. For patients with CHD or other clinical atherosclerotic disease, the target goal for LDL-cholesterol reduction is 100 mg/dL or lower. Maximal dietary therapy should be initiated in patients. Table 5–1 presents serum cholesterol levels and Table 5–2 presents LDL cholesterol levels for U.S. men and women.

Exhibit 5–1 provides the NCEP guidelines for dietary therapy in treatment of high blood cholesterol.

This chapter provides counseling strategies for special low-cholesterol, fat-modified eating patterns to help prevent coronary disease. Good basic nutrition plays a primary role in devising a fat-modified diet pattern. The Food and Nutrition Board has not established a Recommended Dietary Allowance (RDA) for total fat.[3] It does recommend that adequate lipids be incorporated into the diet to provide the body with essential fatty acids and carriers of fat-soluble vitamins. Ingesting 15 to 25 grams of fat per day normally meets this requirement.

Studies in humans and animals show that the requirement for essential fatty acids is fulfilled when 1 to 2 percent of the total caloric intake is provided by linoleic acid.[4] A diet of 1,500 calories can provide 1.5 to 3.0 grams of linoleic acid. This is accomplished easily by using vegetable oils in cooking and salad dressing. Corn, soy, and cottonseed oils each contain 6 to 8 grams of linoleic acid per tablespoon, mayonnaise 6 grams, and margarine 1 to 5 grams.

The United Nations Committee on Dietary Allowances also places a maximum limit on the amount of total polyunsaturated fat consumed in a day. The committee recommends not exceeding 10 percent of dietary calories as polyunsaturated fat.[5]

THEORIES AND FACTS ABOUT NUTRITION AND CORONARY HEART DISEASE

Eating large amounts of cholesterol and fat can cause an elevation in various lipid-carrying particles in the blood, a condition called hyperlipidemia. Hyperlipoproteinemia is a more specific term used to define the class or classes of plasma lipoproteins that are elevated. There is clinical interest in hyperlipopro-

Table 5–1 Mean Serum Cholesterol Levels of Men and Women, SEM, Age-Adjusted Values, Selected Percentiles, Number of Examined Persons, and Estimated Population, by Race and Age: United States, 1978–1980

Race, Age, y	No. of Persons Examined	Estimated Population in Thousands	Mean	SEM	Percentile*								
					5th	10th	15th	25th	50th	75th	85th	90th	95th
Men													
All races†													
20–74	5604	63611	211	1.2	144	156	165	179	206	239	258	271	291
20–24	676	9331	180	1.7	129	136	145	155	176	202	215	227	246
25–34	1067	15895	199	1.5	141	152	159	172	194	220	240	254	275
35–44	745	11367	217	2.0	153	166	173	187	215	244	262	275	293
45–54	690	11114	227	1.8	159	176	182	197	223	255	271	283	303
55–64	1227	9607	229	1.8	164	176	184	198	225	254	277	288	307
65–74	1199	6297	221	1.8	153	167	175	191	217	249	265	279	301
White													
20–74	4883	55808	211	1.2	145	157	166	179	207	239	258	271	291
20–24	581	8052	180	1.8	131	138	146	155	176	202	216	229	244
25–34	901	13864	199	1.7	144	153	161	172	194	220	239	254	273
35–44	653	9808	217	1.8	153	166	173	187	214	244	260	272	291
45–54	617	9865	227	1.8	160	177	181	198	222	254	271	283	303
55–64	1086	8642	230	2.0	164	178	185	190	225	255	278	289	307
65–74	1045	5576	222	2.0	153	167	175	191	217	250	266	281	301
Black													
20–74	607	6102	208	2.5	133	146	156	171	200	238	260	273	301
20–24	79	1043	171	3.7†	…†	128	134	149	170	193	210	211	…†
25–34	139	1546	199	4.1†	129	136	144	163	192	226	248	259	301
35–44	70	1112	218	8.3†	…†	156	168	176	202	238	275	283	…†

continues

45–54	62	1044	229	7.1†	...†	174	184	195	232	261	268	279	...†
55–64	129	801	223	4.8†	157	168	172	183	218	254	271	299	312
65–74	128	555	217	4.2	149	163	173	183	216	244	261	277	299
Age-adjusted values													
All races, 20–74	:	:	211	1.1	:	:	:	:	:	:	:	:	:
White, 20–74	:	:	211	1.1	:	:	:	:	:	:	:	:	:
Black, 20–74	:	:	209	2.5	:	:	:	:	:	:	:	:	:
Women													
All races†													
20–74	6260	69994	215	1.2	143	156	166	179	210	245	266	282	305
20–24	738	9994	184	1.9	132	140	145	157	180	204	216	230	250
25–34	1170	16856	192	1.4	135	145	154	164	188	215	233	243	263
35–44	844	12284	207	1.8	147	158	164	177	202	231	248	260	276
45–54	763	11918	232	2.2	164	178	188	199	228	257	275	290	306
55–64	1329	10743	249	2.0	180	193	203	215	242	277	299	314	336
65–74	1416	8198	246	1.6	173	189	198	214	241	274	295	309	327
White													
20–74	5418	60785	216	1.3	143	156	166	179	210	246	267	282	305
20–24	624	8408	184	2.1	133	140	147	159	181	204	215	230	249
25–34	1000	14494	192	1.5	135	145	153	164	188	215	235	244	261
35–44	726	10584	207	1.9	147	157	164	177	203	231	248	259	277
45–54	647	10369	232	2.6	166	179	188	199	228	257	274	290	308
55–64	1176	9601	249	1.7	180	193	203	215	244	277	298	312	330
65–74	1245	7329	246	1.7	174	190	199	214	242	275	296	309	328

continues

Table 5–1 continued

Race, Age, y	No. of Persons Examined	Estimated Population in Thousands	Mean	SEM	Percentile*								
					5th	10th	15th	25th	50th	75th	85th	90th	95th
Black													
20–74	729	7579	212	3.1	140	154	166	176	205	237	263	279	308
20–24	94	1304	185	4.9†	..†	136	144	156	178	204	220	237	..†
25–34	145	1953	191	4.1†	129	144	156	167	190	212	226	235	267
35–44	103	1415	206	4.5†	143	158	170	175	194	233	254	274	279
45–54	100	1215	230	7.2†	150	172	181	200	226	263	277	291	306
55–64	135	959	251	8.0†	178	185	198	211	233	280	318	336	345
65–74	152	733	243	4.2	173	189	198	211	237	269	290	308	323
Age-adjusted values													
All races, 20–74	...	...	215	1.2	...	...	...	...	...	...	...	...	...
White, 20–74	...	...	215	1.2	...	...	...	...	...	...	...	...	...
Black, 20–74	...	...	214	2.7	...	...	...	...	...	...	...	...	...

*Serum cholesterol values are given in milligrams per deciliter. To convert values to millimoles per liter, multiply by 0.02586.
†Includes data for races not shown separately.
Source: Data taken from *Total Serum Cholesterol Levels of Adults 20–74 Years of Age: United States, 1976–1980, Vital and Health Statistics* by The National Center for Health Statistics, Series II, No. 236, U.S. Department of Health and Human Services Publication, PHS 86-1686.

Table 5–2 Calculated Levels of Serum Low-Density Lipoprotein (LDL) Cholesterol* for Persons† 20 to 74 Years of Age Fasting 12 Hours or More, by Sex and Age: Means and Selected Percentiles, United States, 1976–1980

Sex, Age, y	No. of Persons Examined	Estimated Population in Thousands	Mean	SD	Selected Percentiles								
					5th	10th	15th	25th	50th	75th	85th	90th	95th
Men													
20–74	1037	21262	140	39	80	92	100	113	136	164	181	194	208
20–24	72	1852	109	36	..‡	70	74	88	104	129	149	154	..‡
25–34	174	5186	128	33	76	87	94	108	128	148	161	171	189
35–44	130	3866	145	40	81	96	105	116	138	176	192	203	206
45–54	106	3543	150	36	99	103	112	119	146	171	189	195	211
55–64	267	3943	148	39	84	101	108	118	147	171	191	206	217
65–74	288	2872	149	40	87	105	109	120	144	174	188	199	217
Women													
20–74	1246	27102	141	43	81	91	98	110	136	164	186	199	220
20–24	105	3325	114	33	69	74	83	94	106	136	149	155	179
25–34	194	5517	121	33	72	83	90	98	116	139	154	166	187
35–44	166	4800	129	34	78	90	97	107	126	150	163	171	191
45–54	168	5155	157	45	94	104	116	125	156	184	200	213	226
55–64	282	4644	159	42	101	113	118	129	150	188	205	219	237
65–74	331	3661	162	44	98	109	122	135	158	186	207	226	245

*Serum LDL Cholesterol = Serum Total Cholesterol – HDL Cholesterol – (Triglycerides/5). Persons with a serum triglyceride value greater than 400 mg/dL were excluded.

†Includes other races in addition to black and white.

‡Sample size insufficient to produce statistically reliable results.

Source: Data taken from *Total Serum Cholesterol Levels of Adults 20–74 Years of Age: United States, 1976–1980, Vital and Health Statistics* by The National Center for Health Statistics, Series II, No. 236, U.S. Department of Health and Human Services Publication, PHS 86-1686.

Exhibit 5–1 NCEP Guidelines for Dietary Therapy in Treatment of High Blood Cholesterol

Nutrient	Recommended Intake	
	Step One Diet	*Step Two Diet*
total fat	Less than 30% of total calories	
saturated fatty acids	Less than 10% of total calories	Less than 7% of total calories
polyunsaturated fatty acids	up to 10% of total calories	
monounsaturated fatty acids	10% to 15% of total calories	
carbohydrates	50% to 60% of total calories	
protein	10% to 20% of total calories	
cholesterol	Less than 300 mg/day	Less than 200 mg/day
total calories	to achieve and maintain desirable weight	

Source: N.D. Ernst, et al., "The National Cholesterol Education Program: Implications for Dietetic Practitioners from the Adult Treatment Panel Recommendations." Copyright © The American Dietetic Association. Reprinted by permission from *Journal of the American Dietetic Association,* vol. 88: 1988, p. 1405.

teinemia because of its close association with CHD. Although the etiology of CHD involves a multitude of factors, epidemiological studies have conclusively shown that hypercholesterolemia is a major risk factor for coronary heart disease.[6–15] Many of these studies use a single value of cholesterol at the time of entry into the study. However, multiple measurements of plasma cholesterol concentrations increase the power to identify premature risk for CHD.

Research on Lipoproteins

Although total plasma cholesterol serves as an indicator of CHD, identifying the risk associated with specific particles that carry cholesterol provides even greater diagnostic information. The transport of cholesterol in lipoprotein particles is discussed below.

Before insoluble cholesterol is transported out of the liver cell into the plasma, it must be solubilized by special mechanisms. The liver has developed the capacity to "package" cholesterol into macromolecular complexes in which specific proteins, called apoproteins, interact with phospholipids to bring lipids into soluble form. The resultant particles are called lipoproteins. They contain lipids in their core with unesterified cholesterol (free cholesterol or FC), phospholipids (PL), and apoproteins (aP) in their membrane-like coats.

The major lipoprotein secreted by the liver is very-low-density lipoprotein (VLDL). Newly secreted VLDL contains triglyceride (TG) in its core. Immediately upon entrance into plasma, the basic structure of VLDL begins to alter. First, it acquires more cholesterol esters (CE) in the core. High-density lipoprotein (HDL) appears to transfer CE directly into VLDL, which is altered by lipolypsis of triglyceride through the action of lipoprotein lipase. As hydrolysis proceeds, free fatty acids (FFA) are released, the size of VLDL is reduced, and density increases, resulting in a new category of lipoprotein, designated intermediate-density lipoprotein (IDL). IDL appears to be transformed to LDL, a lipoprotein of lower density. In tissue culture studies, when lipoproteins are added to media cells they can derive most of their cholesterol from uptake of these IDL particles. Figure 5–1 illustrates schematically the mechanisms for cholesterol transport. Brewer provides a more detailed description of lipid and lipoprotein metabolism, including beta-lipoproteins, pre-beta-lipoproteins and alpha-lipoproteins.[16]

Brewer et al.[17] and Eisenberg[18] propose that HDL may protect against atherosclerosis by promoting removal of cholesterol from the peripheral cells (reverse cholesterol transport). In this case it would transport cholesterol from peripheral tissues to the liver. A second mechanism by which HDL might potentially protect against atherosclerosis is by competing with the uptake of LDL by the cells in the arterial wall.[19]

Table 5–2 contains mean cholesterol levels for persons 20 to 74 years of age by race/ethnicity, sex, and age. The normal limits for lipoproteins are described in Table 5–3.

Research on Cholesterol and Fatty Acids and Their Effect on Lipoproteins

Researchers have found that dietary cholesterol is related to morbidity and mortality from coronary heart disease.[20–25] A number of investigators have examined the effect of various fatty acids on lipoprotein levels. All have concluded that a significant portion of the saturated fatty acids should be removed to lower total cholesterol significantly.[26] The investigations have raised questions about what source of energy should replace the saturated fatty acids, with the three major candidates being carbohydrate, polyunsaturated fatty acids, and monounsaturated fatty acids.

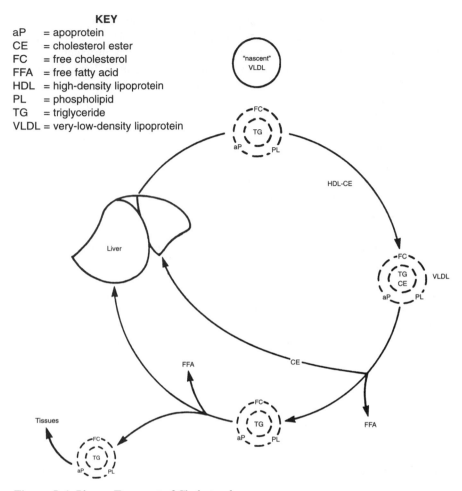

Figure 5–1 Plasma Transport of Cholesterol

In most people, when carbohydrates are substituted for saturated fats, the LDL-cholesterol level will fall about as much as with monounsaturated or polyunsaturated fats.[27–29] If fats are restricted to much below 30 percent of calories and are replaced by carbohydrates, there is a tendency for HDL-cholesterol levels to fall and VLDL-triglyceride levels to rise.[30–33] Many authorities consider these latter changes to be harmless, although there is still some disagreement on this question.[34]

There are two major categories of polyunsaturated fat commonly referred to as omega-6 and omega-3 fatty acids. The major omega-6 fatty acid is linoleic acid. Substitution of foods rich in linoleic acid for those high in saturated fats results

Table 5–3 Summary Recommendations of the Adult Treatment Panel of the National Cholesterol Education Program for Classification of Patients

Classification Based on Total Cholesterol	Classification Based on LDL-Cholesterol
<200 mg/dL (<5.20 mmol/L) desirable blood cholesterol	<130 mg/dL (<3.35 mmol/L) desirable LDL-cholesterol
200–239 mg/dL (5.20–6.15 mmol/L) borderline-high blood cholesterol	130–159 mg/dL (3.35–4.10 mmol/L) borderline-high-risk LDL-cholesterol
≥240 mg/dL (≥6.20 mmol/L) high blood cholesterol	≥160 mg/dL (≥4.15 mmol/L) high-risk LDL-cholesterol

Source: N.D. Ernst, et al., "The National Cholesterol Education Program: Implications for Dietetic Practitioners from the Adult Treatment Panel Recommendations." Copyright © The American Dietetic Association. Reprinted by permission from *Journal of the American Dietetic Association,* vol. 88: 1988, p. 1405.

in a fall in LDL-cholesterol levels.[35–37] Oils rich in linoleic acid include: soybean oil, corn oil, and high-linoleic acid forms of safflower and sunflower seed oils. Fish is the major source of omega-3 fatty acid. At high intakes, it reduces serum triglycerides substantially.[38,39]

Researchers believe that the major component of monunsaturated fat, oleic acid, may cause almost as much of a decrease in LDL-cholesterol levels as the polyunsaturated linoleic acid when either is substituted for saturated fat in the diet.[40–43]

Research on Compliance with Eating Patterns Low in Fat and Cholesterol

Studies aimed at changing dietary habits to include low-cholesterol, fat-modified eating patterns are summarized below.

In the Multiple Risk Factor Intervention Trial (MRFIT), intervention focused on the subjects' developing lifelong shopping, cooking, and eating patterns rather than specifying a structured diet.[44] Individual nutrition counseling with periodic monitoring resulted in significant cholesterol reductions, although risk also declined in the control group.[45] A comprehensive community health–promotion program in North Karelia, Finland, yielded significant reductions in cholesterol in comparison with a reference county where no intervention was implemented.[46] However, the North Karelia Project's design precluded knowledge of which aspects of the health education program instigated the change.

In an evaluation of nutrition education for persons with postmyocardial infarction, Kavetti and Hamalainen found significant improvements with both lecture-discussion and food preparation demonstration strategies. Although neither approach was significantly more effective for stimulating behavior change, this study pointed out the possible importance of organized nutrition education programs for persons with CHD.[47] Several studies have compared the use of educational materials and mass media with interventions augmented by personal contact or counseling by a health professional.[48–59] In each instance, educational programs that included interpersonal methods were more successful.

Several of the programs designed for delivery to groups have engaged social support. For example, Witschi et al. found that family participation improved the magnitude of cholesterol reductions, although the study subjects did not maintain the reductions after the intervention was discontinued.[60] In fact, it has been found repeatedly that improved eating habits and reduced lipid levels do not persist when an intervention is not sustained.[61–63] Bruno et al. were able to attain high continuous participation rates (81 percent) in a worksite program that included six monthly maintenance meetings.[64] The achievement of long-term benefits from dietary interventions on lipids requires further development of booster sessions, self-monitoring techniques, and reinforcement techniques. Glanz summarizes the elements needed to maintain dietary compliance to low-cholesterol, fat-modified diets: enlist social support, maintain periodic contact, encourage self-monitoring, and provide feedback about adherence.[65]

INAPPROPRIATE EATING BEHAVIORS

False information about eating patterns modified for fat and cholesterol can lead to inappropriate eating behaviors.

A common problem many clients face is use of commercial products. Keeping abreast of information on new fat-containing products must be a continuing effort by both nutrition counselors and their clients. Clients and counselors can develop and use a shopping guide to determine whether new products are low or high in fat, as in Exhibit 5–2. This information is based on labels; more specific data can be obtained by writing to the manufacturers.

A frequent problem is the mistaken idea that all vegetable oils are low in saturated fat. A client might exclaim joyously: "This palm oil listed on the label is probably okay on my diet since it is vegetable oil." Unfortunately, palm oil is highly saturated. Another misconception is that eggs alone cause elevated cholesterol levels. A client might state: "As long as I cut out eggs in my diet, I don't need to worry." In fact, foods low in cholesterol and high in saturated fat, such as palm oil and coconut oil, also elevate serum cholesterol.

Some clients feel that certain foods possess strange powers to eliminate cholesterol and therefore lower its concentration in the blood. They see single foods as a panacea. A client might claim: "I eat large amounts of fruits and vegetables so I don't worry about my cholesterol intake." The total diet must be considered

Exhibit 5–2 Low-Fat and Fat-Free Commercial Soups

Below is a list of lower-fat and fat-free commercial soups. Be sure to check the label for the most up-to-date fat gram information.

READY-TO-SERVE SOUPS

Healthy Choice
Broth-based soups
- Bean and Ham
- Beef and Potato
- Chicken with Pasta
- Chicken with Rice
- Country Vegetable
- Hearty Chicken
- Lentil
- Minestrone
- Split Pea with Ham
- Old Fashioned Chicken Noodle
- Vegetable Beef

Cream-based soups
- Chicken Corn Chowder
- Chicken Noodle
- Cream of Mushroom
- New England Clam Chowder
- Turkey with White & Wild Rice

Tomato-based soups
- Chili Beef
- Garden Vegetable
- Tomato Garden

Campbell's
Campbell's Healthy Request Soups
- Tomato
- Bean with Bacon

- Hearty Minestrone
- Chicken Corn Chowder
- Hearty Chicken Noodle
- Hearty Chicken Vegetable
- Hearty Vegetable
- Hearty Vegetable Beef
- New England Clam Chowder
- Southwest Style Vegetable
- Split Pea with Ham
- Tomato Vegetable with Pasta
- Turkey Vegetable with White and Wild Rice

Progresso
- Healthy Classics Chicken Noodle
- Health Classics Lentil
- Healthy Classics New England Clam Chowder
- Healthy Classics Tomato Garden Vegetable
- Vegetable
- Chicken Minestrone
- Ham and Bean
- Macaroni and Bean

Pritikin Soups
- Chicken and Rice
- Hearty Vegetable
- Lentil
- Minestrone
- Split Pea
- Three Bean Chili
- Vegetarian Vegetable

Hain Soups (No Salt Added)
- Chicken Vegetable
- Beef Vegetable
- Garlic and Pasta
- Lentil
- Home Style Naturals Cream of Mushroom
- Split Pea
- Tomato Garden Vegetable

Health Valley
- Black Bean and Vegetables
- Lentil and Carrots
- Bean Vegetable
- Split Pea and Carrots

Pepperidge Farm
- Chicken with Wild Rice
- French Onion

continues

Exhibit 5–2 continued

DRY/INSTANT SOUP MIXES

Fantastic Foods
Hearty Soups
- Cha-Cha Chili
- Country Lentil
- Couscous with Lentils
- Five Bean
- Minestrone
- Jumpin' Black Bean
- Split Pea
- Vegetable Barley

Creamy Soups
- Broccoli & Cheddar
- Corn and Potato Chowder
- Mushroom
- Tomato Rice Parmesano

"Just a Pinch" Cups
- Couscous with Lentils
- Spanish Rice and Beans

Rice and Beans (brown rice/legumes/vegetables and spices):
- Bombay Curry
- Cajun
- Caribbean

- Northern Italian
- Szechuan
- Tex Mex

Couscous Cups (couscous/spices):
- Black Bean Salsa
- Sweet Corn
- Nacho cheddar
- Creole Vegetable

Lipton's
Lipton Recipe Secrets (Mixes can be used to create an entree or complete one dish meal; recipe ideas are included on the packaging)
- Golden Herb with Lemon Soup
- Onion Soup
- Fiesta Herb with Red Pepper Soup
- Savory Herb with Garlic Soup
- Beefy Onion Soup
- Onion-Mushroom Soup
- Beefy-Mushroom Soup

Lipton's Kettle Creations
- Split Pea
- Chicken with Wild Rice

Lipton's Cup-A-Soup
- Chicken Noodle with meat
- Cream of Chicken or Mushroom
- Chicken Vegetable
- Tomato
- Ring Noodle
- Green Pea
- Spring Vegetable

Knorr
Broth-based soups
- Chicken Flavor Vegetable

Hearty soups
- Hearty Lentil
- Navy Bean

Cream-based soups
- Potato Leek

Other low-fat varieties
- Black Bean
- Hearty Minestrone

CONDENSED SOUPS

Campbell's
- Chicken Noodle
- Manhattan Clam Chowder

Campbells Healthy Request: (Soups that can be used to create an entree or a one-dish meal. Recipe ideas are provided on the can label).

Creative Chef Soups
- Cream of Roasted Chicken with Savory Herbs
- Cream of Mushroom with Roasted Garlic and Herbs
- Tomato with Garden Herbs

Campbell's 98% Fat Free Soups

- Reduced Fat Cream of Mushroom
- Reduced Fat Cream of Broccoli
- Reduced Fat Broccoli Cheese

Courtesy of the Women's Health Initiative, 1996, Seattle, Washington.

when assessing fat and cholesterol intake. Single foods do not eliminate the effect of fat and cholesterol in the diet.

Still another erroneous idea is that total fat content does not really matter. As long as a high-fat item is cholesterol free, clients may believe mistakenly that it can be eaten in unlimited quantities. A client might state proudly: "I eat large amounts of peanut butter because it is cholesterol free." This statement is true, but large quantities of fat elevate the caloric level of the diet and can lead to weight gain.

These misconceptions are by no means the only ones that clients voice. They are, however, very common sources of problem eating behaviors. Nutrition counselors see only a small sampling of daily eating behaviors; so if self-reporting methods such as three-day diet diaries are used, it is possible that clients can consume commercial products containing saturated fat without detection for long periods of time.

Clients following fat- and cholesterol-modified eating patterns wrestle with problems of excess. Social pressures can lead clients to eat something they know increases cholesterol, with the familiar alibi: "I just couldn't stop with one bite of that cheesecake at the party last night." These modified eating patterns also may mean a drastic reduction in the amounts of foods clients are accustomed to eating. They may comment: "No one can live on this small amount of meat." Inappropriate eating behaviors may be a direct result of childhood excesses. The stalwart farmer may declare: "I grew up eating three eggs every morning."

Manufacturers have come to the aid of clients who must follow fat-modified diets by providing either "filled" products or nearly fat-free substitutes. The "filled" products are those that may, for example, have animal fat removed and a polyunsaturated fat added. Others may have all animal fat removed, with no polyunsaturated fat replacement. This can leave the product virtually fat free. Unfortunately, in many cases clients anticipate that these new products will be identical in taste to the originals, so frustration and even anger may result when those expectations are not met. In desperation, clients may revert to old eating habits, including products high in animal fat.

Clients equate excesses with the prevention of medical problems: "I use large amounts of oil and margarines extremely high in polyunsaturated fat because I know polyunsaturated fat lowers cholesterol." These inappropriate eating behaviors can lead to excess calories. Clients must learn first to examine ways to reduce saturated fats.

ASSESSMENT OF EATING BEHAVIORS

As in counseling about other eating patterns, knowledge of what the client is currently eating is extremely important. By learning how strict the client's present diet is, the nutrition counselor can tailor dietary intake to lower blood cholesterol. For example, learning that a client currently consumes 600 milligrams of cholesterol a day through a three-day food record may mean that a prescription of 200

milligrams of cholesterol per day with a P/S ratio of 1.0 will lower blood cholesterol dramatically. In contrast, for a client whose intake is 200 milligrams of cholesterol per day, an eating pattern containing 100 milligrams of cholesterol per
day with a P/S ratio of 1.0 may be necessary to lower blood cholesterol. Ideally,
a seven-day record along with a quantified food frequency gives excellent information on current dietary patterns. **Five crucial components of the eating pattern should be assessed:**

1. cholesterol
2. saturated fat
3. polyunsaturated fat
4. monounsaturated fat
5. total dietary fat.

When time is short, Exhibit 5–3 may serve as a quick means of estimating fat
and cholesterol intake. The list can be increased or abbreviated, depending on the
information needed in formulating a dietary pattern.

The review of the dietary data should indicate where a major problem is occurring—cholesterol content, saturated fat content, or both. Identification of where
the major excess lies will lead to a plan for dietary change focused on strategies
to help eliminate the inappropriate patterns.

If nutrition counselors use the brief food frequency monitor in Exhibit 5–3 and
the overall nutritional quality of the diet is in question, clients might fill out a
more detailed, all-inclusive food frequency record to assess the nutrient content
of their diet. Adherence Tool 5–1 is a questionnaire that focuses on food preparation and food patterns, with an emphasis on fat and cholesterol intake.

The fat-related misinformation in the media makes it important to assess the
amount of misinformation a client currently has by asking, "Is this statement true
or false? All vegetable oil helps lower cholesterol." An instrument with a variety
of short true-or-false questions could serve as a basis for discussions of misinformation. Adherence Tool 5–2, Fat Facts or Misfacts, is a short, fun way to discuss misconceptions about the low-cholesterol, fat-controlled eating pattern. This
tool should not be used as a test but as a way of opening a discussion about incorrect ideas the media may have promoted.

As with other eating patterns, assessment of adherence to the low-cholesterol,
fat-controlled eating pattern is important. It may involve seven-day diet records
or very simple check-off systems, as in Adherence Tool 5–3. A check in the box
would indicate adherence with the recommendation of two ounces of meat at
lunch. Analysis of dietary intake from diet diaries can provide valuable information on adherence. Adherence Tools 5–4 and 5–5 provide graphs that illustrate the
client's level of dietary adherence. A survey of food items in the kitchen can
reveal inappropriate cueing that triggers inappropriate eating behaviors. Adher-

Exhibit 5–3 Fat and Cholesterol Intake Monitor

Name _____   Visit No. _____   Date _____

	Amount	Cholesterol (mg)	Total Fat (g)	Saturated Fat (g)	Polyunsaturated Fat (g)	Monounsaturated Fat (g)	Minimum Significant Amount
Eggs							½/mo
Bacon							4 strips/mo
Sausage							2 oz/mo
Meat Lunch							
Dinner							
Luncheon Meat							See sausage
Shrimp							2 oz/mo
Liver, Pork, or Beef							3 oz/6 mo
Liver, Chicken							1 oz/2 mo
Gravy							1 cup/mo
Milk, whole ____							½ cup/wk
2% ____							1 cup/wk
Cheese ____							1 oz/2 wks
Cottage Cheese							½ cup/2 wks
Cream—Light, Sour							1 Tbsp/wk
Heavy							1 Tbsp/mo
Half and Half							1 Tbsp/wk
Nondairy							1 Tbsp/wk
Creamer							

continues

Exhibit 5-3 continued

Food		Yields
Ice Cream	_____	½ cup/mo
Ice Milk	_____	1 cup/mo
Butter	_____	1 tsp/2 wks
Margarine (as spread)	_____	1 tsp/wk
Oil (in cooking)	_____	1 tsp/wk
Salad Dressing	_____	1 tsp/wk
*Breaded Fried Foods	_____	1 Tbsp/wk
*Fried Potatoes	_____	1 tsp/wk
*Baked Products	_____	1 sv/mo
*Snack Foods	_____	1 sv/mo
Chocolate	_____	½ oz/wk
Peanut Butter	_____	1 Tbsp/wk
Nuts	_____	4 Tbsp/mo
Total	_____	

Polyunsaturated fat ÷ saturated fat (P/S) = _____

*For use in calculating:

Yields

3–4" diameter pancakes . . . . 1 tsp fat
1 fried egg . . . . 1 tsp fat
1 Tbsp of salad dressing . . . . 1½ tsp fat
1 oz pan-fried meat, fish, and poultry . . . . ½ tsp fat
1 oz breaded and fried meat, fish, and poultry . . . . . 1 tsp fat
15 pieces of French fried potatoes
  (1½" × ½" × ½") . . . . 2 tsp fat

Yields

½ cup pan-fried potatoes . . . . 2 tsp fat
Cake with frosting (1 piece, 2" × 3" × 2") . . . . 3 tsp fat
Pie (1 piece, 1/7th of 9") . . . . 4 tsp fat
Cookies (4 pieces, 3" diam.) . . . . 3 tsp fat
Doughnuts and sweet rolls (1 piece, 4" diam.) . . . . . . 2 tsp fat
Crackers and chips (excluding
  low-fat crackers) (12 pieces) . . . . 3 tsp fat

Courtesy of Joan Bickel, Karen Smith, Linda G. Snetselaar, and Laura Vailas.

ence Tool 5–6 is an example of a monitoring device that helps identify foods high in fat that are in the client's kitchen. Clients write down the food and check the column corresponding to the type of fat present in the largest quantity.

TREATMENT STRATEGIES

Treatment strategies involve three aspects of compliance: lack of knowledge, forgetfulness, and lack of commitment.

Strategies To Deal with Lack of Knowledge

Meal planning is one way to avoid last-minute decisions and to ensure that clients consistently adhere to the basics of a low-cholesterol, fat-modified diet. Adherence Tool 5–7 provides a format for planning menus. Showing clients how to select foods low in cholesterol and fat is crucial to their eventual success. Counselors might indicate the total cholesterol, saturated fat, polyunsaturated fat, and monounsaturated fat in the original high-cholesterol, high-fat eating pattern. The client's eating pattern can then be compared with one that includes preferred foods but follows a prescription low in cholesterol and fat. Adherence Tool 5–8 is a short list of suggestions for use when dining out, and Adherence Tool 5–9 provides examples of meals eaten at home and in restaurants that are both high and low in cholesterol and fat. Adherence Tool 5–10 shows ranges of P/S ratios for various fats and oils. Demonstrations of the fat content of meals using food models, pats of model margarine and sticks of real margarine provide graphic examples that are lasting images in a client's mind.

With a clear description of the problem, counselors can tailor the diet to specific client needs. Tailoring involves more than simply adapting a standard low-cholesterol, fat-modified diet instruction sheet. A major element is calculating a pattern compatible with the prescription and the client's previous daily eating behavior. A hypothetical example of how tailoring might work in one situation follows:

> Mrs. S. eats seven eggs each week and six ounces of meat a day, drinks only skim milk, and uses four teaspoons of margarine (soft, tub, nondiet) with approximately two teaspoons of Mazola oil. She loves eggs and eats only high-fat meats such as bologna, salami, beef wieners, etc. Based on her blood values and past health history, the dietary prescription agreed upon by the medical team is 200 milligrams of cholesterol, P/S ratio (polyunsaturated fat divided by saturated fat) of 1.0, and total fat 20 to 25 percent of total calories.

Table 5–4 offers a possible dietary pattern designed to incorporate this basic information and still meet the prescription. The table shows how to design a regimen to give success initially because it is tailored to past eating habits. Clients

Table 5–4 Example of a Tailoring Pattern

	Cholesterol*	Total Fat†	Saturated Fat†	Poly-unsaturated Fat†	Mono-unsaturated Fat†
3 eggs/week	91	2.27	.69	.30	.86
4 oz. meat/day	119	15.90	9.00	1.12	5.78
0 dairy (fat)	—	—	—	—	—
3 teaspoons Fleischmann's tub margarine/day		11.20	1.90	3.90	5.20
3 teaspoons Mazola oil/day		14.00	2.00	8.00	4.00
Total	210	43.37	13.59	13.32	15.84
(% of 1,500 calories)		(26%)	(8%)	(8%)	(10%)

*Figures are calculated to the nearest whole number.
†Figures are calculated to the nearest hundredth.
Values were calculated using Jean A.T. Pennington, *Bowes and Church's Food Values of Portions Commonly Used* (Philadelphia: JB Lippincott, 1994). The meat values are a composite score including red meats, poultry, and fish.

should be cautioned that there always will be compromises and changes necessary to meet a specific prescription. For example, an alteration in Mrs. S.'s diet may involve eliminating some of the seven eggs she eats each week. She may need to experiment with low-fat breakfast items such as cereal and English muffins.

Once clients and counselors agree on the pattern, instruction on the diet can begin. This consists of planned steps, beginning with tasks accomplished most easily, and working up to the more difficult ones, a process called staging the diet instruction. For example, Mrs. S. is not a dairy product lover and eats high-fat dairy products only occasionally. Her program would begin by working to eliminate all such products and arranging substitutes. The next step would be changing the amounts and types of meats eaten. Finally, eggs are her "first love" and it will be difficult to eliminate them or to substitute alternate foods. Each of these three changes can be accomplished gradually during separate interviews or telephone conversations. Either way, time should be allowed for the client to experiment with ideas in daily life before moving on to more difficult changes.

Lack of knowledge or confusion from past learning can play a major part in the client's ability to lower blood cholesterol. For example, a man who is asked to lose weight may initially switch from foods that provide polyunsaturated fat to those lower in calories, such as from regular French dressing to low-calorie, fat-free French dressing and from large amounts of margarine to small amounts of diet margarine (which is lower in polyunsaturated fat per teaspoon than regular margarine). The result may be an elevation in blood cholesterol due to a lowering of polyunsaturated fat intake. Several diet diaries may be needed to identify this type of information. The change to small amounts of regular dressing and regular margarine can help in lowering blood cholesterol.

In addition to lack of knowledge, counselors should address misconceptions. A few were covered earlier in this chapter. Others include the following:

- "All beef should be avoided because it is too high in saturated fat." Breeding methods have resulted in low-fat beef cuts that can be used in moderation.
- "All pork is forbidden on low-cholesterol diets." In reality, lean pork is lower in saturated fat than beef.
- "If I fry commercial pork sausage until it's brown, all of the fat is removed." It is impossible to remove all fat from high-fat meats such as pork sausage.
- "I use a lot of nondairy powdered whipped toppings because they contain coconut oil rather than dairy fat." Coconut oil is a highly saturated vegetable oil, so clients should avoid consuming it in large quantities.

To help clear up misconceptions, counselors can provide a list of commercial and noncommercial foods such as that in Exhibit 5–2.

Nutrition counselors can build a resource file of manufactured food products through letters like that in Exhibit 5–4. The letters should be concise, to the point, and specific as to the types of information requested; in Exhibit 5–4, the only interest is fat content. In some instances, additional information on, for example, carbohydrates or protein can be requested.

While information on manufactured products is valuable, clients also need to know how to alter old eating habits on social occasions. In the past, food was considered a symbol of gratitude, love, and celebration on special occasions—associations that can make changing old eating habits at such events very unpleasant or difficult. Telephoning the hostess prior to a social function can help to determine which foods would be best to eat and can aid in avoiding major deviations from the diet prescription.

STRATEGIES TO DEAL WITH FORGETFULNESS

Reminders to eat low-cholesterol, fat-modified foods can take the form of a change in the types of foods clients keep in the refrigerator. Substituting low-fat cheeses and dips for high-fat can serve as a cueing device always to eat appropriately. A reminder on the cupboard door saying, "Don't forget to eat low-fat foods!" can also serve as a cueing device. Notes on the refrigerator to remind the client to call the hostess before a party are valuable cues, too.

Clients for whom diet alone is not enough to bring blood cholesterol levels to within normal range may need to take medications like cholestyramine, a powder that acts as a bile acid sequestrant and thus helps lower blood cholesterol. Clients

Exhibit 5–4 First Step in Building a Resource File

August 11, 1997

Bonnell Soup Company
1000 East Main Street
Anytown, US 99999

Dear Friend:

Since we are involved in counseling many hundreds of patients on cholesterol and fat-modified diets, we often need the assistance of food manufacturers. Determining the exact composition of products allows us to incorporate them into diets, where otherwise they might be prohibited.

Would you please send us your latest figures on the levels of cholesterol, monounsaturated, polyunsaturated, and saturated fatty acids in your Italian Spaghetti with Meatballs? Figures on a per-weight basis are most useful to us.

We would appreciate this information at your earliest possible convenience. Thank you for your help and cooperation.

Sincerely yours,

John Smith, R.D., M.S.
Research Nutritionist

taking cholestyramine may need reminders or cueing devices. A calendar that indicates when medication is taken can also serve as a reminder to take it. Adherence Tool 5–3 provides examples of a one-month and a one-week calendar. This tool can be used to find patterns in the day and time in a week that a client forgets to take medication. For example, Friday lunches may preclude taking medication, resulting in missed doses. A note on the refrigerator saying, "Don't forget to take your noon dose of cholestyramine on Friday" may help. The monthly calendar might be used to observe whether this strategy increases adherence.

Strategies To Deal with Lack of Commitment

Frequent expressions of waning commitment include: "I have more difficulty eating in restaurants than I used to," or "I miss all the 'good' food I used to eat," or "I'm tired of low-fat foods." Responding to these comments with more than information requires careful assessment of the actual problem. Why is commitment declining? Changes in clients' lives can lead to declines in adherence. Is the family in financial hardship? If the family is in danger of losing financial stability, that problem will become a priority. The family that goes through the turmoil of divorce, marriage, remarriage, the addition of a new family member, or the death of a close relative may be at risk for declining adherence and lack of commitment to the medical regimen. Other adherence problems may stem from losing a job or starting a new job.

Rule relaxation may be necessary for a time to help the client through the difficulties of the life change. Exhibit 5–5 is a contract that provides an example of how to deal with this type of problem. Relapse should be discussed with the client as a usual step in the process of behavior change. Ask the client to be specific in discussing what the slip or slips are. Use past data to show how well the client has done over time. Emphasize that current life events will pass and life will go back to its normal phase.

Positive monologues can be important in increasing adherence when commitment is low. By assessing thought processes before and following eating, counselors can observe negative monologues and teach clients to change them to positive monologues. Appropriate improvements in adherence may result. For example, the client who eats a small piece of cheddar cheese may say, "That's it. I blew the diet. It is no use! I just can't stay on this diet. I give up!" With this comment, the client may go into a binge that includes eating three more pieces of cheese. A change from negative to positive might have resulted in this: "I had one small piece of cheese. I know that it is high in saturated fat. I will only have this

---

Exhibit 5–5 Contract

I will not take my cholestyramine for the two days that I am in divorce court (January 21–22, 1997). On January 23, I will begin to take the full dose of medication again and will reward myself by going to a movie on that night. The nutrition counselor will contact me on January 24 at 7:00 PM to check on reestablishing the medication regimen.

If I do not take the full dose of medication on January 23, I forfeit the reward of going to a movie.

Client _____

Nutrition Counselor _____

Physician _____

one piece. I feel great that I was able to stop with this one piece. I will be careful the rest of the day and can still be within the limits of my diet." **Most positive thinking involves positive self-rewards. This type of self-rewarding system can be embellished with positive reinforcement from others.**

The support of the family or significant other is crucial to adherence. Sometimes family members become upset if eating habits must focus on lowering saturated fat. This negative attitude may have an equally negative effect on client adherence. Changes in eating behavior are easier if clients can tell friends and relatives why the new pattern is necessary. For example, clients can explain that cutting down on cholesterol and saturated fats can help prevent coronary heart disease. Such a rationale can encourage helping others who are hosting parties to serve foods that are low in cholesterol and saturated fat. On their own, clients will find that a positive step is to learn to avoid foods that are high in fat and/or cholesterol and to limit their intake to those that are lower in these elements. Exhibit 5–6 shows a food list that allows for holiday treats.

Families can do much to help clients adhere to a fat-modified diet. Nutrition counselors might involve family members in sessions in which the clients are taught food preparation and receive dietary recommendations. However, too much family involvement can pose problems. For example, a quiet hyperlipidemic teenager may have a mother who volunteers all information and allows no verbal contact between client and counselor. The nutrition counselor may decide to see the client alone for parts of the interview or use subtle extinction techniques and nonverbal gestures (e.g., no eye contact) to curb too much involvement by the mother. The counselor might state at the beginning of the interview, "Mrs. J., during today's session I would like to find out from your son what his eating habits are at school. When he has finished, I will ask you to help him in describing eating habits at home." It is important to keep good eye contact with the son to encourage his responses rather than his mother's.

Counselors should instruct the client's friends and other family members (if possible) on how to provide positive reinforcement as a way to improve the individual's adherence to a fat-modified diet. **The following is a checklist that family members might use for positive reinforcement techniques:**

- Praise efforts at decreasing serving sizes of meat, cheese, eggs, and other high-fat, high-cholesterol products.
- Avoid teasing or tempting with high-fat, high-cholesterol foods.
- Record the number of positive and negative comments they make about the diet and try to increase the positive and decrease the negative ones.

Avoid referring to low-cholesterol, fat-modified foods as "different" or "strange."

Exhibit 5–6 Watch the Lights for Eating at Parties

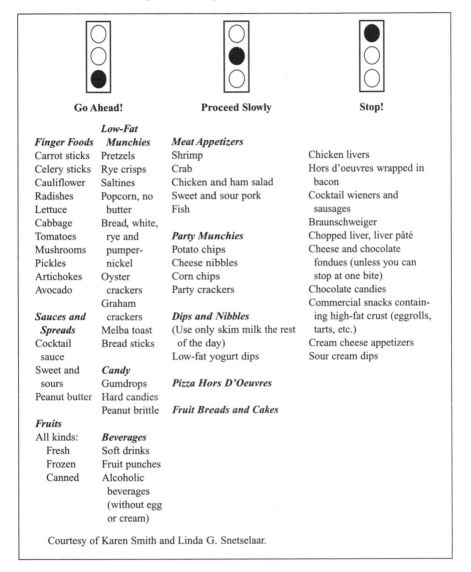

Go Ahead!	**Proceed Slowly**	**Stop!**

Finger Foods	**Low-Fat Munchies**	**Meat Appetizers**	
Carrot sticks	Pretzels	Shrimp	Chicken livers
Celery sticks	Rye crisps	Crab	Hors d'oeuvres wrapped in
Cauliflower	Saltines	Chicken and ham salad	bacon
Radishes	Popcorn, no	Sweet and sour pork	Cocktail wieners and
Lettuce	butter	Fish	sausages
Cabbage	Bread, white,		Braunschweiger
Tomatoes	rye and	**Party Munchies**	Chopped liver, liver pâté
Mushrooms	pumper-	Potato chips	Cheese and chocolate
Pickles	nickel	Cheese nibbles	fondues (unless you can
Artichokes	Oyster	Corn chips	stop at one bite)
Avocado	crackers	Party crackers	Chocolate candies
	Graham		Commercial snacks contain-
Sauces and	crackers	**Dips and Nibbles**	ing high-fat crust (eggrolls,
Spreads	Melba toast	(Use only skim milk the rest	tarts, etc.)
Cocktail	Bread sticks	of the day)	Cream cheese appetizers
sauce		Low-fat yogurt dips	Sour cream dips
Sweet and	**Candy**		
sours	Gumdrops	**Pizza Hors D'Oeuvres**	
Peanut butter	Hard candies		
	Peanut brittle	**Fruit Breads and Cakes**	
Fruits			
All kinds:	**Beverages**		
Fresh	Soft drinks		
Frozen	Fruit punches		
Canned	Alcoholic		
	beverages		
	(without egg		
	or cream)		

Courtesy of Karen Smith and Linda G. Snetselaar.

CONCLUSION

In summary, facilitating adherence to low-cholesterol, fat-modified eating patterns requires clients to have a thorough knowledge of the fat and cholesterol content of foods. Along with increasing clients' knowledge, the nutrition counselor facilitates adherence by providing suggestions for more appropriate cueing devices. Lack of commitment to this eating pattern can cause lapses in dietary adherence. The nutrition counselor has many behavioral strategies available to increase commitment to dietary change.

Review of Chapter 5
(Answers in Appendix H)

1. List six dietary misconceptions and excesses related to low-cholesterol and fat-modified eating patterns that lead to inappropriate eating behaviors.

   a. _____

   b. _____

   c. _____

   d. _____

   e. _____

   f. _____

2. List three of five specific dietary components of a baseline diet that must be assessed before instructing a client on a fat-modified diet.

   a. _____

   b. _____

   c. _____

3. List three strategies that might help the client follow a fat- and cholesterol-controlled eating pattern.

   a. _____

   b. _____

   c. _____

4. The following is an exercise (based on data collected using Exhibit 5–3) to help you apply the ideas just discussed.

   Jim is a 48-year-old mailman who eats all meals at home except for social occasions, in which he participates frequently. He loves meat and rarely eats eggs or dairy products. Tailor an eating pattern to his needs and explain two counseling strategies that might be used to help his dietary adherence on social occasions. The dietary prescription is 200 milligrams of cholesterol with a P/S ratio of 1.0 and 20 percent of the calories coming from fat.

	Cholesterol	Total Fat	Saturated Fat	Polyun- saturated Fat	Mono- unsaturated Fat
___ eggs/week	___	___	___	___	___
___ ounces meat/day	___	___	___	___	___
___ ounces whole milk/day	___	___	___	___	___
___ ___ margarine/day	___	___	___	___	___
___ ___ oil/day	___	___	___	___	___

Total
(% of 2,400   P/S
calories)   (___%)   (___%)   (___%)   ___
Strategies: _____

NOTES

1. National Center for Health Statistics, "Births, Marriages, Divorces, and Deaths for May 1989," *Monthly Vital Statistics Report* 38, no. 5 (Hyattsville, MD: U.S. Department of Health and Human Services, 1989), Publication No. (PHS) 89–11200.

2. "Summary of the Second Report of the National Cholesterol Education Program (NCEP) Expert Panel on Detection, Evaluation and Treatment of High Blood Cholesterol in Adults (Adult Treatment Panel II)," *Journal of the American Medical Association* 269 (1993): 3015–3023.

3. National Research Council, Food and Nutrition Board, *Recommended Dietary Allowances,* 10th ed. (Washington, DC: National Academy of Sciences, 1989), 44–51.

4. R. T Holman et al., "The Essential Fatty Acid Requirements of Infants and the Assessment of their Dietary Intake of Linoleic by Serum Fatty Acid Analysis," *American Journal of Clinical Nutrition* 14 (1964): 70.

5. National Research Council, Food and Nutrition Board, *Diet and Health: Implications for Reducing Chronic Disease Risk. Report of the Committee on Diet and Health, Food and Nutrition Board* (Washington, DC: National Academy Press, 1989), 750.

6. R.S. Renaud and M. de Lorgeril, "Dietary Lipids and Their Relation to Ischaemic Heart Disease: From Epidemiology to Prevention," *Journal of Internal Medicine* 225 (1989): 39–46.

7. J. Stamler and R. Shekelle, "Dietary Cholesterol and Human Coronary Heart Disease: The Epidemiologic Evidence," *Archives of Pathology in Laboratory Medicine* 112 (1988): 1032–1040.

8. R.B. Shekelle and J. Stamler, "Dietary Cholesterol and Ischaemic Heart Disease," *Lancet* 1 (1989): 1177–1179.

9. S.M. Grundy et al., "Workshop on the Impact of Dietary Cholesterol on Plasma Lipoproteins and Atherogenesis," *Arteriosclerosis* 8 (1988): 95–101.

10. D.M. Hegsted and L.M. Ausman, "Diet, Alcohol and Coronary Heart Disease in Men," *Journal of Nutrition* 118 (1988): 1184–1189.

11. K. Liu et al., "Dietary Lipids, Sugar, Fiber and Mortality from Coronary Heart Disease: Bivariate Analysis of International Data," *Arteriosclerosis* 2, no. 3 (1982): 221–227.

12. D. Kromhout et al., "The Inverse Relation between Fish Consumption and 20-Year Mortality from Coronary Heart Disease," *New England Journal of Medicine* 312 (1985): 1205–1209.

13. T.L.V. Ulbricht and D.A.T. Southgate, "Coronary Heart Disease: Seven Dietary Factors," *Lancet* 338 (1991): 985–992.

14. D. Steinberg et al., "Antioxidants in the Prevention of Human Atherosclerosis: Summary of the Proceedings of a National Heart, Lung, and Blood Institute Workshop: September 5–6, 1991, Bethesda, Maryland," *Circulation* 85, no. 6 (1992): 2338–2345.

15. K.F. Gey et al., "Inverse Correlation Between Plasma Vitamin E and Mortality from Ischemic Heart Disease in Cross-Cultural Epidemiology," *American Journal of Clinical Nutrition* 53 (1991): 326S–334S.

16. H.B. Brewer, Jr., "Lipid and Lipoprotein Metabolism," in *Drug Treatment of Hyperlipidemia*, ed. B.M. Rifkind (New York: Marcel Dekker, 1991), 1–15.

17. H.B. Brewer, Jr., et al., "High Density Lipoproteins: An Overview," in *Report of the High-Density Lipoprotein Methodology Workshop*, ed. K. Lippel (Washington, DC: U.S. Department of Health, Education and Welfare, NIH Publication No. 79-1661, 1979), 29–42.

18. S. Eisenberg, "High-Density Lipoprotein Metabolism," *Journal of Lipid Research* 25 (1984): 1017–1058.

19. Eisenberg, "High-Density Lipoprotein Metabolism."

20. P.M. Clifton et al., "Relationship between Sensitivity to Dietary Fat and Dietary Cholesterol," *Arteriosclerosis* 10 (1990): 394–401.

21. M.B. Katan and A.C. Beynen, "Characteristics of Human Hypo- and Hyperresponders to Dietary Cholesterol," *American Journal of Epidemiology* 125 (1987): 387–399.

22. M.B. Katan et al., "Congruence of Individual Responsiveness to Dietary Cholesterol and to Saturated Fat in Humans," *Journal of Lipid Research* 29 (1988): 883–892.

23. M.B. Katan et al., "Differences in Individual Responsiveness of Serum Cholesterol to Fat-Modified Diets in Man," *European Journal of Clinical Investigation* 18 (1988): 644–647.

24. Grundy, "Workshop on the Impact of Dietary Cholesterol on Plasma Lipoproteins and Atherogenesis."

25. S.L. Connor and W.E. Connor, "The Importance of Dietary Cholesterol in Coronary Heart Disease," *Preventive Medicine* 12 (1983): 115–123.

26. S.M. Grundy and M.A. Denke, "Dietary Influences on Serum Lipids and Lipoproteins," *Journal of Lipid Research* 31 (1990): 1149–1172.

27. S.M. Grundy, "Comparison of Monounsaturated Fatty Acids and Carbohydrates for Lowering Plasma Cholesterol," *New England Journal of Medicine* 314 (1986): 745–748.

28. S.M. Grundy et al., "Comparison of Monounsaturated Fatty Acids and Carbohydrates for Reducing Raised Levels of Plasma Cholesterol in Man," *American Journal of Clinical Nutrition* 47 (1988): 965–969.

29. H.N. Ginsberg et al., "Reduction of Plasma Cholesterol Levels in Normal Men on an American Heart Association Step 1 Diet or a Step 1 Diet with Added Monounsaturated Fat," *New England Journal of Medicine* 322 (1990): 574–579.

30. Grundy, "Comparison of Monounsaturated Fatty Acids and Carbohydrates for Lowering Plasma Cholesterol."

31. J.T. Knuiman et al., "Total Cholesterol and High Density Lipoprotein Cholesterol Levels in Populations Differing in Fat and Carbohydrate Intake," *Arteriosclerosis* 7 (1987): 612–619.

32. E.A. Brinton et al., "A Low-Fat Diet Decreases High Density Lipoprotein (HDL) Cholesterol Levels by Decreasing HDL Apolipoprotein Transport Rates," *Journal of Clinical Investigation* 85 (1990): 144–151.

33. C.E. West et al., "Boys from Populations with High-Carbohydrates Intake Have Higher Fasting Triglyceride Levels Than Boys from Populations with High-Fat Intake," *American Journal of Epidemiology* 131 (1990): 271–282.

34. National Cholesterol Education Program, *Second Report of the Expert Panel on Detection, Evaluation, and Treatment of High Blood Cholesterol in Adults* (Bethesda, MD: National Institutes of Health, National Heart, Lung, and Blood Institute, NIH Publication No. 93-3095, II-8, September 1993).

35. A. Keys et al., "Serum Cholesterol Response to Changes in the Diet. IV. Particular Saturated Fatty Acids in the Diet," *Metabolism* 14 (1965): 776–787.

36. D.M. Hegsted et al., "Quantitative Effects of Dietary Fat on Serum Cholesterol in Man," *American Journal of Clinical Nutrition* 17 (1965): 281–295.

37. R.P. Mensink and M.B. Katan, "Effects of Dietary Fatty Acids on Serum Lipids and Lipoproteins: A Meta-Analysis of 27 Trials, *Arteriosclerosis and Thrombosis* 12 (1992): 911–919.

38. W.S. Harris, "Fish oils and Plasma Lipid and Lipoprotein Metabolism in Humans: A Critical Review," *Journal of Lipid Research* 30 (1989): 785–807.

39. W.E. Connor, "Hypolipidemic Effects of Dietary Omega-3 Fatty Acids in Normal and Hyperlipidemic Humans: Effectiveness and Mechanisms," in *Health Effects of Polyunsaturated Fatty Acids in Seafoods*, ed. A. Simopoulos, et al. (Orlando, FL: Academic Press, 1986), 173–210.

40. Mensink and Katan, "Effects of Dietary Fatty Acids on Serum Lipids and Lipoproteins: A Meta-Analysis of 27 Trials."

41. D.M. Dreon et al., "The Effects of Polyunsaturated Fat vs Monounsaturated Fat on Plasma Lipoproteins," *Journal of the American Medical Association* 262 (1990): 2462–2466.

42. E.M. Berry et al., "Effects of Diets Rich in Monounsaturated Fatty Acids on Plasma Lipoproteins—Jerusalem Nutrition Study: High MUFAs and High PUFAs," *American Journal of Clinical Nutrition* 53 (1991): 899–907.

43. A.W. Caggiula et al., "The Mutiple Risk Factor Intervention Trial (MRFIT). VI. Intervention on Blood Lipids," *Preventive Medicine* 10 (1981): 1269–1272.

44. T.A. Dolecek et al., "A Long-Term Intervention Experience: Lipid Responses and Dietary Adherence Patterns in the Multiple Risk Factor Intervention Trial," *Journal of the American Dietetic Association* 86 (1986): 752–798.

45. Multiple Risk Factor Intervention Trial Research Group, "Multiple Risk Factor Intervention Trial: Risk Factor Changes and Mortality Results," *Journal of the American Medical Association* 248 (1982): 1465–1477.

46. A. McAlister et al., "Theory and Action for Health Promotion: Illustrations from the North Karelia Project," *American Journal of Public Health* 72 (1982): 43–50.

47. R.L. Kavetti and H. Hamalainen, "Long-Term Effect of Nutrition Education on Myocardial Infarction Patients: A 10-Year Follow-Up Study," *Nutrition Metabolism and Cardiovascular Disease* 3 (1993): 185–192.

48. A.C. Buller, "Improving Dietary Education for Patients with Hyperlipidemia," *Journal of the American Dietetic Association* 72 (1978): 277–281.

49. R.F. Heller et al., "Secondary Prevention after Acute Myocardial Infarction," *American Journal of Cardiology* 72 (1993): 759–762.

50. M. Stern et al., "Results of a Two-Year Health Education Campaign on Dietary Behavior," *Circulation* 54 (1976): 826–833.

51. World Health Organization European Collaborative Group, "European Collaborative Trial of Multifactorial Prevention of Coronary Heart Disease: Final Report on the 6-Year Results," *Lancet* 2 (1986): 869–872.

52. G. Rose, "European Collaborative Trial of Multifactorial Prevention of Coronary Heart Disease," *Lancet* 1 (1987): 747–751.

53. L. Wilhelmsen et al., "The Multifactor Primary Prevention Trial in Goteborg, Sweden," *European Heart Journal* 7 (1986): 279–288.

54. J.W. Farquar et al., "Effects of Communitywide Education on Cardiovascular Disease Risk Factors: The Stanford Five-City Project," *Journal of the American Medical Association* 264 (1990): 359–365.

55. J. Tuomilehto et al., "Decline in Cardiovascular Mortality in North Karelia and Other Parts of Finland," *British Medical Journal* 293 (1986): 1068–1071.

56. E. Engblom et al., "Exercise Habits and Physical Performance during Comprehensive Rehabilitation after Coronary Artery Bypass Surgery," *European Heart Journal* 13 (1992): 1053–1059.

57. G. Schuler et al., "Regular Physical Exercise and Low-Fat Diet: Effects of Progression of Coronary Artery Disease," *Circulation* 86 (1992): 1–11.

58. N.D. Barnard et al., "Adherence and Acceptability of a Low-Fat, Vegetarian Diet among Patients with Cardiac Disease," *Journal of Cardiopulmonary Rehabilitation* 12 (1992): 423–431.

59. W.L. Haskell et al., "Effects of Intensive Multiple Risk Factor Reduction on Coronary Atherosclerosis and Clinical Cardiac Events in Men and Women with Coronary Artery Disease: The Stanford Coronary Risk Intervention Project (SCRIP)," *Circulation* 89 (1994): 975–990.

60. J.C. Witschi et al., "Family Cooperation and Effectiveness in a Cholesterol-Lowering Diet," *Journal of the American Dietetic Association* 72 (1978): 384–389.

61. R.S. Reeves et al., "Effects of a Low Cholesterol Eating Plan on Plasma Lipids: Results of a Three-Year Community Study," *American Journal of Public Health* 73 (1983): 873–877.

62. Stern et al., "Results of a Two-Year Health Education Campaign on Dietary Behavior."

63. Witschi et al., "Family Cooperation and Effectiveness in a Cholesterol-Lowering Diet."

64. R. Bruno et al., "Randomized Controlled Trial of a Nonpharmacological Cholesterol Reduction Program at the Worksite," *Preventive Medicine* 12 (1983): 523–532.

65. K. Glanz, "Nutrition Education for Risk Factor Reduction and Patient Education: A Review," *Preventive Medicine* 14 (1985): 721–752.

Adherence Tool 5–1: Client Questionnaire for Cholesterol- and Fat-Controlled Eating Patterns

The following questionnaire is a monitoring device that has been designed to efficiently collect patient information in clinical nutrition programs. It has several functions.

Initially, it is a useful screening device or test of motivation. Individuals who may not take time to fill it out probably won't take time to participate fully in the behavioral diet and cholesterol modification programs.

Secondly, the answers to these questions can be of great use to the therapist during the initial interviews and later during the nutrition sessions. The weight history allows a systematic look at the clients' own views of their weight problems (if there are any), and at some of the environmental influences they feel are important to their eating habits. The history of past attempts to make changes in eating patterns, the lengths of time they have stayed in dietary modification programs, and the reasons for past failure can all be useful. Also, their report of mood changes during previous periods of dieting can help you anticipate and deal with problems that might arise during treatment.

The questions about social and family history provide additional information that is of use medically: for example, the cause of parental death and the family weight history.

In most states the information contained in this questionnaire is confidential. Without **written** approval from the clients, this information cannot be divulged to interested individuals, physicians, insurance companies, or law enforcement agencies.

Sources: Adapted from J.M. Ferguson, *Learning To Eat: Behavior Modification for Weight Control*, with permission of Bull Publishing Company, © 1975. Questions 50–56 are reprinted from "Food Preparation Questionnaire" with permission of Nutrition Coordinating Center, University of Minnesota.

Adherence Tool 5–1   continued

Name:_____ Sex: M F Age:____ Birthdate:_____

Address: _____ Home phone: _____

_____ Office phone: _____

WEIGHT HISTORY

1. Indicate on the following table the periods in your life when you have been overweight. *If you have never been overweight, skip to question 15.* Where appropriate, list your maximum weight for each period and number of pounds you were overweight. Briefly describe any methods you used to lose weight in that five-year period (e.g., diet, shots, pills). Also list any significant life events you feel were related to either your weight gain or loss (e.g., college tests, marriage, pregnancies, illness).

Age	Maximum Weight	Pounds Overweight	Methods Used To Lose Weight	Significant Events Related to Weight Change
Birth				
0–5				
6–10				
11–15				
16–20				
21–25				
26–30				
31–35				
36–40				
41–45				

Age	Maximum Weight	Pounds Overweight	Methods Used To Lose Weight	Significant Events Related to Weight Change
46–50				
51–55				
56–60				
61–65				

2. Your present weight＿＿＿＿＿ Height ＿＿＿＿＿

3. Describe your present weight (check one)

＿＿ Very overweight

＿＿ Slightly overweight

＿＿ About average

4. Are you dissatisfied with the way you look at this weight? (check one)

＿＿ Completely satisfied

＿＿ Satisfied

＿＿ Neutral

＿＿ Dissatisfied

＿＿ Very dissatisfied

5. At what weight have you *felt* your best or do you think you would feel your best?＿＿＿＿＿

6. How much weight would you like to lose? ＿＿＿＿＿＿＿＿＿＿＿＿＿

7. Do you feel your weight affects your daily activities? (check one)

＿＿ No effect

＿＿ Some effect

＿＿ Often interferes

＿＿ Extreme effect

8. Why do you want to lose weight at this time? ＿＿＿＿＿＿＿＿＿＿

＿＿＿＿＿＿＿＿＿＿＿＿＿＿＿＿＿＿＿＿＿＿＿＿＿＿＿

continues

Adherence Tool 5–1   continued

9. What are the attitudes of the following people about your attempt(s) to lose weight?

	Negative (They disapprove or are resentful)	Indifferent (They don't care or don't help)	Positive (They encourage me and are understanding)
Husband			
Wife			
Children			
Parents			
Employer			
Friends			

10. Do these attitudes affect your weight loss or gain?   Yes_____   No_____

   If yes, please describe: _____

   _____

   _____

11. A number of different ways of losing weight are listed below. Please indicate which methods you have used by filling the appropriate blanks.

	Ages Used	Number of Times Used	Maximum Weight Lost	Comments (Length of Time Weight Loss Maintained; Successes; Difficulties)
TOPS (Take Off Pounds Sensibly)				
Weight Watchers				
Pills				
Supervised Diet				
Unsupervised Diet				
Starvation				
Behavior Modification				
Psychotherapy				
Hypnosis				
Other				

12. Which method did you use for the longest period of time? _____

_____

13. Have you had a major mood change during or after a significant weight loss? Indicate any mood changes on the following checklist.

	Not at All	A Little Bit	Moder- ately	Quite a Bit	Extremely
a. Depressed, sad, feeling down, unhappy, the blues	___	___	___	___	___
b. Anxious, nervous, restless, or uptight all the time	___	___	___	___	___
c. Physically weak	___	___	___	___	___
d. Elated or happy	___	___	___	___	___
e. Easily irritated, annoyed, or angry	___	___	___	___	___
f. Fatigued, worn out, tired all the time	___	___	___	___	___
g. A lack of self-confidence	___	___	___	___	___

14. What usually goes wrong with your weight-loss programs? _____

_____

_____

_____

15. How *physically* active are you? (check one)

___ Very active   ___ Average   ___ Very inactive

___ Active   ___ Inactive

16. What do you do for physical exercise and how often do you do it?

Activity (for example, swimming, jogging, dancing)	**Frequency** (daily, weekly, monthly)

continues

Adherence Tool 5–1   continued

MEDICAL HISTORY

17. When did you last have a complete physical examination? _____

18. Who is your current doctor? _____

19. What medical problems do you have at the present time? _____

    _____

    _____

20. What medications, vitamins or mineral preparations, or drugs do you take regularly? _____

    _____

    _____

    Attach label if available.

21. List any medications, drugs, or foods you are allergic to: _____

    _____

    _____

    _____

22. List any hospitalizations or operations. Indicate how old you were at each hospital admission.

    Age   Reason for hospitalization

    _____   _____

    _____   _____

    _____   _____

23. List any serious illnesses you have had that have not required hospitalization. Indicate how old you were during each illness.

    Age   Illness

    _____   _____

    _____   _____

    _____   _____

24. Describe any of your medical problems that are complicated by excess weight.

    _____

    _____

    _____

25. How much alcohol do you usually drink per week? _____

26. List any psychiatric contact, individual counseling, or marital counseling that you have had or are now having.

     Age   Reason for contact and type of therapy

_____   _____

_____   _____

_____   _____

SOCIAL HISTORY

27. Circle the last year of school attended:

   1 2 3 4 5 6 7 8   9 10 11 12   1 2 3 4   M.A.   Ph.D.

    Grade School   High School   College

    Other _____

28. Describe your present occupation _____

_____

29. How long have you worked for your present employer? _____

30. Present marital status (check one):

_____ Single

_____ Married

_____ Divorced

_____ Widowed

_____ Separated

_____ Engaged

31. Answer the following questions for each marriage:

Date of marriage	_____	_____	_____
Date of termination	_____	_____	_____
Reason (death, divorce, etc.)	_____	_____	_____
Number of children	_____	_____	_____

32. Spouse's Age _____ Weight _____ Height _____

continues

Adherence Tool 5–1   continued

33. Describe your spouse's occupation _____
_____

34. Describe your spouse's weight (check one):

___ Very overweight   ___ Slightly underweight

___ Slightly overweight   ___ Very underweight

___ About average

35. List your children's ages, sex, heights, weights, and circle whether they are overweight, average, or underweight. Include any children from previous marriages, whether they are living with you or not.

Age	Sex	Weight	Height	Overweight			Underweight	
___	___	___	___	very	slightly	average	slightly	very
___	___	___	___	very	slightly	average	slightly	very
___	___	___	___	very	slightly	average	slightly	very
___	___	___	___	very	slightly	average	slightly	very
___	___	___	___	very	slightly	average	slightly	very

36. Who lives at home with you? _____
_____

FAMILY HISTORY

37. Is your father living?__Yes__No   Father's age now, or age at and cause of death _____
_____

38. Is your mother living?__Yes__No   Mother's age now, or age at and cause of death _____
_____

39. Describe your father's occupation_____

40. Describe your mother's occupation _____

41. Describe your father's weight while you were growing up (check one). If you have never been overweight skip to question 50.

___ Very overweight   ___ Slightly underweight

___ Slightly overweight   ___ Very underweight

___ About average

42. Describe your mother's weight while you were growing up (check one).

____ Very overweight

____ Slightly overweight

____ About average

____ Slightly underweight

____ Very underweight

43. List your brothers' and sisters' ages, sex, present weights, heights, and circle whether they are overweight, average, or underweight.

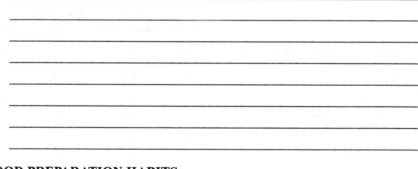

Age	Sex	Weight	Height		Overweight		Underweight	
___	__	____	_____	very	slightly	average	slightly	very
___	__	____	_____	very	slightly	average	slightly	very
___	__	____	_____	very	slightly	average	slightly	very
___	__	____	_____	very	slightly	average	slightly	very
___	__	____	_____	very	slightly	average	slightly	very

44. Please add any additional information you feel may be relevant to your current eating habits. This includes interactions with your family and friends that might sabotage a dietary modification program, and additional family or social history that you feel might help us understand your dietary habits.

_____

_____

_____

_____

_____

_____

_____

_____

FOOD PREPARATION HABITS

45. Do you salt your food at the table? (check one)

____ always

____ occasionally

____ never

continues

Adherence Tool 5–1   continued

46. If you add salt, how would you rate yourself in terms of amount of salt added at the table? (check one)

____ light

____ moderate

____ heavy

47. Do you use a salt substitute at the table such as Lite, Lo-Salt, or No-salt? (check one)

____ always

____ occasionally

____ never

If used, specify brand name: _____

48. Do you regularly use other salt seasonings at the table such as Accent, onion salt, or garlic salt? (check one)

____ Yes

____ No   Specify kind(s):_____

49. Check whether salt or salt substitute is usually added in *preparing* the following foods:

	Salt	Salt Substitute	Seasoning Salts	None
Pasta, such as noodles, macaroni	[ ]	[ ]	[ ]	[ ]
Rice	[ ]	[ ]	[ ]	[ ]
Potatoes	[ ]	[ ]	[ ]	[ ]
Other vegetables	[ ]	[ ]	[ ]	[ ]
Meat	[ ]	[ ]	[ ]	[ ]
Fruit	[ ]	[ ]	[ ]	[ ]
Other (e.g., coffee)	[ ]	[ ]	[ ]	[ ]
specify _____	[ ]	[ ]	[ ]	[ ]
_____	[ ]	[ ]	[ ]	[ ]

If salt substitute, specify kind/brand _____

50. Are the following table and cooking fats used (check one)?

Butter   ____ yes   (Specify: ____ regular,   ____ unsalted)

                        ____ no

Margarine   ____ yes   (Specify: ____ regular,   ____ unsalted)

                        ____ no

Specify brand(s):

_____   ____stick   ____tub   ____diet   ____spread

_____   ____stick   ____tub   ____diet   ____spread

_____   ____stick   ____tub   ____diet   ____spread

Vegetable oil (such as corn, soy, safflower, sunflower, etc.) (circle one)

___ yes   (Specify types and/or brands used: _____)

___ no   ___ _____

_____

Spray shortening (such as Pam)

___ yes   (Specify brand: _____)

___ no   _____

_____

Solid shortening (such as Crisco, Spry, Fluffo, etc.) (circle one)

___ yes   (Specify types and/or brands used:_____)

___ no   _____

_____

Other cooking fats (such as lard, bacon drippings, salt pork, poultry fat, etc.) (circle one)

___ yes   (Specify _____)

___ no   _____

_____

continues

Adherence Tool 5–1   continued

51. Check the fat most often used in preparing each of the following foods:

	Butter	Margarine	Spray shortening	Oil, such as Wesson, Mazola	Vegetable shortening such as Crisco, Fluffo, Spry	Bacon fat	Lard	Chicken fat	Beef suet	None
Eggs, fried	[ ]	[ ]	[ ]	[ ]	[ ]	[ ]	[ ]	[ ]	[ ]	[ ]
Eggs, scrambled	[ ]	[ ]	[ ]	[ ]	[ ]	[ ]	[ ]	[ ]	[ ]	[ ]
French toast	[ ]	[ ]	[ ]	[ ]	[ ]	[ ]	[ ]	[ ]	[ ]	[ ]
Cornbread	[ ]	[ ]	[ ]	[ ]	[ ]	[ ]	[ ]	[ ]	[ ]	[ ]
Potatoes, mashed	[ ]	[ ]	[ ]	[ ]	[ ]	[ ]	[ ]	[ ]	[ ]	[ ]
Potatoes, french fried	[ ]	[ ]	[ ]	[ ]	[ ]	[ ]	[ ]	[ ]	[ ]	[ ]
Potatoes, pan fried	[ ]	[ ]	[ ]	[ ]	[ ]	[ ]	[ ]	[ ]	[ ]	[ ]
Greens	[ ]	[ ]	[ ]	[ ]	[ ]	[ ]	[ ]	[ ]	[ ]	[ ]
Other vegetables	[ ]	[ ]	[ ]	[ ]	[ ]	[ ]	[ ]	[ ]	[ ]	[ ]
White beans, pinto	[ ]	[ ]	[ ]	[ ]	[ ]	[ ]	[ ]	[ ]	[ ]	[ ]
Gravy	[ ]	[ ]	[ ]	[ ]	[ ]	[ ]	[ ]	[ ]	[ ]	[ ]
White sauce	[ ]	[ ]	[ ]	[ ]	[ ]	[ ]	[ ]	[ ]	[ ]	[ ]
Pie crust	[ ]	[ ]	[ ]	[ ]	[ ]	[ ]	[ ]	[ ]	[ ]	[ ]

52. Indicate the most *usual* method of preparing each of the following. If you fry any of them, comment on whether the item is dipped in flour or batter or breaded before frying and what fat is used for frying. Also check whether gravy is prepared.

Item	Method of Cooking (e.g., pan frying, broiling, deep frying)	Kind of Fat Used (if any)
Hamburger		
Steaks		
Chops		
Poultry		
Fish		
Shellfish (shrimp, etc.)		
Liver		
Other, specify		

53. Do you use gravy on meats? (check one)

    ___ Yes   ___ No

54. If you prepare gravies, do you usually use (check one):

    ___ cornstarch   ___ flour

    Is the liquid usually (check one):   ___ milk   ___ water   ___ other

    (Specify: _____)

55. Indicate how much fat is usually trimmed from the meat before cooking or eating (check one):

    ___ trim most   ___ trim some   ___ usually don't trim

continues

Adherence Tool 5–1   continued

56. Check the salad dressing *most often* used with the following salads: (Specify brand)

	Mayonnaise-Type (Such as Miracle Whip, Spin Blend)	Regular Mayonnaise (Such as Hellmann's, Kraft)	Imitation Mayonnaise (Such as Bright Day)	Weight Watchers' Mayonnaise	Other—Specify as French, Italian, Ranch-style, etc. Also Specify Creamy, Clear, Lo-Cal, etc.
Potato salad					
Cole slaw					
Tossed salad					
Macaroni salad					
Other (specify)					

Adherence Tool 5–2:   Fat Facts or Misfacts (Monitoring Device)

	True	False
1. All vegetable oil helps lower cholesterol.	_____	_____
2. Saturated fat is found only in animal products.	_____	_____
3. Hydrogenation is a beneficial process that makes fat less saturated.	_____	_____
4. Cholesterol is found in some peanut butter.	_____	_____
5. Cholesterol is found in all animal products.	_____	_____
6. All foods that are high in saturated fat are also high in cholesterol.	_____	_____

Adherence Tool 5–3:   One-Month and One-Week Calendar (Monitoring Device)

ONE-MONTH CALENDAR

Sun.	Mon.	Tues.	Wed.	Thur.	Fri.	Sat.
1 ✔	2	3 ✔	4 ✔	5	6 ✔	7 ✔
8	9	10	11	12	13	14
15	16	17	18	19	20	21
22	23	24	25	26	27	
28	29	30	31	1	2	3

month of _____ 19 ____   If you have any questions, please call: _____

ONE-WEEK CALENDAR

NAME: _____

ATTN:_____   THANK YOU!

Adherence Tool 5–4: Graphs of Dietary Intake of Sterols and Fats (Monitoring Device)

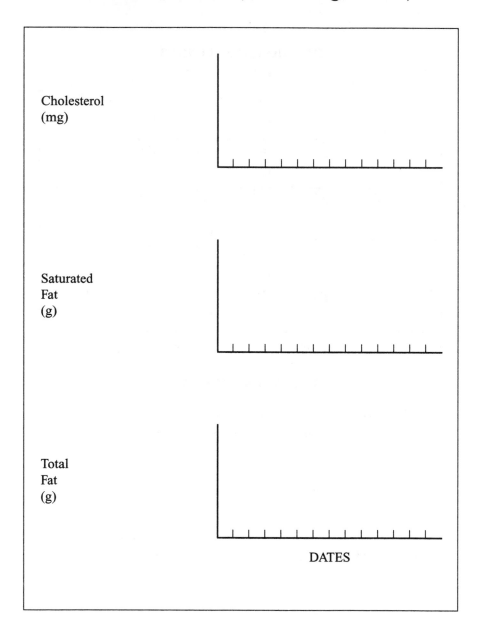

Adherence Tool 5–5: Graphs of Serum Lipid Values (Monitoring Device)

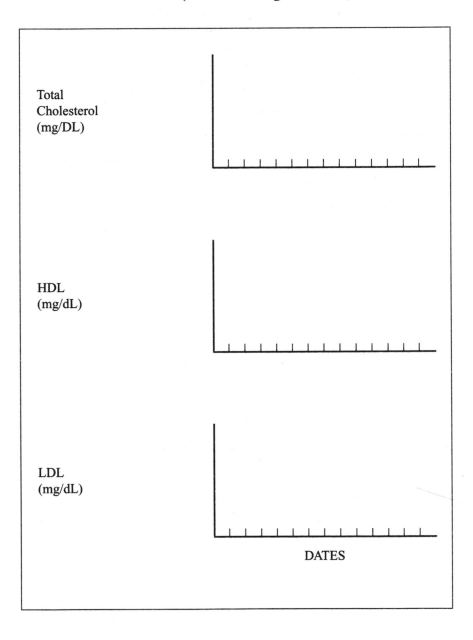

Total
Cholesterol
(mg/DL)

HDL
(mg/dL)

LDL
(mg/dL)

DATES

Adherence Tool 5–6: Pantry Survey
(Monitoring Device)

Food	Saturated Fat (Hydrogenated Vegetable Fat)	Poly-unsaturated Fat	Mono-unsaturated Fat

Adherence Tool 5–7: Client Meal Planning Chart (Informational Device)

Meal planning can help you in keeping your fat and cholesterol intake low. Before your next visit, plan three days of meals that avoid foods high in fat and cholesterol.

	Day 1	Day 2	Day 3
Breakfast			
Snack			
Lunch			
Snack			
Dinner			
Snack			

Adherence Tool 5–8:   Tips for Dining in Restaurants (Informational Device)

Select from the following suggestions:

Appetizers

Clear soup (bouillon, fat-free consomme), fruits or vegetables, juices, seafood cocktail (except shrimp), oysters, or clams on the half-shell. (Be sure to count the seafood as part of your meat allowance.)

Salads

Lettuce and other vegetables, fruits, fruit and cottage cheese (use as part of milk allowance), gelatin. Use lemon juice, vinegar and oil, French dressing, or mayonnaise as your dressing.

Entree

Baked, broiled, or roasted fish, poultry, lean meat, cottage cheese.

Vegetables

All vegetables prepared without butter, meat fat, or cream sauce.

Potatoes and Substitutes

Baked or broiled without dressing, mashed if made without butter, plain rice, macaroni, or spaghetti.

Desserts

Fresh or canned fruits, fruit compotes, sherbert, gelatin, unfrosted angel food cake.

Beverages

Coffee or tea (without cream), carbonated beverages, fruit juices, milk (as allowed), and alcoholic beverages (unless not allowed because of medical problems).

Breakfast Cereals

All cereals without coconut, served with allowed milk.

Miscellaneous

Nuts (except walnuts and filberts), honey, jam, syrup, hard candy, marshmallows, gumdrops, hard fruit drops, jellybeans, mints (no chocolate or bon bons), condiments, and seasoning, as allowed.

Avoid

Combination dishes, fried or creamed foods, foods made with whole milk products, butter, cheese, or gravy. Do not eat pastries (sweet rolls, pies, cakes, cookies, doughnuts, waffles), fatty meats (bacon, sausage, luncheon meats), cream soups, or potato or corn chips.

Inquire about the fat and other ingredients used in menu items. Then give specific instructions regarding the methods of preparation of your selection.

Adherence Tool 5–9: Comparing High-Cholesterol, High-Fat Menus with Low-Cholesterol, Low-Fat Menus (Informational Device)

HIGH-CHOLESTEROL, HIGH-FAT MENU (AT HOME)

Breakfast 1

Egg (1)
Bacon (2 strips)
Toast (2 slices)
Blue Bonnet Stick Margarine
(2 teaspoons)
Milk, Whole (8 ounces)
Orange Juice (4 ounces)

Lunch 1

Bologna (1 ounce)
Bread (2 slices)
Mayonnaise (1 tablespoon)
Blue Bonnet Stick Margarine
(2 teaspoons)
Potato Chips (1 cup)
Mr. Goodbar (1 bar)
Milk, whole (8 ounces)

Dinner 1

Roast Beef (5 ounces)
Mashed Potatoes (½ cup)
Corn (½ cup)
Bread (2 slices)
Blue Bonnet Stick Margarine (6 teaspoons)
Cherry Cobbler (1 cup)
Ice Cream (½ cup)
Milk, whole (8 ounces)

continues

Note: Nutrient values are taken from a variety of sources including Jean A.T. Pennington, Bowes and Church's *Food Values of Portions Commonly Used* (Philadelphia: J.B. Lippincott, 1994), labels and Nutrient Data System (NDS), University of Minnesota. Actual calculations for individual eating patterns could include a variety of data tables currently available to the nutrition counselor.

Adherence Tool 5–9 continued

Breakfast 1

	Amount	Cholesterol (mg)	Total Fat (g)	Saturated Fat (g)	Polyunsaturated Fat (g)	Monounsaturated Fat (g)	P/S Ratio
Egg	1	213	5.30	1.60	.70	2.00	
Bacon	2 strips	11	6.24	2.20	.74	3.30	
Toast	2 slices	—	—	—	—	—	
Blue Bonnet Stick Margarine	2 tsp.	—	5.33	1.00	1.00	1.33	
Milk, whole	8 oz.	34	8.15	5.08	.29	2.78	
Orange juice	4 oz.	—	—	—	—	—	
TOTAL		258	25.02	9.88	2.73	9.41	.28

Lunch 1

	Amount	Cholesterol (mg)	Total Fat (g)	Saturated Fat (g)	Polyunsaturated Fat (g)	Monounsaturated Fat (g)	P/S Ratio
Bologna	1 slice (23 g)	13	6.52	2.68	.24	3.60	
Bread	2 slices	—	—	—	—	—	
Mayonnaise	1 Tbsp.	8	10.96	1.60	5.70	3.10	
Blue Bonnet Stick Margarine	2 tsp.	—	5.33	1.00	1.00	1.33	
Potato Chips	1 cup	8	8.60	3.42	1.02	4.16	
Mr. Goodbar	1 bar	10	16.10	9.00	.80	5.70	
Milk, whole	8 oz.	34	8.15	5.08	.29	2.78	
TOTAL		73	55.66	22.78	9.05	20.67	.40

Dinner 1

	Amount	Cholesterol (mg)	Total Fat (g)	Saturated Fat (g)	Polyunsaturated Fat (g)	Monounsaturated Fat (g)	P/S Ratio
Roast Beef (medium fat)	5 oz.	130	21.10	9.15	5.50	6.45	
Mashed Potatoes*	½ cup	—	—	—	—	—	
Corn*	½ cup	—	—	—	—	—	
Bread	2 slices	—	—	—	—	—	
Blue Bonnet Stick Margarine	6 tsp.	—	16.00	3.00	3.00	4.00	
Cherry Cobbler*	1 cup	—	—	—	—	—	
Ice Cream	½ cup	30	7.16	4.46	.27	2.43	
Milk, whole	8 oz.	34	8.15	5.08	.29	2.78	
TOTAL		194	52.41	21.69	9.06	15.66	.42

Fat used in these recipes was figured into the amount of Blue Bonnet margarine.

Total Daily Intake—Diet 1

	Cholesterol (mg)	Total Fat (g)	Saturated Fat (g)	Polyunsaturated Fat (g)	Monounsaturated Fat (g)	P/S Ratio
Diet 1	525	133.09	54.35	20.84	45.74	.38
Percent of 2,770 Calories*		43%	18%	7%	15%	
Recommendations	200	25%	8.3%	8.3%	8.3%	1.00

*All calorie values here and on the following pages are estimates and may include fat-free foods not listed.

continues

Adherence Tool 5–9   continued

HIGH-CHOLESTEROL, HIGH-FAT MENU (IN A RESTAURANT)

Breakfast 2

Egg McMuffin (1)
Orange Juice (4 ounces)
Milk, whole (8 ounces)

Lunch 2

Big Mac (1)
Fries (regular)
Milk, whole (8 ounces)
Apple Pie (1)

Dinner 2

Tenderloin (1)
Fries (regular)
Milk, whole (8 ounces)

Breakfast 2

	Amount	Choles-terol (mg)	Total Fat (g)	Saturated Fat (g)	Polyun-saturated Fat (g)	Monoun-saturated Fat (g)	P/S Ratio
Egg McMuffin	1	226	11.20	3.80	1.30	6.10	
Orange Juice	4 oz.	—	—	—	—	—	
Milk, whole	8 oz.	34	8.15	5.08	.29	2.78	
TOTAL		260	19.35	8.88	1.59	8.88	.18

Lunch 2

	Amount	Choles-terol (mg)	Total Fat (g)	Saturated Fat (g)	Polyun-saturated Fat (g)	Monoun-saturated Fat (g)	P/S Ratio
Big Mac	1	103	32.40	10.10	1.50	20.90	
Fries, regular	1	12	17.10	7.20	.70	9.20	
Milk, whole	8 oz.	34	8.15	5.08	.29	2.78	
Apple Pie	1	12	14.80	4.80	.90	9.10	
TOTAL		161	72.45	27.18	3.39	41.98	.12

continues

Adherence Tool 5–9 continued

Dinner 2

	Amount	Choles-terol (mg)	Total Fat (g)	Saturated Fat (g)	Polyun-saturated Fat (g)	Monoun-saturated Fat (g)	P/S Ratio
Tenderloin	1	90	24.99	6.42	5.55	13.02	
Fries, regular	1	12	17.10	7.20	.70	9.20	
Milk, whole	8 oz.	34	8.15	5.08	.29	2.78	
TOTAL		136	50.24	18.70	6.54	25.00	.35

Total Daily Intake—Diet 2

	Choles-terol (mg)	Total Fat (g)	Saturated Fat (g)	Polyun-saturated Fat (g)	Monoun-saturated Fat (g)	P/S Ratio
Diet 2	557	142.04	54.76	11.52	75.86	.21
Percentage of 2,500 Calories		51%	20%	4%	27%	—
Recommendations	200	25%	8.3%	8.3%	8.3%	1.00

LOW-CHOLESTEROL, LOW-FAT MENU (AT HOME)

Breakfast 3
English Muffin (1)
Canadian Bacon (1 ounce)
Milk, skim (8 ounces)
Fleischmann's Tub Margarine (2 teaspoons)
Orange Juice (4 ounces)

Lunch 3

Turkey (1 ounce)
Bread (2 slices)
Miracle Whip (1 teaspoon)
Chips (½ cup)
Zucchini Cake (1 serving)
Milk, skim (8 ounces)

Dinner 3

Fish (5 ounces)
Mashed Potatoes (½ cup)
Corn (½ cup)
Tossed Salad (1 cup)
Dressing (1 tablespoon)
Fleischmann's Tub Margarine (1 teaspoon)
Sherbert (½ cup)
Milk, skim (8 ounces)

continues

Adherence Tool 5–9   continued

Breakfast 3

	Amount	Choles-terol (mg)	Total Fat (g)	Saturated Fat (g)	Polyun-saturated Fat (g)	Monoun-saturated Fat (g)	P/S Ratio
English Muffin	1	—	—	—	—	—	
Canadian Bacon	1 oz.	25	2.84	.87	.28	1.69	
Milk, Skim	8 oz.	5	.44	.29	.02	.13	
Fleischmann's Tub Margarine	2 tsp.	—	6.00	1.00	2.67	1.67	
Orange Juice	4 oz.	—	—	—	—	—	
TOTAL		30	9.28	2.16	2.97	3.49	1.4

Lunch 3

	Amount	Choles-terol (mg)	Total Fat (g)	Saturated Fat (g)	Polyun-saturated Fat (g)	Monoun-saturated Fat (g)	P/S Ratio
Turkey	1 oz.	22	1.10	.33	.26	.51	
Bread	2 slices	—	—	—	—	—	
Miracle Whip	1 tsp.	1	1.63	.24	.88	.51	
Chips	½ cup	—	4.67	.59	2.72	1.36	
Zucchini Cake	1 sv.	—	4.67	.59	2.72	1.36	
Milk, Skim	8 oz.	5	.44	.29	.02	.13	
TOTAL		28	12.51	2.04	6.60	3.87	3.2

Dinner 3

	Amount	Choles-terol (mg)	Total Fat (g)	Saturated Fat (g)	Polyun-saturated Fat (g)	Monoun-saturated Fat (g)	P/S Ratio
Fish (6%)	5 oz.	113	5.70	1.50	1.32	2.88	
Mashed Potatoes	½ cup	—	3.78	.69	1.68	1.41	
Corn	½ cup	—	3.78	.69	1.68	1.41	
Tossed Salad	1 cup		—	—	—	—	
Dressing	1 Tbsp.		4.67	.61	1.87	2.19	
Fleischmann's Tub Margarine	1 tsp.		3.00	.50	1.33	.83	
Sherbert	½ cup		—	—	—	—	
Milk, Skim	8 oz.	5	.24	.14	.00	.10	
TOTAL		118	21.17	4.13	7.88	8.82	1.91

Total Daily Intake—Diet 3

	Choles-terol (mg)	Total Fat (g)	Saturated Fat (g)	Polyun-saturated Fat (g)	Monoun-saturated Fat (g)	P/S Ratio
Diet 3	176	42.96	8.33	17.45	16.18	2.09
Percent of 1,923 Calories		20%	4%	8%	8%	
Recommendations	200	25%	8.3%	8.3%	8.3%	1.00

Adherence Tool 5–9   continued

LOW-CHOLESTEROL, LOW-FAT MENU (IN A RESTAURANT)

Breakfast 4
Apple Danish (1)
Orange Juice (4 ounces)
Milk, skim (8 ounces)

Lunch 4

McChicken (1)
Orange Drink (12 ounces)
Strawberry Sundae (1)

Dinner 4

Broiled Cod (13 ounces)
Baked Potato (1)
Tossed Salad (2 cups)
Dressing (1 tablespoon)
Fleischmann's Tub Margarine (2 teaspoons)
Fresh Fruit Compote (1 cup)
Milk, skim (8 ounces)

Breakfast 4

Amount	Choles-terol (mg)	Total Fat (g)	Saturated Fat (g)	Polyun-saturated Fat (g)	Monoun-saturated Fat (g)	P/S Ratio
Apple Danish	1	25	17.90	3.50	2.00	10.80	
Orange Juice	4 oz.	—	—	—	—	—	
Milk, Skim	8 oz.	5	.44	.29	.02	.13	
TOTAL		30	18.34	3.79	2.02	10.93	.58

Lunch 4

Amount	Choles-terol (mg)	Total Fat (g)	Saturated Fat (g)	Polyun-saturated Fat (g)	Monoun-saturated Fat (g)	P/S Ratio
McChicken	1	43	28.60	5.40	11.60	11.40	
Orange Drink	12 oz.	—	—	—	—	—	
Strawberry Sundae	1	5	1.10	.60	—	.40	
TOTAL		48	29.70	6.00	11.60	11.80	1.93

continues

Adherence Tool 5–9   continued

Dinner 4

	Amount	Cholesterol (mg)	Total Fat (g)	Saturated Fat (g)	Polyunsaturated Fat (g)	Monounsaturated Fat (g)	P/S Ratio
Broiled Cod (6%)	3 oz.	68	3.84	.87	1.26	1.71	
Baked Potato	1	—	—	—	—	—	
Tossed Salad	2 cups	—	—	—	—	—	
Dressing	1 Tbsp.	—	4.54	.71	2.60	1.23	
Fleischmann's Tub Margarine	2 tsps.	—	6.00	1.00	2.67	1.67	
Fresh Fruit Compote	1 cup	—	—	—	—	—	
Milk, Skim	8 oz.	5	.44	.29	.02	.13	
TOTAL		73	14.82	2.87	6.55	4.74	2.28

Total Daily Intake—Diet 4

	Cholesterol (mg)	Total Fat (g)	Saturated Fat (g)	Polyunsaturated Fat (g)	Monounsaturated Fat (g)	P/S Ratio
Diet 4	151	62.86	12.66	20.35	27.47	1.60
Percent of 2,455 Calories		23%	5%	8%	10%	
Recommendations	200	25%	8.3%	8.3%	8.3%	1.00

Adherence Tool 5–10: P/S Ratios of Various Fats and Oils (Informational Device)

	Oils and Margarines		Nuts		Other Fats
	8.0	Safflower oil	8.0	8.0	Safflower mayonnaise
	7.0	Sunflower oil Walnut oil	7.0	7.0	
	6.0		6.0	Sunflower seeds Walnuts 6.0	
Helps Raise P/S Ratio	5.0	Corn oil	5.0	5.0	Sandwich spread
	4.0	Soybean/Cotton-seed oil (Wesson, Crisco, etc.)	4.0	4.0	Mayonnaise Salad dressing (Miracle Whip type)
	3.0	Soybean oil Sesame oil	3.0	Pecans, Pumpkin seeds, Chestnuts, Almonds 3.0	Imitation mayonnaise
Has Little Effect on P/S Ratio	2.0	Peanut oil	2.0	Peanuts, Mixed nuts, Brazil nuts, Filberts, Hazel-nuts 2.0	Peanut butter
	1.0	Olive oil	1.0	Pistachio nuts Cashews 1.0	Crisco shortening, Avocado, Olives
Has Negative Effect on P/S Ratio	0.0	Palm oil Coconut oil	0.0	Macadamia nuts	Carob coated candy, Bacon, Butter, Chocolate, Coconut
				0.0	

Note: P/S = polyunsaturated fat ÷ saturated fat.
Courtesy of Pat Pace, R.D., M.S., Baylor University.

CHAPTER 6

Nutrition Counseling in Treatment of Diabetes

CHAPTER OBJECTIVES

1. Identify factors that contribute to common inappropriate behaviors associated with carbohydrate-, protein-, and fat-controlled eating patterns.

2. Identify specific nutrients to emphasize in assessing a baseline eating pattern before providing dietary instruction.

3. Identify strategies to help combat inappropriate eating behaviors.

4. Generate strategies to deal with clients following carbohydrate-, protein-, and fat-controlled eating patterns.

5. Recommend dietary adherence tools for clients on carbohydrate-, protein-, and fat-controlled eating patterns.

NUTRITION AND DIABETES

The publication of results from the Diabetes Control and Complications Trial has pointed to the importance of intensive therapy, including dietary eating pattern control, in delaying progression of diabetic retinopathy, nephropathy, and neuropathy in patients with insulin-dependent diabetes mellitus.[1] Providing appropriate eating patterns for clients with diabetes can be a challenge. All dietary factors, both amount and content, must be carefully controlled, yet the client must be allowed a reasonable selection of foods. This chapter is designed to provide potential solutions to problems encountered in working with clients with diabetes.

The American Dietetic Association and the American Diabetes Association provide basic goals for medical nutrition therapy in persons with diabetes:

- Achieve and maintain near-normal blood glucose levels.
- Achieve optimal blood lipid levels.
- Include appropriate calories.
- Prevent, delay, or treat nutrition-related risk factors or complications such as hypoglycemia, short-term illness, exercise-related problems, renal disease, autonomic neuropathy, hypertension, and cardiovascular disease.
- Improve or maintain overall health through optimal nutrition.[2,3]

Diet for treatment of diabetes falls into two categories based on whether the client has insulin-dependent diabetes mellitus (IDDM) or non-insulin–dependent diabetes mellitus (NIDDM).

This chapter provides information on theories and facts about NIDDM and IDDM. The effects of specific nutrients, sweeteners, alcohol, and exercise on blood glucose levels are described. Methods and means of managing diabetes through glucose monitoring, insulin regimens, and dietary intervention are reviewed. Adherence to diabetic eating patterns is covered in a section describing research in this area. Also included are eating behaviors that are inappropriate for optimum compliance with diabetic eating patterns. Methods for assessing eating patterns prior to instruction on a diabetic dietary recommendation are described. The chapter discusses treatment strategies for lack of knowledge related to general dietary modifications that affect blood glucose levels and lack of knowledge regarding fat intake and weight gain. Strategies designed to deal with forgetfulness and lack of commitment are also provided.

THEORIES AND FACTS ABOUT NUTRITION AND NON-INSULIN–DEPENDENT DIABETES

The person with NIDDM is usually obese and has peripheral resistance to insulin. The treatment of choice is caloric restriction with resulting weight loss, which allows decreased insulin resistance and reduced and normalized blood glucose levels. The single most important goal in managing a person with obesity and NIDDM is to achieve and maintain desirable body weight by reducing total energy intake to levels below energy expenditure. With the loss of weight, blood glucose levels normalize.

The macronutrient composition of the diet for the person with NIDDM is less important than for the person with IDDM. For weight reduction, the diet should be adequate in nutrients but restricted in calories. For persons on diets very low in calories and suboptimal in micronutrients, a vitamin and mineral supplement is appropriate. For persons who cannot adhere to a weight-loss diet, insulin or oral agents may be necessary to lower blood glucose levels. Such persons are usually insulin insensitive and respond poorly to exogenous insulin. The oral agents function in two ways to lower blood glucose levels: (1) they increase insulin release from the beta cells and (2) increase the sensitivity of cell receptor sites. Of the three oral agents, tolbutamide (Orinase) is the weakest; tolazamide (Tolinase) and chlorpropamide (Diabinese) are more potent. Second-generation oral hypoglycemic agents include glyburide and glipizide.

The sulfonylurea compounds all circulate bound to plasma albumin and are metabolized in the liver and then excreted by the kidneys. Some of the metabolites produced in the liver also have hypoglycemic effects. The presence of hepatic or renal disease is a contraindication for the use of oral agents. In persons with IDDM, these drugs are absolutely contraindicated. For these drugs to be effective, the patient must be able to produce endogenous insulin.

In a person with obesity and NIDDM who is treated with oral agents, regularity of meals and the relationship of meals to physical activity are important. Irregular exercise and eating patterns can lead to periods of severe hypoglycemia. Weight loss is the key to achieving control in NIDDM.

New drugs that affect digestion of foods may also be important in alleviating problems in persons with NIDDM. Acarbose, a starch blocker, is currently in clinical use outside the United States and is under review in this country. Acarbose is an alpha-glucoside hydrolase inhibitor that has hypoglycemic effects by blocking the digestion of starches, sucrose, dextrin, and maltose to absorbable monosaccharides. Absorption of glucose and other monosaccharides is not affected. The net result is a decrease in the postprandial rise in plasma glucose levels.[4]

THEORIES AND FACTS ABOUT NUTRITION AND INSULIN-DEPENDENT DIABETES

Insulin-dependent persons have complete beta cell failure, cannot produce insulin, are prone to ketoacidosis, and require exogenous insulin. Therapy revolves around insulin, diet, and exercise. Currently, research on IDDM is flourishing.[5–7] Diet is known to be important in controlling plasma glucose abnormalities and preventing hypoglycemia.[8,9]

Effective insulin treatment to avoid extremely high and low blood glucose levels requires a standardized daily regimen of food intake. Several factors in dietary control are important: (1) timing of meals, (2) dietary composition, (3) caloric intake, and (4) level and regularity of physical activity.

Even if a client is following an intensive regimen in which each meal is covered with regular insulin, timing and regularity of meals are important. Practitioners view each person as an individual, taking lifestyle, physical activity, and insulin administration into consideration. They stress a regular eating and exercise pattern as a goal for clients receiving insulin. Inconsistency in meals or exercise makes regulation of insulin doses difficult and can frequently lead to highs and lows in blood sugars.

Controversy exists with regard to the best nutrient distribution for dietary prescription. The American Dietetic Association recommends the following nutrient distribution:

1. Individuals should receive 10 to 20 percent of daily calories from protein with no less than adult Recommended Dietary Allowance (RDA) (0.8 g/kg/day) with evidence of nephropathy; adjust for very young children, pregnant and lactating women, and some elderly persons.
2. Individualize the percentage of daily calories from fat, based on the nutrition assessment and treatment goals. For those older than two years, saturated fat is less than 10 percent of daily calories. This value drops to less than 7 percent with elevated low-density lipoprotein (LDL). Polyunsaturated fat is up to 10 percent of total calories. Most of the total fat should be monounsaturated fat. Total fat varies with treatment goals: approximately 30 percent (<10 percent saturated fat) is recommended for normal weight persons with normal lipids and less than 30 percent (<7 percent saturated fat) is recommended for obese persons with elevated LDL levels.
3. Individualize the percentage of daily calories from carbohydrate, based on the patient's eating habits. The percentage of daily calories from carbohydrate can be devised after the protein and fat goals have been met. The percentage and distribution will vary with insulin regimens and treatment goals.[10,11]

These recommendations are general, flexible requirements. The major goal should be to normalize blood sugars with glycosylated hemoglobin (HbA1c) in the normal range. (See Table 6–1 and "Blood Glucose Monitoring" below for a detailed discussion of HbA1c.)

EFFECTS OF SPECIFIC NUTRIENTS, SWEETENERS, ALCOHOL, AND EXERCISE ON BLOOD GLUCOSE LEVELS

Carbohydrates

Digestible Carbohydrate

Traditionally, dietary recommendations focused on use of complex carbohydrate and minimization of simple carbohydrate, assuming that the latter was absorbed rapidly and thus produced swings in blood glucose.[12,13] Subsequent studies demonstrated significantly different blood glucose and insulin responses to different types of simple and complex carbohydrates.[14,15] Other factors such as how

Table 6–1 Glycemic Control for People with Diabetes

Biochemical Index	Nondiabetic	Goal	Action Suggested
Preprandial glucose (mg/dL)	<115	80–120	<80, >140
Bedtime glucose (mg/dL)	<120	100–140	<100, >160
Hemoglobin A1c (%)	<6	<7	>8

Notes: Values are for nonpregnant individuals. "Action suggested" depends on individual patient circumstances. Hemoglobin A1c is referenced to a nondiabetic range of 4.0–6.0% (mean 5.0%; standard deviation 0.5%).* In the Diabetes Control and Complications Trial, the experimental group had glycosylated hemoglobins of approximately 7.0% and the standard group 9.0%.†

* "American Diabetes Association Position Statement: Standards of Medical Care for Patients with Diabetes Mellitus," *Diabetes Care*, Vol. 17, pp. 616–624, 1994.

† The Diabetes Control and Complications Research Group, "The Effect of Intensive Treatment of Diabetes on the Development and Progression of Long-Term Complications in Insulin-Dependent Diabetes Mellitus," *The New England Journal of Medicine*, Vol. 329, pp. 977–986, 1993.

---

quickly the food is eaten, how much is eaten, the way in which the food has been processed and cooked, and the combination of foods eaten have a major effect.

Carbohydrate is the general name for chemical compounds having the empirical form $C_n(H_2O)_n$. Digestible dietary carbohydrate has traditionally been classified as *simple* (monosaccharides, disaccharides, and oligosaccharides) or *complex* (polysaccharides). Most foods do not fall into just one category, but are a combination. In human nutrition the monosaccharides of most importance are the six-carbon sugars—glucose, fructose, and galactose. Glucose, also known as dextrose or corn sugar, is present in sweet fruits such as berries, grapes, pears, and oranges and in certain vegetables, notably corn and carrots. Relatively large amounts occur in honey as well. Dextrose from corn syrup is often used commercially as a sweetener in prepared foods. Fructose, also called levulose or fruit sugar, is also found in most fruits and vegetables. Galactose is not found free in foods, although it is a major constituent of the principal carbohydrate in milk, lactose.

Disaccharides are formed when two monosaccharides are chemically bonded together. When glucose and fructose are bonded, sucrose, or table sugar, results. It is found in most fruits and vegetables and is a major component of brown sugar, maple sugar, and molasses. Many processed foods are sweetened with sucrose. When glucose and galactose are bonded, the disaccharide lactose results. Lactose, the only significant carbohydrate of animal origin, is found in milk and milk products. Maltose is another important disaccharide that results when two identical glucose units bond. Maltose is found in germinating seeds, some breakfast cereals, and fermented products, such as beer.

Oligosaccharides are next in complexity, containing between three and ten monosaccharide units. The oligosaccharides, stachyose and raffinose occur in small amounts in legumes such as kidney beans and lentils and, although believed to be inert metabolically, they are acted on by bacteria in the lower small intestine and colon and may cause increased flatus production.

The term *polysaccharide* denotes the combination of a number of monosaccharides. Polysaccharides of plant origin are commonly known as starches, of which there are several types. Different carbohydrate-containing foods (for example, corn, wheat, and apples) have different starches, each genetically determined. For example, amylose is a plant starch in which hundreds of glucose units are combined to form one long, straight chain. Amylopectin is another plant starch, also composed solely of glucose units, but arranged in branched chains. Various plants contain both amylose and amylopectin, although in different proportions.

The most abundant polysaccharide (and probably the most common organic molecule on earth) is cellulose, a component of plant cell walls. The body cannot digest cellulose because the human digestive system does not have the capacity to break the cellulose linkage structure. The amylose structure, however, is readily digested. In summary, small structural distinctions make the difference in how each molecule behaves and is used.

The one animal polysaccharide, glycogen, is not present in the food supply to an appreciable extent. Although it is stored as an energy source in some animal tissue (muscle and liver), it disappears with the death of the animal, leaving only negligible amounts in foods such as liver and fresh shellfish. The significance of glycogen for humans is its manufacture by the body during the course of glucose metabolism.[16]

During digestion, even large molecules of carbohydrate, such as starch, are eventually hydrolyzed to monosaccharides. Through enzymatic activity and chemical activity involving gastric acid, dietary carbohydrate is converted to the three monosaccharides (Figure 6–1).

In diabetes management, one of the most controversial topics is the type of dietary carbohydrate consumed. In the past, a commonly accepted belief was that because sugars are smaller molecules, they are more rapidly digested and absorbed than complex carbohydrates. Researchers believed that the larger molecules of complex carbohydrate took longer to be absorbed, resulting in a slower and more moderate rise in blood glucose levels. Patients were advised to avoid simple carbohydrate and encouraged to increase their intake of complex carbohydrate. In the 1970s and 1980s, researchers began to challenge this dietary dogma, asserting that glycemic changes were not related solely to the molecular structure of the carbohydrate consumed.[17–19]

Several investigators have conducted research in people with diabetes indicating that glycemic response is not related solely to the molecular structure of the

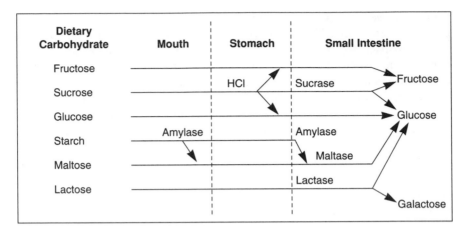

Figure 6–1 Schematic Diagram of Carbohydrate Digestion. *Source:* From P.A. Kreutler, *Nutrition in Perspective*, 2nd ed. Copyright © 1987 by Allyn and Bacon. Reprinted by permission.

carbohydrate consumed. Bantle and his coworkers found no differences in metabolism of glucose between diets containing predominantly starch or simple sugar in patients with type I or type II diabetes.[20–22] Additional research shows no adverse effects of sucrose on glycemia.[23–29]

Although much research is still necessary to explain fully how carbohydrates affect diabetic control, research has provided some very interesting clues.[30] Over the years, studies point to the following factors in the relationship of complex carbohydrates and their effect on blood glucose values:

- nature of the starch
- protein-starch interaction
- antinutrients other than fiber
- physical form
  1. cooking method
  2. particle size (blending, grinding, etc.)

Crapo and coworkers studied the glycemic and insulin responses to a group of carbohydrate-containing foods, including bread, rice, potato, and corn, of normal and glucose-intolerant volunteers. Their findings indicated that the differences in responses to these foods are related to differences in the digestibility of starches.[31–34] Studies have also shown that, because of its chemical structure, amylopectin can be digested more quickly than amylase. The glucose chains of amylose are bound by hydrogen bonds, making them less available for amylitic attack than amylopectin, which has many branched chains of glucose.[35] Indeed, raw legume starch (high in amylose) is less digestible than cornstarch in rats.[36]

An interaction between the protein and starch in food may also influence the digestibility and blood glucose response to the starch.[37] Anderson et al. found that removing protein from flour increased its digestibility.[38]

In addition to the starch and protein components of foods, antinutrients (natural enzyme inhibitors, lectins, phytates, and tannins) may affect starch digestibility and the blood glucose response. Enzyme inhibitors, lectins, and phytates were shown to produce hypoglycemia and decreased growth in rats.[39–43] Furthermore, antinutrients may inhibit starch digestion in the gastrointestinal tract.[44–47]

The physical form of complex carbohydrates also affects blood glucose responses. A greater rise in blood glucose was reported after consumption of cooked as opposed to raw starches. Researchers found that raw plant foods produced lower blood glucose responses than did cooked plant foods.[48–50] Researchers have looked at moist and dry heat methods of cooking. Jenkins found that drying cooked red lentils in a warm oven for 12 hours resulted in significantly enhanced glycemic response and rate of in vitro digestion as compared with lentils boiled 20 minutes.[51]

The size of the starch particle is also important in starch digestibility. Digestibility increased when beans were ground first and then cooked as opposed to when they were cooked first and then ground.[52] O'Dea and others found that the blood glucose response to whole apples increased when apples were blended to a puree or when the juice was extracted.[53–55]

Indigestible Carbohydrate

Fiber is carbohydrate that is not hydrolyzed by human digestive enzymes. It consists of plant cell walls composed mostly of three polysaccharides—cellulose, pectic substances, and hemicellulose—as well as noncarbohydrate lignin. Fiber is a component of plant foods only; it is not found in foods of animal origin.

It is important to draw a clear distinction between the effects of purified fiber added to a diet and fiber naturally present in food. In general, the viscous, water-soluble fibers, such as guar and pectin (purified fiber), have been most effective in flattening postprandial glycemia in normal and diabetic volunteers and reducing urinary glucose loss in diabetic subjects. Part of this action may stem from the ability of these fibers to slow gastric emptying and reduce the rate of small intestinal absorption, possibly by increasing the thickness of the unstirred water layer immediately adjacent to the small intestinal absorptive surface.

Fiber naturally occurring in foods may reduce the rate of small intestinal digestion by impeding the penetration of the food by digestive enzymes, as may viscous forms of fiber. However, disruption of the normal relationship of starch and fiber, as in the milling of wheat products, may greatly reduce any effect the fiber might have on postprandial glycemia.

Concerns have been raised about the vitamin and mineral status of people who change from an habitually low-fiber diet to a diet of higher fiber content. Studies of vitamin and mineral status in adult subjects on high-fiber diets have not found evidence of deficiency.[56-58] Two populations at greatest risk, children[59-61] and pregnant women,[62,63] also have shown no harmful effects of fiber. Another population at risk is the elderly. Studies have not been done to evaluate mineral malabsorption in this age group. Use of high-fiber diets in this group should be approached with caution.[64] Use of high-fiber diets in persons with gastroparesis is contraindicated.[65]

Many natural food fiber/diabetes studies report improvement in glucose control.[66-68] One limiting factor in these studies is the difficulty in knowing what caused this improvement—the fiber component of the diet or other simultaneous changes in macronutrient content. Anderson indicates that most of the reduction in insulin requirements for lean diabetic patients eating high-carbohydrate fiber diets may be related to the 70 percent carbohydrate and 12 percent fat content, with only a small role assigned to fiber content.[69] Studies that have included the soluble-fiber supplements guar and pectin have demonstrated improved glucose control.[70,71] By contrast, insoluble-fiber supplements such as wheat bran and cellulose have usually produced no significant change.[72-73]

The amounts of dietary fiber were high in studies showing improved glycemic control. These high amounts (more than 50 grams per day) would be difficult to achieve for most persons in the Western world. The 1994 recommendations for persons with diabetes do not suggest high-fiber diets for one reason, because the levels necessary to improve glycemic control would be difficult to obtain from foods.[74-75]

Classifying Carbohydrates Using the Glycemic Index

As stated earlier, researchers have found variations in blood sugars when specific foods within the categories of simple and complex carbohydrate were tested for post-ingestion blood glucose excursions. Wolever and his colleagues provided one method of classifying foods according to their effect on blood glucose levels.[76]

In theory, the higher the glycemic index value, the higher the blood glucose values would be expected to rise after the ingestion of the food. Results of early glycemic index research proved contrary to previous beliefs about the effect of carbohydrate on blood glucose levels. For example, researchers were surprised to find that instant potatoes had a higher glycemic index of 120 than ice cream with 69 (Table 6–2).

As a class, legumes are the foods that produce the flattest glycemic response, which is thought to be due to the slow release of carbohydrate during digestion

Table 6–2 Glycemic Index of Selected Foods

Food	Glycemic Index	Food	Glycemic Index
Breads		**Legumes**	
White	100	Kidney beans, canned	74
Whole meal	100	Lentils, green, canned	74
Pumpernickel	68	Baked beans, canned	70
Pasta		Kidney beans, dried	43
Spaghetti, white,		Lentils, green, dried	36
boiled 15 min	67	Soybeans, canned	22
Spaghetti, brown,		Soybeans, dried	20
boiled 15 min	61	**Fruit**	
Spaghetti, white,		Banana	84
boiled 5 min	45	Orange juice	71
Cereal Grains		Orange	59
Millet	103	Apple	52
Rice, brown	81	Apple juice	45
Rice, instant, boiled 1 min	65	**Sugars**	
Barley, pearled	36	Maltose	152
Breakfast Cereals		Glucose	138
Cornflakes	121	Sucrose	83
Puffed wheat	110	Lactose	57
Shredded wheat	97	Fructose	26
Porridge oats	89	**Dairy Products**	
"All Bran"	74	Ice cream	69
Root Vegetables		Yogurt	52
Potato, instant	120	Skim milk	46
Potato, mashed	98	Whole milk	44
Potato, new/white, boiled	80	**Snack Foods**	
Potato, sweet	70	Corn chips	99
Vegetables		Potato chips	77
Carrots, cooked	92		
Peas, frozen	74		

Source: Data from TMS, Wolever. *World Review of Nutrition Dietetics,* Vol. 62, pp. 120–185, copyright © 1990.

rather than to slowed carbohydrate absorption.[77–78] **The glycemic index (GI) is defined as:**

$$GI = 100 \times F/R$$
$$F = \text{test food}$$
$$R = \text{reference food (bread)}$$

Retrospective studies have shown that when diet GI is decreased, improved blood glucose results.[79,80]

The GI concept is not widely accepted as a method of diabetes meal planning. Tools for patient education have not been developed. However, clients may wish to emphasize foods within food groups that demonstrate lower glycemic indexes (lentils and beans). Raw and unpeeled foods have also been associated with lower glycemic response. However, foods should not be eliminated or included in the meal plan based solely on lower GI value.[81] Any change in the diet creates counterchange; therefore, counselors must always consider the total diet and its appropriateness for an individual.

Fat

The fat content of the diet is important for individuals with diabetes from two standpoints. First, diabetic persons have a two to three times greater incidence of atherosclerosis and risk of death from cardiovascular disease than do nondiabetic persons, with an expected reduction in lifespan of five to seven years.[82] Lower saturated fat, cholesterol, and total fat may help avoid coronary complications. Second, a study by O'Dea of persons with type II diabetes showed that the coingestion of fat with a carbohydrate meal reduced the postprandial glucose response to carbohydrate load but had no effect on insulin response.[83] The mechanism of action is poorly understood. One possibility is that glucose absorption from the small intestine is delayed because of the fat-induced delay in gastric emptying.

Although fat has been associated with decreased gastric emptying, the addition of fat to a carbohydrate load does not necessarily alter its effect on blood glucose levels. Studies on the effect of fat on blood glucose levels showed varying responses.[84] One study showed that fat has no impact on digestion rates or blood glucose responses.[85] Others found a reduction in postprandial blood glucose responses when a saturated fat (butter) was eaten with carbohydrate, without an associated decrease in insulin response.[86,87] One study showed no significant changes in acute postprandial glucose responses and insulin levels when subjects ingested amounts of fat smaller than those described in the studies above. However, the subjects demonstrated a large impairment of carbohydrate tolerance following a standard meal eaten four hours after the high-fat breakfast.[88] The exact mechanism behind this effect is unclear. Ferrannini and his coworkers demonstrated an inhibition of insulin-stimulated glucose utilization when plasma-free fatty acids were elevated.[89]

Brackenridge stresses that food combinations can alter rates of carbohydrate digestion and absorption, modifying the pattern of glucose rise after a meal.[90] When this occurs, although the total amount of glucose released into the bloodstream may be unchanged, the postprandial glucose rise can be delayed or blunted. This reaction will change insulin demand and availability. Exhibit 6–1 shows two meals with identical carbohydrate content; however, both fat and fiber are very different. These two meals may produce significantly different 2-hour postprandial glucose levels. Postmeal glucose testing will provide data to determine the optimal size and timing of the premeal insulin bolus for specific meals.

Protein

Protein is also important in the diabetic person's diet. Approximately 58 percent of animal protein intake may eventually be converted to glucose, but at a much slower rate than carbohydrate.[91–93] High-protein diets have been recommended for the treatment of diabetes and may be associated with beneficial effects in some people with diabetes, but these diets have not yet been investigated scientifically. Concern about high-protein diets seems to center on the

---

Exhibit 6–1 Isocarbohydrate Meals

	Item	*CHO (g)*	*Fat (g)*	*Fiber (g)*
Meal 1:	8 oz orange juice	27	0	<1
	2 slices white bread	26	2	2
	2 oz part-skim cheese	2	8	<1
	1 oz puffed rice cereal	13	0	<1
	4 oz skim milk	6	0	<1
	Black coffee	0	0	0
	Total	**74**	**10**	**~4**
Meal 2:	1 apple (3/lb)	18	1	3
	2 slices bran bread	26	4	6
	2 tsp soft margarine	1	10	<1
	½ cup 100% Bran	23	2	13
	4 oz low-fat milk	6	3	<1
	Total	**74**	**~20**	**~22**

Source: Reprinted from B. Brackenridge, "Carbohydrate Counting for Diabetes Therapy," in *Handbook of Diabetes Medical Nutrition Therapy*, M.A. Powers, ed., p. 262. Copyright © 1996, Aspen Publishers, Inc.

increased fat and cholesterol content that accompanies such diets unless food choices are made carefully. High-protein diets are contraindicated in diabetic patients with renal disease in predialysis states.

Calories

The caloric content of the diet is very important, as the majority of persons with IDDM initially lose a significant amount of weight. A diet must be adequate in calories for normal growth and development in pediatric age groups and for desirable body weight in adults. In the pregnant diabetic individual, caloric intake must be adjusted for normal growth and development of the fetus. Excess weight can lead to insulin resistance. Chapter 4 discusses strategies to aid in decreasing calories.

Sweeteners

Many alternatives are open to diabetic persons who want to use nonglucose-containing sweeteners. Three low-calorie sweeteners currently approved for use in the United States are acesulfame potassium, aspartame, and saccharin. Low-calorie sweeteners with approval or reapproval pending include alitame, cyclamate, and sucralose.

Acesulfame Potassium

Acesulfame potassium is 200 times sweeter than sucrose, is heat stable, and blends well with other nutritive and nonnutritive sweeteners. Studies using both humans and animals have shown that acesulfame potassium is not metabolized nor does it accumulate in the body. Because it is not metabolized, it has no caloric value. It has no effect on blood glucose, cholesterol, total glycerol, or free glycerol levels.[94] In terms of safety, no adverse effects were documented even at administered doses of 1,000 times higher than anticipated maximum dietary intake by humans. It has been deemed safe for all segments of the population.[95,96] In one packet of sweetener, equivalent to the sweetness of two teaspoons of sugar, there are only 10 milligrams of potassium (1 medium-sized banana = 440 milligrams potassium).

Aspartame

Aspartame has a slow onset of a sweet taste that is sustained over time. It is stable in dry foods but decomposes on prolonged exposure to high temperatures or in liquid form. Aspartame is metabolized in the gastrointestinal tract to aspartic acid, phenylalanine, and methanol. The aspartic acid is primarily used for energy through conversion to CO_2 in the Krebs cycle. The phenylalanine is primarily incorporated into body protein, either unchanged or as tyrosine. The methyl group is hydrolyzed by intestinal esterases to methanol. The metabolism of aspartame is the same as that of its equivalent natural components. The individual components are rapidly metabolized and do not accumulate at recommended intakes.[97] It would be extremely difficult to consume amounts large enough to accumulate to toxic levels because the body continuously clears the byproducts from the system.[98,99] Aspartame in the amount of 2.7 grams per day does not affect blood glucose control.[100] The Food and Drug Administration (FDA) has found aspartame to be a safe sweetener for the general population, including pregnant women and children. One qualifier is that persons who do not tolerate phenylalanine should avoid aspartame-containing products.[101]

Saccharin

Saccharin is a white, crystalline powder synthesized from toluene. It is approximately 300 times sweeter than sucrose. Despite many claims that saccharin has a bitter aftertaste, it continues to be a popular tabletop sweetener. Saccharin is only slightly soluble in water and is stable under many conditions. It is synergistic with other sweeteners, such as aspartame. The continued use of saccharin is due at least in part to its long shelf life, low price, and thermal stability. Saccharin is not metabolized and is excreted unchanged, primarily by the kidneys in the urine.[102] Researchers have found that "as a group, users of artificial sweeteners (saccharin and cyclamates) have little or no excess risk of cancer of the lower urinary tract."[103] The American Medical Association reviewed experimental data and reaffirmed its stand that saccharin should continue to be available as a food additive.[104] Both the American Dietetic Association and the American Diabetes Association have stated that saccharin poses no health hazard.[105,106]

Sweeteners Pending FDA Approval

Alitame. Alitame is a dipeptide-based amide formed from 1-aspartic acid and d-alanine. It is 2,000 times sweeter than sucrose. It is stable at high temperatures and over a broad pH range and less stable in lower ranges (acids). It can be used in sodas, fruit drinks, baked goods, confections, and tabletop sweeteners.[107] Alitame is metabolized to its two proteins and other components. The amino acids are metabolized and the remainder excreted unchanged.

Cyclamate. Cyclamate, a derivative of cyclohexylsulfamic acid, is 30 times sweeter than sucrose. It enhances the sweetness of other sweeteners, is heat stable, mitigates the bitter aftertaste of saccharin when saccharin is the second sweetener, increases the product's stability or shelf life, and usually reduces product cost.[108] Cyclamate is metabolized in the digestive tract, and its byproducts are secreted by the kidneys. Its primary metabolite is cyclohexylamine, which some scientists believe may be more toxic than clyclamate. Cyclohexylamine is formed from the nonabsorbed cyclamate by bacteria in the gastrointestinal tract. Not all persons are able to metabolize cyclamate, and those who do only metabolize a portion of what is consumed.[109] It has been shown that cyclamate has no significant effect on blood glucose.[110] The FDA continues to review data for other safety issues in addition to carcinogenicity (such as genetic damage and testicular atrophy).[111] However, the safety of cyclamate for human use has been supported.[112]

Sucralose. Sucralose is 600 times sweeter than sucrose. It is made from sugar by selectively substituting three chlorine atoms for three hydroxyl groups on the sugar molecule. It has a similar taste profile to sugar with no unpleasant aftertaste, and it has no calories. It is stable in solutions and at varying pH levels and temperatures. It can be used in cooking and baking. Sucralose is essentially non-metabolized. It passes rapidly through the body without being broken down. It is not digested in the gastrointestinal tract and only a small amount (about 15 percent of that ingested) is absorbed through the small intestine. The remainder passes through the digestive system unchanged and is excreted in the feces. Sucralose does not accumulate in any tissues and is not actively transported across the blood-brain barrier to the central nervous system, across the placental barrier, or from the mammary gland into breast milk.[113] Studies indicate that sucralose can be used safely by everyone, including pregnant and lactating women, children, and persons with type I and type II diabetes.[114] Also sucralose does not promote tooth decay.[115] The FDA is currently reviewing the petition to use sucralose in 15 food and beverage categories.[116]

Alcohol

Alcohol intake may cause hypoglycemia because the enzyme most common in alcohol metabolism, alcohol dehydrogenase (ADH), inhibits gluconeogenesis in the liver. In a fasting person, 2 ounces of distilled liquor may result in hypoglycemia. In a fed person, with well-controlled diabetes, moderate alcohol intake of either 8 ounces of regular beer, 4 ounces of dry wine, or 2 ounces of distilled liquor along with a meal does not seem to affect the blood glucose level dramatically.[117] Individuals who have had just a small food intake may experience hypoglycemia within 6 to 36 hours after alcohol ingestion.[118] Self-monitoring blood glucose levels before and after alcohol intake and a meal enables the person to predict potential hypoglycemia and prevent it from occurring.

Alcohol has been shown to cause hyperglycemia in the fed state due to glycogenolysis in the liver and peripheral insulin resistance.[119] The rise in blood glucose depends on the quantity of alcohol consumed and the amount of liver glycogen stores available.[120]

Intoxication can result in decreased competence in administering insulin or other hypoglycemic agents or lack of ability to time and plan meals appropriately. In addition, alcohol intoxication can mask the symptoms of hypoglycemia and impede appropriate treatment. Another potential metabolic consequence of alcohol ingestion is elevated plasma triglyceride levels. Because diabetes is associated with an increased incidence of hypertriglyceridemia, nutrition counselors should consider the effect of alcohol on plasma triglyceride levels in the dietary therapy of any diabetic client. It would seem prudent to curtail alcohol ingestion significantly in clients with preexisting elevations of plasma triglyceride. The caloric content of the alcohol must be considered and included in the diabetic meal plan if it is to be consumed. Finally, because alcohol intake may cause hypoglycemia, clients should be warned about and given strategies to deal with this potential problem.[121]

In summary, persons with diabetes should avoid alcohol abuse. Counselors can explain the specific risks for people with diabetes. Moderate ingestion of alcohol is the key for diabetic individuals, with caution regarding its effect on caloric balance, control of plasma triglyceride levels, and reduced reaction time.

Exercise

Exercise can modulate the body's sensitivity to insulin and increase peripheral glucose use resulting in improved metabolic control for those with diabetes. **The goals of an exercise program for individuals with diabetes are**

1. to maintain or improve cardiovascular fitness to prevent or minimize the long-term cardiovascular complications of diabetes
2. to improve flexibility, which is impaired as muscle collagen becomes glycated
3. to improve muscle, which may deteriorate as a result of neuropathy and which uses glucose as fuel
4. to ensure that persons with IDDM can participate safely in and enjoy physical or sports activities
5. to assist in glucose management and weight control in people with NIDDM
6. to allow individuals with diabetes to experience the same benefits and enjoyment that people without diabetes gain from a regular exercise program.[122]

The questions about nutritional issues that are still unanswered make it impossible to quantify definitively the ideal macronutrient content of the diabetic diet. It is the nutrition counselor's responsibility to review dietary intake and look at corresponding blood sugars to determine possible alterations in matching insulin and diet for future occasions. The field is developing rapidly and, as new facts have emerged from research, nutritional recommendations have been revised. As researchers continue to make advances, new data will help to define the components of the optimal diet.

MANAGEMENT OF DIABETES

To manage diabetes, counselors must understand blood glucose testing, insulin types and their effect on blood glucose levels, and management schemes.

Blood Glucose Monitoring

Methods are available for accurate and convenient self-measurement of blood glucose. In one, a small drop of blood is obtained from the finger with a device called an autolet and placed on a strip (Chemstrip or Dextrostick). An enzymatic reaction takes place to cause the strip to change color, indicating the amount of glucose in the blood. The stick is read through comparison with a color chart or by a machine, the glucometer. Thorough instruction in monitoring is crucial and should be given by trained medical personnel. Home blood glucose monitoring that is completed incorrectly may not reflect actual blood glucose levels.

Monitoring blood glucose levels requires measurement in the fasting state and then two or three hours after breakfast, lunch, and dinner. The fasting blood glucose level is a guide to the effectiveness of overnight control of diabetes. The postprandial blood glucose values indicate how well insulin matches the foods eaten at meals. The goal is to prevent hyperglycemia and hypoglycemia after a meal. When multiple injections of regular insulin are given, it is preferable to measure blood glucose levels before each meal (preprandially) (30 minutes before a meal at approximately the time of an injection or a bolus) rather than two hours after a meal. For clients who are willing, measurement 30 minutes before and 2 hours after a meal may give information that helps in normalizing blood glucose levels. Changes in insulin regimens are based on these blood glucose determinations, usually on a pattern of blood sugars over a period of three days.

In addition to blood glucose monitoring, the measurement of glycosylated hemoglobin indicates the degree of long-term control of diabetes. Glucose in the blood reacts with free amino groups in proteins in a stable and irreversible nonenzymatic process called glycosylation. Thus glucose is attached to the protein for the life of the protein. Hemoglobin, one of several proteins exhibiting glycosylation, has a life span of 100 to 120 days. The percentage of glycosylated hemoglobin in the blood reflects the time-averaged blood glucose levels from the preceding two to three months.[123-126] Table 6–1 (see p. 185) indicates optimum levels for glycosylated hemoglobin.

In persons with IDDM, it is important to document ketones in the urine. When blood glucose levels are out of control or when clients are acutely ill, ketone bodies can be important early warning signs of impending diabetic ketoacidosis. On sick days, it is important for clients to take insulin, test their blood glucose frequently, test their urine for ketones, and try to eat their usual amount of carbohydrate, divided into smaller meals and snacks. If blood glucose levels rise above 250 mg/dL, all of the usual amount of carbohydrate is not necessary. Frequent fluid intake is also recommended.

Types of Insulin

Diet and insulin must be matched closely to achieve normalized blood glucose levels. The insulin preparations available today fall into four categories:

1. *Rapid short-acting insulin* (insulin analog, named lispro)—peaks in five minutes and is eliminated from circulation in less than two hours.
2. *Short-acting insulin*—peaks in three to four hours and lasts six to eight hours. Included in this category are Regular and Semilente insulin.
3. *Intermediate-acting insulin*—peaks 8 to 10 hours after injection and lasts 18 to 24 hours. NPH (neutral-protamine Hagedorn) and Lente are intermediate-acting insulins.
4. *Long-acting insulin*—peaks 14 to 16 hours after injection and has some effect for up to 36 hours. Protamine zinc (PZI) and Ultralente are long-acting insulins.

The newest of the four insulins described above is lispro (Hamalog). It allows persons with diabetes to inject a dose and eat. This eliminates the need for injecting regular insulin 30 minutes prior to a meal. Without this time lag, patients have increased flexibility in food choices and a spontaneity that they are not afforded with regular insulin on injection regimens.

Insulin manufacturers have developed premixed ratios of NPH and regular insulin. The most commonly prescribed premixed insulin is 70/30 (70 percent NPH and 30 percent regular, a standard based on the two-thirds to one-third guideline). Also available is 50/50 insulin, which can reduce postprandial hyperglycemia and the risk of subsequent hypoglycemia.

Multiple daily injection (MDI) therapy and the constant subcutaneous infusion insulin (CSII) pump provide the dietitian with a wealth of flexibility in dietary recommendations. Timing of meals, dietary composition, caloric content of the diet, and physical activity are immensely important to the successful use of MDI or CSII. Teamwork among physician, nurse, and dietitian is crucial to success. During the Diabetes Control and Complications Trial, subjects in the experimental study group (following an intensive management protocol) had the option of using either MDI therapy, consisting of three or more injections per day, or the CSII pump.

Regular insulin is used in the CSII pump, which is attached to the abdomen subcutaneously with a needle. From a syringe attached to the pump, insulin flows through tubing to the needle injection site. The pump is a kind of computer that, when programmed, allows insulin to enter the body much as the pancreas slowly maintains a constant insulin level throughout the day. The pump also allows the client to increase the amount of insulin in a bolus at each meal, which also mimics the normally functioning pancreas. A basal dose of insulin is programmed into the computer-like pump to provide a constant, small dose of regular insulin at all times. Meals are covered by bolusing or pushing a button on the pump with the appropriate number (shown in a window) that coincides with the correct units of regular insulin to match a meal.

MDI therapy is similar to the pump concept in that regular insulin is injected via syringe to cover each meal. Basal needs are usually met with NPH, frequently given at supper or bedtime for overnight control, or with one to two injections of Ultralente insulin given before breakfast or before both breakfast and supper.

DIETARY INTERVENTION

Both CSII and MDI therapy require the use of a dietary exchange pattern, which should be based upon individual needs and preferences (for example, for cardiovascular problems, The American Heart Association's recommendations as discussed in Chapter 5 may be necessary). The exchange list shown in Adherence Tool 6–6 includes only items preferred by one particular client. Each food is placed in a category with items that have approximately equivalent carbohydrate, protein, and fat contents. For persons on the pump or MDI, an additional step that allows more flexibility without sacrificing accuracy is carbohydrate counting or counting total available glucose.

The major rationale for using carbohydrate counting is that dietary carbohydrate is the main determinant of meal-related insulin demand. Although the absolute glucose excursion and rate of glucose appearance differ among individual carbohydrate foods,[127] it is estimated that 90 to 100 percent of digestible dietary carbohydrate enters the bloodstream as glucose in the first few hours after a meal.[128] This system recognizes that only a portion of fat and protein are metabolized to glucose and that overall these nutrients yield much less glucose than does an equal amount of carbohydrate.[129] When fat and protein intake are relatively consistent from day to day, the basal or intermediate-acting insulin present between meals is adjusted to handle the glucose released by their metobolism. A quite precise estimate of the insulin demand created by a particular meal or snack can, therefore, be derived by simply counting the grams of carbohydrate it contains.

The basic meal plan for a patient who uses carbohydrate counting is composed of gram totals of carbohydrate to be consumed at each planned meal and snack. There are two ways to develop such a plan.[130] The preferred method for patients with type I diabetes is to base the plan on the client's current eating habits. An average or usual meal pattern can be identified using several days of food records provided by the client. This pattern can then be translated into the carbohydrate gram equivalent that is consumed at each meal or snack. This approach can also be used for patients with type II diabetes, with adjustments to the usual intake negotiated to match intake with available insulin (endogenous or exogenous) as needed. Any desirable changes to improve overall nutritional intake or to address specific risk factors are negotiated on an incremental basis as education progresses.

Alternatively, a carbohydrate plan can be derived from an estimated or calculated calorie prescription by multiplying the desired caloric intake by the desired proportion of carbohydrate and dividing the resulting value by 4. For example, a client is estimated to require 2,000 calories for weight maintenance and the goal is for the client to consume 50 percent of calories as carbohydrate. Multiply 2,000 calories by 0.5 and divide the resulting value (1,000) by 4 calories/gram of carbohydrate. The total daily carbohydrate allowance would be 250 grams. This total allowance is then distributed among the day's meals and snacks with attention to the client's preferences for meal size and composition, and subsequently fine-tuned on the basis of blood glucose results.

The next step is to calculate premeal doses of regular insulin using the insulin-to-carbohydrate ratio. For persons with diabetes, there is an identifiable ratio between grams of carbohydrate eaten and the number of units of insulin required. This ratio can be used to calculate the appropriate premeal dose of insulin (bolus) for any meal or snack of known carbohydrate content. The ratio varies significantly from client to client: from as little as 5 grams of carbohydrate per unit of insulin up to 20 grams. The 150-pound jogger with type 1 diabetes may require only one unit of insulin for each 20 grams of carbohydrate, while the 200-pound woman with type 2 diabetes may require one unit of insulin for each 10 grams of carbohydrate. In the Diabetes Control and Complications Trial in Iowa, persons with type 1 diabetes usually required one unit of premeal bolus of regular insulin for each 10 to 15 grams of carbohydrate. In general, the lower the total daily insulin dose, the greater the number of grams of carbohydrate covered by a single unit of insulin. The precise ratio for each person should be individually determined.

The total available glucose (TAG) system[131] is based on research described by Munro and Allison in their classic text, *Mammalian Protein Metabolism,* Volume I, in which these authors discuss the gluconeogenic properties of certain proteins.[132] The amino acids that are definitely gluconeogenic are rapidly degraded to intermediates of glycolysis of the tricarboxylic acid cycle. Amino acids that give irregular results when administered in a large single dose are relatively slowly degraded, either because of the low activity of the enzymes of intermediary metabolism or because of the slow absorption. The high yield of glucose on feeding proteins indicates that the conversion of protein to carbohydrate in dogs can be maximal. Munro and Allison identify amino acids as rapidly gluconeogenic, variably gluconeogenic, and nongluconeogenic.

Lusk reported in 1928 that meat protein yields 58 grams of glucose per 100 grams of protein metabolized.[133] He also studied the gluconeogenic effects of casein, whose amino acid composition is similar to that of mixed meat protein.

The calculated maximum yield of casein is 57 grams of glucose per 100 grams of protein. This idea has resulted in the use of a fixed number (TAG) for each meal as a way of controlling blood sugars. The number is derived from calculations with exact figures of carbohydrate and animal protein, found in *Bowes and Church's Food Values of Portions Commonly Used.*[134] For example, cooked beef cubed steak weighs 3½ ounces (100 grams), contains 0.0 grams of carbohydrate, 28.6 grams of animal protein, and 14.4 grams of fat.

To calculate TAG, the following formula is used:
0.0 grams of carbohydrate plus (28.6 grams of animal protein × 0.58) equals TAG.

The conversion factor for animal protein is the value discovered in Lusk's animal studies. TAG is a value that approximates the amount of ingested glucose that will be available for cell use. Lusk also found that about 10 percent of fat is converted to carbohydrate. Some nutritionists add in this value for a total TAG calculation.[135] In an attempt to simplify calculations, this value, usually low if diets include 30 to 35 percent of calories from fat, is not used here. By giving each meal a total figure for TAG, individuals can vary intake of fat without going over the recommended grams of TAG. **TAG for each exchange is as follows:**

- 1 fruit exchange = 15 grams of TAG
- 1 meat exchange = 4 grams of TAG
- 1 vegetable exchange = 5 grams of TAG
- 1 bread exchange = 15 grams of TAG
- 1 milk exchange = 17 grams of TAG

Table 6–3 shows calories, carbohydrate, protein, and fat values for each exchange. Appendix 6–A and Appendix 6–B show exchange groups with amounts of food equivalent to one exchange. Exhibit 6–2 provides a sample bolus calculation by different methods.

There are several guidelines to follow to cover intake (TAG) with insulin. One unit of regular insulin covers approximately 10 to 15 grams of TAG, depending upon the individual. For one person, one unit of insulin may cover 11 grams of TAG, with normal blood glucose values resulting; for a second person, one unit of regular insulin may cover 9 grams of TAG. For each person, the ratio of TAG to insulin depends on the time of day and physical activity. The ratio may be different at breakfast than at lunch or supper. As a general rule of thumb, a person with diabetes should wait 30 minutes before eating a meal after bolusing or injecting regular insulin (Table 6–4). Exhibit 6–3 contains tips for adjusting insulin.

There are several cautions in using TAG and carbohydrate counting. These values do not take into consideration the fat or vegetable protein calories for TAG or fat and total protein for carbohydrate counting. Clients may consume a diet very

Table 6–3 Summary of the 1995 Exchange Lists

List	Carbohydrate (g)	Protein (g)	Fat (g)	Calories
Carbohydrates				
Starch	15	3	1 or less	80
Fruit	15	—	—	60
Milk				
Skim	12	8	0–3	90
Low-fat	12	8	5	120
Whole	12	8	8	150
Other carbohydrates	15	Varies	Varies	Varies
Vegetables	5	2	—	25
Meat/meat substitutes				
Very lean	—	7	1	35
Lean	—	7	3	55
Medium fat	—	7	5	75
High fat	—	7	8	100
Fat	—	—	5	45

Source: Data from *Exchange Lists for Meal Planning*, copyright © 1995, The American Dietetic Association and the American Diabetes Association.

high in calories but have normal blood glucose levels. Even though the TAG system and carbohydrate counting allow for flexibility, a low-fat diet that emphasizes nutrient adequacy is very important. One last qualifying statement is important. Munro and Allison stated that, while it is possible to determine whether an amino acid can cause a net increase of carbohydrate, it cannot be predicted whether this gluconeogenic effect is significant.[136] TAG in combination with a standard exchange system can result in good blood glucose control in compliant persons.

Exhibit 6–2 Sample Bolus Calculation by Different Methods

Patient:	37-year-old woman, 112 lb		
Estimated Ratio:	15 g carbohydrate (CHO) per unit insulin **or**		
	1 interchange per unit of insulin		

	Method of Carbohydrate Counting		
Sample Meal	*Gram Counting*	*Exchanges*	*TAG*
1 ham sandwich	36 g CHO	2 starch = 30 g	36 g CHO + 12.6 g CHO (21 g protein x 0.6)
4 oz serving bean soup	11 g CHO	½ starch = 8 g	11 g CHO + 1.8 g CHO (3 g protein x 0.6)
Green salad	5 g CHO	Free	5 g CHO
8 oz low-fat milk	12 g CHO	1 milk = 12 g	12 g CHO + 4.8 g CHO (8 g protein x 0.6)
3 fresh apricots	12 g CHO	1 fruit = 15 g	12 g CHO
Total carbohydrate	**76 g**	**65 g**	**95.2 g**
Calculated premeal dose of short-acting insulin or bolus	5.1 U[a]	4.3 U[a]	6.3 U[a,b]

[a]Doses containing fractional units can be given by pump; for injections with syringe or pen, round dose to nearest whole unit.

[b]In patients using systems such as total available glucose (TAG) that account for dietary protein in the bolus insulin dose calculation, total daily insulin doses will not be different, as compared with the same patient using simply carbohydrate counting. However, different basal insulin rates or insulin-to-carbohydrate ratios may be derived under the TAG approach because of the different way in which premeal doses are being determined.

Source: Reprinted from B. Brackenridge, "Carbohydrate Counting for Diabetes Therapy," in *Handbook of Diabetes Medical Nutrition Therapy*, M.A. Powers (Gaithersburg, MD: Aspen Publishers, 1996), 259.

Table 6–4 Timing Boluses To Cover Snacks or Meals That Are Very High in Fiber, Fat, or Simple Sugars as Compared with Usual Snacks or Meals

Time of Bolus	Usual Meal	High in Fiber	High in Fat	High in Simple Sugars
15 Minutes		X	X	
30 Minutes	X			
45 Minutes				X

Facilitating control in the client with type 1 diabetes mellitus requires understanding the time-action curves of all insulin preparations. The DCCT used 38 different insulin regimens, including the usual combinations such as ultralente with NPH or NPH three times a day, to achieve specified blood glucose targets.[137] Figure 6–2 visually depicts the time-action curves of various combination insulin regimens. Information on these time-action curves is essential to ensure appropriate meal planning. The goal is to match foods and their specific amounts to be eaten at the best times in order to prevent glycemic excursions. The dietitian must be involved as a strategic member of the team to maximize blood glucose control. Problem solving for common blood glucose patterns is summarized in Table 6–5, providing a generic basis for alterations in meal composition, amounts, and timing.

The constant *subcutaneous infusion insulin pump's* effect is schematically shown in Figure 6–3. The amount of insulin given to cover each meal varies for each individual. It takes time and constant supervision by a physician to find the right match of insulin for TAG to achieve normal blood glucose levels. For example, at breakfast three units of regular insulin may be given to cover 45 grams of TAG, equivalent to one unit of insulin for every 15 grams of TAG (45 grams TAG ÷ 3 units of regular insulin = 15 grams of TAG per unit of regular insulin). If this client were to plan an increase in food intake at this meal to 60 grams of TAG or an increase of 15 grams over the recommended TAG, one extra unit of insulin will be needed. At lunch this client boluses two units of regular insulin for every 66 grams of TAG, which equals one unit of insulin for every 33 grams of TAG (66 grams of TAG ÷ 2 units of regular insulin = 33 grams of TAG per unit of regular insulin). If the client planned to eat only 33 grams of TAG at lunch, a bolus of one unit of insulin would cover the decreased intake. At dinner nine units of regular insulin are given to cover 81 grams of TAG, or one unit of insulin for every 9 grams of TAG (81 grams of TAG ÷ 9 units of regular insulin = 9 grams of TAG per unit of regular insulin). If 47 grams of TAG were planned for dinner, this client could bolus with 5.2 units of regular insulin (47 grams of TAG ÷ 9 grams of TAG per unit of regular insulin = 5.2 units of insulin).

Exhibit 6–3 Adjusting Insulin

Nutrition counselors should keep the following in mind as they help patients with diabetes to problem solve to reach target blood glucose values.

1. Make sure target blood glucose ranges have been set or negotiated with the patient. Otherwise, the patient has no idea what is to be accomplished. An old saying applies: "If you don't know where you're going, any road will get you there!"

2. Fix the fasting first. Because blood glucose levels will stay in about the same range or elevate throughout the day for those with NIDDM, getting the fasting blood glucose level normalized sets the tone for the rest of the day, provided the patient continues to eat appropriately.

3. Look to the previous medication dose when solving a problem time of day. For example, if there is a high midafternoon blood glucose pattern and the morning shot of NPH/regular insulin was the last administration, perhaps more NPH is required.

4. Do not be reactionary. Observe patterns of blood glucose levels versus responding to one or two isolated values. Practitioners may want to discard the lowest and highest values as outliers when perusing blood glucose logs. Allow a new regimen (an increase or decrease in food, medications,

or activity) to be tried for at least three days before considering another change.

5. Do not automatically blame the diet. Just because you are a dietitian does not mean that diet is the only aspect of diabetes care you must consider. Timing of meals and medications, poor fluid intake, site selection and rotation for insulin administration, activity changes, acute stress, illness, or other medications can account for out-of-range blood glucose values.

6. Change only one or two things at a time when modifying the diet so that the effectiveness of each change can be documented separately. If too many components are altered at once, the cause cannot be determined because it is confounded by other variables.

7. Correct the basal rates first. For those on intensive therapy (MDI or CSII), boluses of regular insulin can only be accurately determined if basal insulin (Lente, NPH, Ultralente, or basal rate on an insulin pump) is correct. Similarly, insulin-to-carbohydrate ratios cannot be refined unless basal rates have been correctly adjusted. Basal rates are correct when the individual with diabetes can skip a meal and the blood glucose remains stable (hypoglycemia or hyperglycemia does not occur).

Source: Reprinted from S.L. Thom, "Diabetes Medications and Delivery Methods," in *Handbook of Diabetes Medical Nutrition Therapy*, ed. M.A. Powers, p. 102, © 1996, Aspen Publishers, Inc.

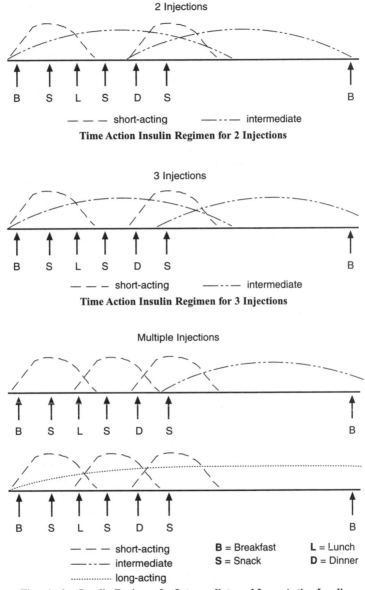

Figure 6–2   Time-Action Curves of Various Combination Insulin Regimens. *Source:* Reprinted with permission from *Physician's Guide to Insulin-Dependent (Type I) Diabetes,* 1988. Copyright © 1994 by American Diabetes Association.

Table 6–5 Common Problem Patterns Found from Blood Glucose Monitoring

Problem	Potential Cause*	Potential Solutions
High fasting glucose	Insulin resistance,† insufficient insulin available overnight, rebound hyperglycemia overnight (Somogyi effect), Dawn Phenomenon	Adjust P.M. intermediate- or long-acting insulin dose or time Weight reduction to reduce insulin resistance
High glucose after breakfast	Inadequate insulin produced or injected to cover breakfast, peak insulin action not at anticipated time	Adjust time or dose of short-acting A.M. insulin Decrease size of breakfast or adjust amount of breakfast carbohydrate or divide breakfast into two smaller morning meals
Insulin reactions (hypoglycemia) before lunch	Insufficient breakfast for A.M. short-acting insulin or peak action later than anticipated time	Adjust time, type, or dose of A.M. short-acting insulin Add morning snack or increase breakfast
Insulin reactions (hypoglycemia) in afternoon	Excessive A.M. intermediate-acting insulin, skipping or inadequate lunch	Adjust time, type, or dose of A.M. intermediate-acting insulin Add afternoon snack or increase lunch
High glucose in afternoon	Inadequate insulin produced or intermediate-acting A.M. insulin is insufficient for need, or excessive snack or lunch	Adjust time or dose of P.M. insulin Add afternoon snack or increase lunch
High glucose at night after evening meal	Inadequate insulin produced or insufficient insulin to cover dinner, or evening meal too large	Adjust time, or dose of P.M. insulin Reduce size of meal or alter meal composition (↓ carbohydrate)
Insulin reactions (hypoglycemia) at night	Excessive amount of insulin or insufficient dinner meal or evening snack	Adjust time, type, or dose of evening or bedtime insulin Increase dinner and/or snack carbohydrate

*In addition to food and insulin, other factors may affect blood glucose (e.g., exercise, sick days, infection).

†Insulin resistance associated with obesity is likely to result in high glucose levels throughout the day.

Source: Adapted from Powers MA, Barr P, Franz M, Holler H, Wheeler ML, Wylie-Rosett J. *Nutrition Guide for Professionals: Diabetes Education and Meal Planning,* p. 6, copyright © 1989, American Dietetic Association/American Diabetes Association.

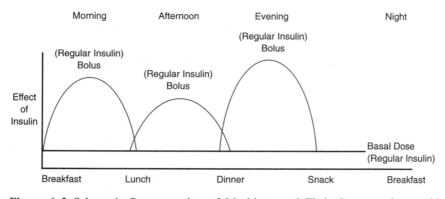

Figure 6–3 Schematic Representation of Mealtimes and Their Correspondence with Insulin Delivered by the Constant-Infusion Insulin Pump.

RESEARCH ON ADHERENCE TO EATING PATTERNS CONTROLLED FOR CARBOHYDRATE, PROTEIN, AND FAT

Adherence to a prescribed dietary plan is one of the most important aspects of diabetes management and perhaps the most difficult for clients to learn or with which to comply. Researchers have found that many clients do not understand or follow their diabetic diet regimens.[138] As a solution to this problem, clinicians are beginning to advocate highly individualized, flexible approaches to diet management that can accommodate individual eating habits and preferences.[139]

A number of studies have examined correlates of diabetic diet noncompliance, including knowledge, health values, and social and cultural factors.[140–142] None of these studies provides a clear, unified direction for diabetic nutrition education, but when reviewed in combination, they emphasize the need for comprehensive interventions that include social support, promotion of self-care and active participation, and emphasis on how (as well as why) to follow the dietary eating pattern.[143] Because of the complexity of the optimal educational approach, few studies have rigorously evaluated the effectiveness of strategies to improve dietary adherence among clients with diabetes.

Wiensier et al. achieved excellent compliance with an individualized diet prescription, frequent follow-up and feedback, and social support in a controlled trial of an experimental diabetic diet.[144] However, there have been few controlled educational experiments. One found that a group program was more effective than individual bedside teaching.[145] Another demonstrated that a programmed learning unit that reduced the amount of professional time needed resulted in knowledge increases comparable to those achieved after a longer individual counseling session.[146] Dunn et al. found that a comprehensive program resulted in knowledge gains.[147] The Webb et al. study of a multimethod group program demonstrated the program's effects in improving adherence to the carbohydrate and fat composition of the diet, as well as glycemic control.[148] Because of the generally accepted comprehensive approach to diabetes education, along with the complex self-care regimens prescribed for clients with diabetes, it is unlikely that research can tell nutritionists exactly which educational strategies contribute the most to diet adherence. Self-monitoring of blood glucose is a technology that has been found acceptable to clients and effective for improving glycemic control.[149–152] Unfortunately, the investigators of this strategy did not collect dietary data to discern the behavioral effects of self-monitoring; nor did they employ a control group receiving similar management without glucose self-monitoring.

Several implications for practice emerge from the studies reviewed here and the published commentaries of clinicians. Most important, dietary adherence is best when the diet is tailored to the individual client. The education plan should also be tailored, as seen in Slowie's case studies.[153] Comprehensive educational diagnosis tools have been developed, and validated knowledge tests toward this end are available.[154] Computerized dietary analysis with simple recommendations as part of a printout can provide both assessment and feedback.[155]

Social support from family members as well as other clients with diabetes is important in facilitating lifestyle changes.[156] Schwartz et al. found a higher percentage of abnormal blood glucose control measures (fasting blood glucose values and HbA1c) in individuals with many recent life events. These researchers felt that social support may decrease the individual's isolation and help deal with life events, with resulting improved control.[157] Frequent follow-up, feedback (including glucose self-monitoring), and behavioral methods such as contingency contracting and self-reinforcement can improve outcomes.[158–160] A large number of print and audiovisual instructional aids are available through health agencies, the American Diabetes Association, and commercial sources. Educational materials must be appropriate for the comprehension level of program participants; a mismatch can impede understanding of the regimen.[161]

Researchers who studied compliance with accuracy in describing food portions found that men with diabetes underestimated chicken portions (i.e., ate portions that were larger than estimated) by an average of 30 to 40 percent and underestimated rice portions (i.e., ate portions that were smaller than estimated) by an average of 25 to 35 percent.[162] In another study, clients with diabetes (24 with IDDM and 184 with NIDDM) were asked what factors contributed to nonadherence to their diabetic regimens. Standardized questions revealed few differences between type I and type II participants on the level of reported adherence or reasons for nonadherence. Subjects reported adhering least well to dietary and physical activity components of the regimen. Open-ended questions revealed that the most common reasons for dietary nonadherence were the situational factors of eating out at restaurants and inappropriate food offers from others. These researchers suggested that diabetes education programs should inform clients of high-risk situations and provide training in covert modeling and behavioral rehearsal to enhance assertive skills.[163,164]

INAPPROPRIATE EATING BEHAVIORS

Most persons with IDDM complain about the lack of spontaneity in their new eating patterns. The joy of eating seems to rely partially on the element of surprise, but one very important way to normalize blood sugars is to keep the eating pattern consistent from day to day. This is one of the most difficult dilemmas facing the client with IDDM. Without consistency in the eating pattern, changes in insulin levels are difficult to adjust and dangerous.

A second common problem involves social eating. The major problem is knowing how to count foods with unknown ingredients. Secondary, but also important, is the ability to avoid large quantities of foods that elevate blood glucose levels. As do many clients on new eating patterns, the insulin-dependent person initially finds the diet new and exciting. Adherence to diet and control of blood glucose levels are excellent. With time, the newness of the diet diminishes and the desire to be "like everyone else" can overcome the desire to achieve good control or normalized blood glucose levels.

ASSESSMENT OF EATING BEHAVIORS

A thorough initial assessment is crucial to future dietary success. Assessing the client's prior experience with dieting and on diabetic eating patterns is very important. Many persons with type I diabetes have followed weight-loss diets in the past, even though one of the initial symptoms of diabetes is weight loss. Some younger diabetic persons may have never followed a diet. If this is the case, setting the stage for successful adherence to diet is crucial.

Carefully assessing daily eating patterns is important. Time may not allow for food record collection, but a thorough diet history or quantified food frequency may provide some useful information on past eating habits. Counselors should attend to variations in eating patterns. For example, a clue to potential problems with weekend blood sugars is dietary patterns that are very different from weekday patterns.

The diet history can also give the counselor a good impression of nutrient intake. Many persons, particularly teenagers, may be eating diets low in calcium, iron, or vitamin A and C. Fat intake may be high, with a large portion coming from saturated fat. Cholesterol intake may also be high. In addition to a quantified food frequency or diet history, the Client Eating Questionnaire for Low-Calorie Eating Patterns in Treating Obesity, Adherence Tool 4–1 in Chapter 4, may be useful in identifying past and present weight loss and resulting dietary behaviors. Once the client begins the new eating pattern, food records can be very helpful. The food record in Adherence Tool 6–1 might be used in assessing adherence to the new eating pattern.

Throughout the initial assessment phase, family support is crucial to eventual success. For adolescents, positive support without overbearing dictation of rules is important. For older clients, positive support from spouse or significant others should be assessed.

Prior knowledge about foods is also important. Some persons who are newly diagnosed may have a variety of misconceptions about a diabetic eating pattern. "I can no longer eat carbohydrates," is one common fallacy. Counselors should determine whether the client has followed a previous diet with an exchange pattern that might conflict with the new diabetic exchange pattern. Some concepts learned in Weight Watchers may no longer apply. Some clients may begin using only commercial foods labeled "dietetic." Counselors should assess each client's understanding of what is eliminated in "dietetic" products. Frequently fat, not carbohydrate, is reduced, leaving a product that may be high in simple sugars. Once a client is instructed on the new eating pattern, frequent and consistent assessment of adherence to the pattern is important. This may involve diet records, 24-hour recalls on the phone (if possible, for three days to one week), or short diet records requiring simple check-off systems, such as Adherence Tool 6–2. This tool can be used to help clients monitor and avoid snacking if it is not a part of the recommended regimen. Tracking eating behaviors with a graph may be helpful. If the recommendation for TAG is 40 at breakfast, 40 at lunch, and 60 at dinner, graphing intake over one month's time may be helpful. Adherence Tool 6–3 shows an example of a graph in which TAG for breakfast is represented by a line. One heavy horizontal line represents the desired TAG for this meal.

Dietary nonadherence will be reflected in biochemical data such as blood glucose and glycosylated hemoglobin levels. Graphing these two parameters can illustrate trends. For example, drawing a graph of weekly blood sugar and glycosylated hemoglobin levels once every three months will show difficult weeks and "in-control" weeks (see Adherence Tool 6–4). Adherence Tool 6–5 allows the client to make a check mark when boluses are administered 30 minutes prior to a meal. Assessing what might have happened to cause changes in blood sugars may be the first step to changes in adherence.

TREATMENT STRATEGIES

Problems with following diabetic eating patterns fall into three categories: lack of knowledge, forgetfulness, and lack of commitment. This section provides suggestions for strategies to deal with lack of knowledge and cueing devices to help solve problems of forgetting. Lack of commitment, the most difficult problem to solve, is obvious from repeated highs and lows in blood sugars, elevated glycosylated hemoglobins, or both, in spite of information given to help correct the situation.

Strategies To Deal with Lack of Knowledge

Lack of Knowledge Related to General Dietary Modifications That Affect Blood Glucose

To begin a nutrition counseling session appropriately, counselors must provide the client with adequate information. The counselor should design an instructional plan to provide information on a diabetic eating pattern, including one week of intensive dietary counseling, possibly a three-day hospital stay, while the client is beginning the new diet pattern. Additional information is given in subsequent visits one month apart. Information should be given in small amounts, with practice time included in each session to allow the client to complete exercises with the nutrition counselor. This valuable practice is a way of setting the stage for behaviors that will be required in daily life.

Tailoring is once again very important to diet adherence (see Adherence Tool 6–6). Ideally each client should receive a diet pattern that fits the individual's lifestyle. A computer can be used to create an individual exchange list and dietary pattern. For the person with diabetes, this type of tailoring makes for less work in learning many food items, provides greater detail, and can stimulate learning because it creates a feeling of ownership.

In teaching the concept of TAG, counselors should use concrete and tailored examples (see Exhibit 6–4). Adherence Tools 6–7 and 6–8 provide practice and tips on using TAG. Adherence Tools 6–9 to 6–11 help the client practice calculating TAG and exchanges in recipes. In applying TAG, clients need a basic understanding of weighing and measuring (see Adherence Tool 6–12). For clients who want to take home information about TAG, Adherence Tools 6–13 and 6–14 are helpful. Written as well as verbal advice is important.

Meal planning is also extremely important. Adherence Tool 6–15 provides practice in planning a menu using a new eating pattern.

Counselors should emphasize the importance of knowing the contents of commercial products. Adherence Tool 6–16 provides practice in reading labels.

Exhibit 6–4 Teaching TAG

---

1. Give an example:

Exchange	TAG	
2 Fruit	= 30	
1 Bread	= 15	
1 Meat	= 4	
1 Fat	= 0	
	49	= TAG at breakfast

2. Describe clearly what the client can eat:

Breakfast	Breakfast TAG	
	Carbohydrate (grams) +	Animal Protein (grams) × 0.58
1 large apple	30.0	—
(197 grams)	—	
1 slice of bread	11.7	—
1 teaspoon margarine	—	—
1 ounce Canadian bacon	—	+ (5.6 grams × 0.58 = 3.3)
	41.7	+ 3.3 = 45.0 grams of TAG

The same example can be used with exchanges only:

Breakfast	Breakfast Exchanges
1 large apple	2 Fruit
1 slice of bread	1 Bread
1 teaspoon margarine	1 Fat
1 ounce Canadian bacon	1 Meat

If clients frequently eat in restaurants, counselors should select the menus from a few favorite places, calculate TAG for a meal, have the client bolus, and actually visit the restaurant with the client. If problems arise, the counselor can guide the client through the meal.

After presenting crucial information in a way that tailors the eating pattern to each person, counselors must stage changes in eating habits to coincide with recommendations. Clients can find it difficult to follow all dietary restrictions immediately. Focus on the least difficult problem first, while asking clients to continue to follow all restrictions to the greatest degree possible. In addition, work closely with clients and let them decide which problem is the least difficult. An example of this type of staging with information follows:

Client: "I think learning the specific amounts of foods in each of these exchange categories will be difficult."

Nutrition counselor: "Let's begin slowly, taking each category one week at a time. Continue to look up amounts for the categories you must follow, but learn amounts of your favorite foods in one category by reviewing them daily over a one-week period."

Client: "That sounds more manageable!"

Lack of Knowledge Related to Fat Intake and Weight Gain

Lack of knowledge about foods can make a crucial difference in weight gain for insulin-dependent persons. Many clients are upset by the initial and frequently steady weight gain that results when blood glucose levels normalize; weight gain occurs because calories, no longer being lost in the urine, are used for energy and, eventually, weight gain. Many clients misuse the idea that fat contributes little to elevations in blood glucose. They think that if fat is "free," it may be used to add to meals when a TAG limit or exchange pattern is "used up" in a day.

Table 6–6 illustrates the case of one client whose blood glucose levels were normal on the average but whose fat intake was causing significant climbs in weight based on monthly determinations. The diet was checked very carefully to determine where caloric intake might be contributing to weight gain. This client was doing everything requested in terms of following exchanges and TAG for breakfast. Blood glucose levels were normal, but unfortunately weight and blood cholesterol levels were up because the breakfast eaten contained 127 more calories than the recommended meal. Blood low-density lipoprotein cholesterol levels were up, mainly because of the extremely high intake of saturated fat (the recommended amount of saturated fat is 3.86 grams; actual consumption was up to 14.40 grams).

Following in-depth dietary instruction on the fat and saturated fat content of certain foods, this client can alter intake to reduce weight and blood cholesterol levels. Table 6–7 indicates recommended intake and actual intake after instruction. The figures show that TAG is actually a bit low in the low-fat meal. A suggestion might be to add 4.6 grams of carbohydrate, or approximately 5 grams ($\frac{1}{3}$ fruit exchange). Table 6–8 compares nutrient intake for the recommended high- and low-fat diets. It clearly illustrates how careful instruction on fat content of foods can minimize eventual problems with weight gain and increases in low-density lipoprotein cholesterol.

Table 6–6 Recommended and Actual Fat Consumption before Instruction

RECOMMENDED BREAKFAST PATTERN

Breakfast	Carbohydrate (g)	Protein (g)	Fat (g)	TAG
1 Meat	—	7	5	4
2 Bread	30	4	—	30
3 Fat	—	—	15	—
2 Fruit	30	—	—	30
	60	11	20	64

464 kilocalories
3.86 grams saturated fat
5.19 grams polyunsaturated fat

ACTUAL HIGH-FAT BREAKFAST

Breakfast	Carbohydrate (g)	Protein (g)	Fat (g)	TAG
1 ounce sausage (28 grams)	0.5	4.0	8.1	2.8
2 muffins (40 grams)	32.0	6.2	8.0	32.0
4 teaspoons margarine	—	—	16.4	—
1 large apple (197 grams)	30.0	0.4	0.7	30.0
	62.5	10.6	33.2	64.8

591 kilocalories
14.40 grams saturated fat
2.68 grams polyunsaturated fat

Source: Reprinted with permission from J.A.T. Pennington and H.N. Church, *Bowes and Church's Food Values of Portions Commonly Used*, copyright © 1995, Lippincott-Raven Publishers.

Table 6–7 Recommended and Actual Fat Consumption after Instruction

RECOMMENDED BREAKFAST PATTERN

Breakfast	Carbohydrate (g)	Protein (g)	Fat (g)	TAG
1 Meat	—	7	5	4
2 Bread	30	4	—	30
3 Fat	—	—	15	—
2 Fruit	30	—	—	30
	60	11	20	64

464 kilocalories; 3.86 grams saturated fat; 5.19 grams polyunsaturated fat

ACTUAL LOW-FAT BREAKFAST

Breakfast	Carbohydrate (g)	Protein (g)	Fat (g)	TAG
1 ounce Canadian bacon (28 grams)	—	5.6	2.00	3.2
1 English muffin (57 grams)	26.2	4.5	1.10	26.2
4 teaspoons margarine	—	—	11.34	—
1 large apple (197 grams)	30.0	0.4	0.70	30.0
	56.2	10.5	15.14	59.4

403 kilocalories; 2.67 grams saturated fat; 5.14 grams polyunsaturated fat

Source: Reprinted with permission from J.A.T. Pennington and H.N. Church, *Bowes and Church's Food Values of Portions Commonly Used*, copyright © 1995, Lippincott-Raven Publishers.

Table 6–8 Comparison of Recommended versus High- and Low-Fat Diets

Nutrients (g)	Recommended Diet	High-Fat Diet	Low-Fat Diet
Carbohydrate	60.00	62.5	56.2
Protein	11.00	10.60	10.50
Fat	20.00	33.20	15.14
Saturated Fat	3.86	14.40	2.67
Polyunsaturated Fat	5.19	2.68	5.14
Kilocalories	464.00	591.00	403.00

Figure 6–6 shows two weight graphs for a client. One indicates an increase in weight following high fat intake. The second shows how weight comes down with a change in the fat content of the diet. Clear instructions on monitoring blood glucose levels is essential. A client who is not monitoring appropriately or is guessing at blood glucose levels can be counseled to increase or decrease insulin and dietary intake inappropriately.

For persons on the constant subcutaneous infusion insulin (CSII) pump, eating three meals a day is very important. Snacking can lead to problems, as Exhibit 6–5 shows. This example illustrates several rules. First, clients on the CSII pump must limit meals to three a day or at least keep three hours between meals. Second, timing boluses is extremely important. In most cases, clients should give an injection or punch in a bolus on the pump 30 minutes before eating. The blood glucose of 60 at 5:00 PM indicates a timing problem: insufficient time (five minutes) between bolus and snack. The candy bar caused a rise in blood glucose before the regular insulin could have an effect. By the time the insulin peaked, the effect of the candy bar was gone, resulting in low blood glucose. Third, it is important to cover snacks with adequate amounts of regular insulin. Exhibit 6–5 shows insufficient amounts of insulin given to cover both snacks. In this case, assume that one unit of insulin covers 10 grams of TAG. (Remember, in reality the ratio of insulin to TAG varies for different times of day and different persons.) The bedtime snack was very high in fat and fiber. Timing was changed to allow for high fat and fiber intake, but the bolus for the bedtime snack did not sufficiently cover TAG (assuming one unit of insulin for every 10 grams of TAG, one unit of insulin will not cover 64 grams of TAG). Some clients may not need to

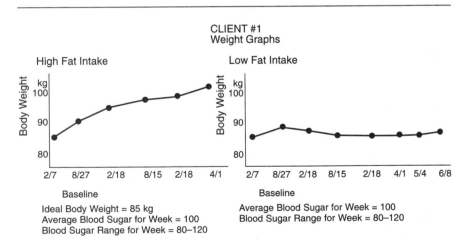

CLIENT #1
Weight Graphs

High Fat Intake   Low Fat Intake

Baseline   Baseline

Ideal Body Weight = 85 kg   Average Blood Sugar for Week = 100
Average Blood Sugar for Week = 100   Blood Sugar Range for Week = 80–120
Blood Sugar Range for Week = 80–120

Figure 6–6 Weight Graphs

Exhibit 6–5 Meal, Blood Glucose, and Insulin Diary, #1

Blood Glucose Levels	*Actual Intake*			
	Breakfast (10:30 AM) Nothing Eaten			
Pre-Lunch (10:30 AM) Blood Glucose = 100 mg/dL Recommended Insulin Given				
	Lunch (11:00 AM) Recommended Pattern Followed			
Pre-Afternoon Snack (2:55 PM) No Blood Glucose Taken Insulin Given = 2 Units Regular Insulin				
	Afternoon Snack (3:00 PM) 2-ounce Snicker's Candy Bar			
	Carbohydrate	Protein	Fat	Kilocalories
	33.0	6.0	13.0	270
Pre-Dinner (5:00 PM) Blood Glucose = 60 mg/dL Took glucose tablet				
	Dinner (5:30 PM) Recommended Dietary Pattern Followed			
Pre-Bedtime Snack (9:45 PM) No Blood Glucose Taken Insulin Given = 1 Unit Regular Insulin				
	Bedtime Snack (10:00 PM) Popped Corn (6 cups) + 5 tablespoons margarine			
	Carbohydrate	Protein	Fat	Kilocalories
	64.2	10.8	34.2	607.8

cover bedtime snacks with regular insulin, but the client in Exhibit 6–5 has very high nighttime blood sugars if regular insulin is not used to cover the snack.

Table 6–4 provides a rough guide for timing boluses on the CSII pump. These times are helpful when covering a snack (if necessary) that is very different in fat and/or fiber content from the usual snack. Changing the timing of a bolus may help to allow for increased digestion time such as 15 minutes instead of 30 minutes for popped corn with a large amount of fat. In addition, allowing three hours between meals can prevent one bolus of regular insulin from affecting the bolus

Exhibit 6–6 Meal, Blood Glucose, and Insulin Diary, #2

Blood Glucose Levels	*Actual Intake*

Breakfast (9:30 AM)
  Blood Glucose = 100
  Recommended Insulin Given	

	Breakfast (10:00 AM) Recommended Pattern Followed

Prelunch (11:00 AM)
  Blood Glucose = 285
  Extra Dose of Regular Insulin Given	

	Lunch (11:30 AM) Recommended Pattern Followed

Postlunch (12:30 PM)
  Blood Glucose = 45 (REACTION)
  Treated with Glucose Tablets	

that follows. Exhibit 6–6 illustrates this idea. In this example the regular insulin bolus for breakfast peaks too close to the peak of the lunch bolus, resulting in a reaction at 12:30 PM. The prelunch blood glucose is actually postprandial breakfast glucose. Because the prelunch blood glucose is high, extra insulin is given to adjust for it, which brings blood glucose levels down. With extra insulin for lunch and less than three hours between breakfast and lunch, the regular insulin peaks are too close, resulting in hypoglycemia.

In summary, many of the difficulties encountered by clients with type I diabetes can be eliminated through monitoring (via diary) and thus identifying problems contributing to poor adherence. Basic early instruction on diet is crucial. Tailoring the regimen helps eliminate certain problems with later backsliding. For example, although fat intake may be of minor significance in altering blood glucose values, it is important to eventual weight gain. Information about fat is important. Three basic rules for clients on the CSII pump or MDI are also important:

1. Limit meals to three a day and/or allow three hours between meals.
2. Bolus or inject insulin 30 minutes prior to eating (or 5 minutes for lispro).
3. Cover diet intake with adequate amounts of insulin.

Strategies To Deal with Forgetfulness

Cueing devices can help persons with IDDM remember to bolus or inject insulin on time. Reminders on the refrigerator to give insulin 30 minutes before eating are important. If a morning or evening dose is a problem, signs on the mirror in the bathroom can cue clients.

A simple calendar requiring check marks can help the client who constantly forgets to bolus or inject insulin 30 minutes before a meal. Adherence Tool 6–5 is an example of a monthly monitoring device that, if placed in a visible area and used as a daily recording device, could serve as a cue. The same calendar might serve as a reminder of problems for clients who eat in restaurants frequently. A star might remind clients to plan for a restaurant meal by calling the restaurant to find out what is on the menu and ask questions to determine what is in a recipe. By planning ahead, clients can select food appropriately with little effort while in the restaurant. Most people can save favorite restaurant menus and calculate exchange or TAG values for favorite selections. Extra care and effort initially can make eating in restaurants more enjoyable.

Strategies To Deal with Lack of Commitment

Most insulin-dependent persons enter periods of low commitment to keeping blood glucose leveis normal. This can be evidenced in a variety of ways. One is "bouncing" blood glucose levels that have a roller coaster appearance when graphed. Another is relatively good blood glucose levels with high glycosylated hemoglobin levels. This may indicate problems with high blood sugars at night, but it can also signal fabricated glucose values. A third clue to lack of commitment is the client who comes in saying, "I just want to have one day where I don't have to worry about blood glucose levels, fingersticks, diet, and exercise."

The extract that follows illustrates the thoughts that are familiar to many persons with diabetes. This monologue was written by a person with diabetes and illustrates the dilemma that occurs in trying to lead a normal life and be in control at all times.

So you begin on the perfection side. Your whole world revolves around your diabetes. You weigh and measure and time everything. You learn to eat when you're not hungry. You learn not to eat when you are hungry. You do everything right, and you have reactions anyway. There is never a break. There is never a vacation from your diabetes.

Even one slight deviation from perfection causes you to panic. You just know something horrible is going to happen. You're going to go into a coma and die like everyone keeps telling you. But then you realize nothing really bad happened. You don't even feel bad physically. So you ease up just a little on the strictness of the requirements. You allow yourself a little more freedom. You realize you're not even having as many reactions. You're not quite as uptight about doing things perfectly.

But you do begin to feel a little guilty, especially when people tell you about diabetics who were on the imperfect side and they died. But really you're doing fine. You begin to experiment—see how far you can push your limits. You find you feel awful here, and you have more reactions. So you find a very comfortable place somewhere in the middle. You still structure things, and you don't just eat anything you want to. But your world allows other things besides diabetes now. And then it happens: PROBLEMS accompanied by GUILT compounded by FEAR or more PROBLEMS. You're told that there never was a middle ground. Either you are all the way over on the perfection side, or you are totally on the imperfection side. And your problems are evidence that you are as far over on the imperfection side as you can possibly be. So everyone tells you that you could avoid more problems IF you will just switch back to the perfection side. So you switch back. But you are human. There are other things to think about besides diabetes. You make choices. Now what? You know you're really on the imperfection side. But you must try to convince everyone that you're on the perfection side, because you find out that family and friends will nag you if they find out that you are imperfect And your doctors don't really want to know you're not perfect. They only want to hear how perfectly their regimen is working. So you live a normal life. You learn to take tests only when you know they're going to be perfect; or if you take a test that isn't perfect you simply don't record it. MORE GUILT!

You eat only what's on your diet when you're with others. But when you're by yourself you find the only thing you can think about eating is anything that's forbidden. You "pig out."

You make sure your random blood sugars are in the perfect range when you visit the doctor. You learn to be so good at deception that you begin to wonder just where you really are in your control. You realize you've even been deceiving yourself. How good has your control really been? You feel fine. Your A1c's are good. You've had very few reactions, and the tests that you take for your own knowledge are mostly good. And then it happens: MORE PROBLEMS.

Now everyone knows that you really weren't perfect. So they remind you that it's your own fault. If you had just been perfect the problems would never have happened. So now what? You just learn to live with not only the physical pain, but the GUILT that comes with it for the rest of your life. Or until someone comes along who is not afraid that your humanness will make her a failure. She listens. She hears you. Then she speaks magic works: "IT'S NOT YOUR FAULT!" It takes a while for the word to sink in. The layers of guilt have been building for years. But then it hits you. You can let go of all the guilt. It's honestly okay to be HUMAN. But best of all you know that someone understands you and accepts you just the way you are. And because she cares, you know you don't have to face your problems alone. Then the pain isn't so hard to live with.[165]

A problem with lack of commitment is not solved with recipes, information on the nutrient content of a commercial product, or more telephone contact without appropriate intervention. The following dialogue illustrates one possible initial approach to dealing with lack of commitment. Strategies include open questions to identify the problem, paraphrasing, empathy, and contracting.

> *Client:* "I just want to have one day without diabetes, without fingersticks, and without dietary calculations. Living with diabetes is not like other tasks in life. You can't say, 'I worked hard and now I am finished. I did a good job.' Diabetes is forever!"
>
> *Nutrition counselor:* "You have thought about this for a long time. Can you describe why you feel this way now and initially you seemed to be more enthusiastic?" (Open Question)
>
> *Client:* "When you first start treating your diabetes, it's fun and exciting. You feel better for the first time in a long while. You feel in control. You are given responsibility for diet and fingersticks and exercise."
>
> *Nutrition counselor:* "You're sort of in a honeymoon phase." (Paraphrase)
>
> *Client:* "Yes, exactly. But things change. Your friends get tired of hearing about how well you are doing. They don't give you as much positive reinforcement for your labor. In fact they seem to get tired of hearing you talk about your disease and how well you are doing. Without this support, you get tired of doing everything well."
>
> *Nutrition counselor:* "So you need to have some kind of reward for your efforts, but your friends don't always come through." (Paraphrase and Empathy)
>
> *Client:* "Yes."
>
> *Nutrition counselor:* "Let's try to list a few ways that you can provide positive reinforcement for yourself. What things in your life really make you feel good?"
>
> *Client:* "Well, I like to read. I love to watch MTV. I like eating pizzas."
>
> *Nutrition counselor:* "Great, let's set up a contract. Whenever you have blood sugars on three consecutive preprandial sticks between 100 and 130 in a day, you can reward yourself with one of these fun things. We will even figure out how to count pizza. I can help by calling the restaurant. Let's write the contract." (See Exhibit 6–7.)

As with other diets, lack of commitment may be a direct result of a change in life events. Clients who go through a divorce may blame their preoccupation with diabetes care, resulting in changes in the care taken to follow a dietary regimen.

Exhibit 6–7 Contract

I will reward myself each day for preprandial blood sugars between 100 and 130 on three consecutive occasions in a day. The following things will be used as rewards:
1. Going to the library for a good novel
2. Watching MTV
3. Eating three slices of a Pizza Hut Canadian Bacon Pizza containing approximately 63 grams of TAG.

If my blood sugars are not between 100 and 130 preprandially, I will not receive any of the above three rewards.

    (*Nutrition counselor*) will call me each Friday at 10:00 AM at work to check on my progress.

Patient _____

Nutrition Counselor_____

    Significant family changes such as marriage or remarriage, birth of a child, or death of a close relative can have devastating effects on blood sugars. In one family the husband, Mr. X, was on an insulin pump. His father died of complications of the disease. Following his death, the client's wife began looking at the disease differently. She felt that she should not have married someone with a disease so devastating and was concerned about her children eventually being diagnosed with diabetes. For several months, Mr. X's blood glucose values were uncontrolled and his attitude toward his care was very casual. His wife finally sought psychiatric care, and Mr. X's dietary adherence began to improve.

    Job-related changes can also affect blood glucose values. The loss of a job and beginning of a new one can cause schedule changes that make lunch hours less predictable or stimulate snacking. One woman who began babysitting in her home snacked every time the children ate. Her blood glucose values were very high and occasionally low from insulin boluses taken too close together. Another woman moved from a secretarial position to a job in a bakery. Everyone snacked on doughnut holes at 10:00 AM, and she joined the group. Loss of a job can make matters other than diabetes care a higher priority.

    The insulin-dependent person who is diagnosed with another disease, such as heart disease, may become very discouraged. One man stated, "I am too young to have to worry about both diabetes and heart disease." Frequently another illness may require added dietary restrictions that complicate the regimen and make it more difficult to follow, adding stress to an already complicated life situation.

    One of the positive aspects of good adherence and normalized blood glucose levels is fewer symptoms. When a client can connect diet with positive, healthful feelings there is a great deal of incentive to work hard for good dietary adherence. Reminding clients how well they felt while they were strictly following the new eating pattern may be enough to change lack of commitment to enthusiasm. In some cases, planning a one-week menu may help the client cut back on dietary calculations and worry just before a meal. After planning the menu with the nutrition counselor on several occasions, clients may begin planning on their own, allowing for more spontaneity and fewer calculations for the rest of the week.

Counselors can involve family members in helping with diet by asking them to reinforce good dietary behaviors. They might even participate in signing a contract. With the client, the counselor can make a list of stressful events that take place in one week and ask the family to assist in making certain times of the day less stressful. The children might help with laundry or pack a sack lunch.

In some cases, constructive confrontation may be beneficial to increasing dietary commitment. For example:

Nutrition counselor: "I really thought we were doing well in working together on dietary problems. (Personal Relationship Statement) I see your glycosylated hemoglobin has gone up one whole point. Your diet records also show an increase in snacking." (Description of Behavior)

Client: "I know I just don't have any motivation. I really want to do well."

Nutrition counselor: "You seem to be saying two things: (1) you want to do well, and (2) you just don't care. (Description of Feelings and Interpretation of Client's Situation) Am I right?"

Client: "Yes." (Understanding Response)

Nutrition counselor: "How do you feel about what I am saying?" (Perception Check)

Client: "I'm trying to do two things, and I feel like a failure all the time. Sometimes I just say I might as well give up, and I do. I don't check my blood sugars or I check them at times when I know they are good and write those numbers down. Then I just throw my hands up in despair and say what's the use and start snacking."

Nutrition counselor: "Good, you seem to be able to talk about exactly what you are feeling and that's pretty low sometimes. (Interpretive Response and Constructive Feedback) Would you be willing to do a diary of your thoughts?"

Client: "What's that?"

Nutrition counselor: "It's not difficult. Just record what you think in a few sentences every time you eat. Use this form (Appendix G). We will talk about your thought diary when you come to the next visit."

Client: "I will try to record before and after each meal, but may miss on weekends."

Nutrition counselor: "Record as often as you can. This is to help you. I do not want it to become a burden."

At the next visit, the discussion could revolve around how to replace negative thoughts with positive thoughts, such as "I only ate one small cracker. I won't eat any more. I'm doing great today."

Strategies to deal with lack of commitment are very important to a client's long-term success with a diabetic regimen. Identifying changes in life events can signal eventual problems. Many strategies to deal with these changes are included in this chapter and focus on identifying positive support persons and appropriate use of constructive confrontation.

Review of Chapter 6
(Answers in Appendix H)

1. List three factors that are commonly associated with carbohydrate-modified diets and lead to inappropriate eating behaviors:
   a. _____
   b. _____
   c. _____

2. List two nutrients to emphasize in collecting baseline information on diets for persons with diabetes.
   a. _____
   b. _____

3. Identify four strategies to help combat inappropriate eating behaviors when working with clients on new diabetic eating patterns:
   a. _____
   b. _____
   c. _____
   d. _____

4. The following describes a problem situation with a client who has been instructed on a diabetic diet. Identify a strategy that might help solve this client's problem and explain your reason for selecting it.

   Mr. J. has been placed on a diabetic diet. During nutrition assessment you found that he has most difficulty with afternoon snacks. At his company during break, everyone eats frosted cupcakes, candy bars, or jellybeans. (a) What further questions would you ask to elicit more information? (b) What strategies would you use to help alleviate the problem? (c) Why did you choose these strategies?

   a. _____
   b. _____
   c. _____

NOTES

1. The Diabetes Control and Complications Research Group, "The Effect of Intensive Treatment of Diabetes on the Development and Progression of Long-Term Complications in Insulin-Dependent Diabetes Mellitus," *New England Journal of Medicine* 329 (1993): 977–986.

2. American Diabetes Association, "American Diabetes Association Position Statement: Nutrition Recommendations and Principles for People with Diabetes Mellitus, *Diabetes Care* 17 (1994): 519–522.

3. American Dietetic Association, "Nutrition Recommendations and Principles for People with Diabetes Mellitus," *Journal of the American Dietetic Association* 94 (1994): 504–506.

4. J.A. Balfour and D. McTavish, "Acarbose: An Update of Its Pharmacology and Therapeutic Use in Diabetes Mellitus," *Drugs* 46 (1993): 1025–1054.

5. Diabetes Control and Complications Trial, "The Effect of Intensive Treatment of Diabetes on the Development and Progression of Long-Term Complications in Insulin-Dependent Diabetes Mellitus."

6. L.M. Delahanty and B.N. Halford, "The Role of Diet Behaviors in Achieving Improved Glycemic Control in Intensively Treated Patients in the Diabetes Control and Complications Trial," *Diabetes Care* 16 (1993): 1453–1458.

7. The Diabetes Control and Complications Trial Research Group, "Nutrition Interventions for Intensive Therapy in the Diabetes Control and Complications Trial: Implications for Clinical Practice," *Journal of the American Dietetic Association* 93 (1993): 758–767.

8. American Diabetes Association, "American Diabetes Association Position Statement: Nutrition Recommendations and Principles for People with Diabetes Mellitus."

9. American Dietetic Association, "Nutrition Recommendations and Principles for People with Diabetes Mellitus."

10. American Diabetes Association, "American Diabetes Association Position Statement: Nutrition Recommendations and Principles for People with Diabetes Mellitus."

11. American Dietetic Association, "Nutrition Recommendations and Principles for People with Diabetes Mellitus."

12. P.A. Crapo et al., "Plasma Glucose and Insulin Responses to Orally Administered Simple and Complex Carbohydrates," *Diabetes* 25 (1976): 741–747.

13. J.W. Anderson and K. Ward, "Long-Term Effects of High Carbohydrate, High Fiber Diets on Glucose and Lipid Metabolism: A Preliminary Report on Patients with Diabetes," *Diabetes Care* 1 (1978): 77–82.

14. P.A. Crapo et al., "Postprandial Hormone Responses to Different Types of Complex Carbohydrates in Individuals with Impaired Glucose Tolerance," *American Journal of Clinical Nutrition* 33 (1980): 1723–1728.

15. P.B. Geil, "Complex and Simple Carbohydrates in Diabetes Therapy," in *Handbook of Diabetes Medical Nutrition Therapy*, ed. M.A. Powers (Gaithersburg, MD: Aspen Publishers, Inc., 1996), 304.

16. S.L. Thom, "Diabetes Medications and Delivery Methods," in *Handbook of Diabetes Medical Nutrition Therapy*, ed. M.A. Powers (Gaithersburg, MD: Aspen Publishers, Inc., 1996), 95.

17. Crapo et al., "Plasma Glucose and Insulin Responses to Orally Administered Simple and Complex Carbohydrates."

18. P.A. Crapo et al., "Postprandial Glucose and Insulin Responses to Different Complex Carbohy-drates," *Diabetes* 26 (1977): 1178–1183.

19. Crapo et al., "Postprandial Hormone Responses to Different Types of Complex Carbohydrates in Individuals with Impaired Glucose Tolerance."

20. J.P. Bantle et al., "Postprandial Glucose and Insulin Responses to Meals Containing Different Carbohydrates in Normal and Diabetic Subjects," *New England Journal of Medicine* 309 (1983): 7–12.

21. J.P. Bantle et al., "Metabolic Effects of Dietary Fructose and Sucrose in Types I and II Diabetic Subjects," *Journal of the American Medical Association* 256 (1986): 3241–3246.

22. J.P. Bantle et al., "Metabolic Effects of Dietary Sucrose in Type II Diabetic Subjects," *Diabetes Care* 16 (1993): 1301–1305.

23. G. Slama et al., "Sucrose Taken During a Mixed Meal Has No Additional Hyperglycemic Action over Isocaloric Amounts of Starch in Well-Controlled Diabetics," *Lancet* 2 (1984): 122–125.

24. F. Bornet et al., "Sucrose or Honey at Breakfast Have No Additional Acute Hyperglycemic Effect over an Isoglucidic Amount of Bread in Type II Diabetic Patients," *Diabetologia* 28 (1985): 213–217.

25. C. Abraira and J. Derler, "Large Variations of Sucrose in Constant Carbohydrate Diets in Type II Diabetes," *American Journal of Medicine* 84 (1988): 193–200.

26. G. Forlani et al., "Hyperglycemic Effect of Sucrose Ingestion in IDDM Patients Controlled by Artificial Pancreas," *Diabetes Care* 12 (1989): 296–298.

27. J.E. Wise et al., "Effect of Sucrose-Containing Snacks on Blood Glucose Control," *Diabetes Care* 12 (1989): 423–426.

28. A.L. Peters et al., "Effect of Isocaloric Substitution of Chocolate Cake for Potato in Type I Dia-betic Patients," *Diabetes Care* 13 (1990): 888–892.

29. E. Loghmani et al., "Glycemic Response to Sucrose-Containing Mixed Meals in Diets of Chil-dren with Insulin-Dependent Diabetes Mellitus," *Journal of Pediatrics* 119 (1991): 531–537.

30. T.M.S. Wolever and R.G. Josse, "The Role of Carbohydrate in the Diabetes Diet," *Medicine, Exercise, Nutrition, and Health* 2 (1993): 84–99.

31. Crapo et al., "Plasma Glucose and Insulin Responses to Orally Administered Simple and Com-plex Carbohydrates."

32. A. Coulson et al., "Effect of Source of Dietary Carbohydrate on Plasma Glucose and Insulin Responses to Test Meals in Normal Subjects," *American Journal of Clinical Nutrition* 33 (1980): 1279–1282.

33. Crapo et al., "Postprandial Hormonal Responses to Different Types of Complex Carbohydrate in Individuals with Impaired Glucose Tolerance."

34. A. Coulson et al., "Effect of Differences in Sources of Dietary Carbohydrate on Plasma Glucose and Insulin Responses to Meals in Patients with Impaired Carbohydrate Tolerance," *American Journal of Clinical Nutrition* 34 (1981): 2716–2720.

35. R.M. Sandstedt et al., "The Digestibility of High Amylose Corn Starches. The Apparent Effect of the AE Gene on Susceptibility to Amylose Action," *Cereal Chemistry* 39 (1962): 123–131.

36. P. Geervani and R. Theophilus, "Influence of Legume Starches on Protein Nutrition and Avail-ability of Lysine and Methionine to Albino Rats," *Journal of Food Science* 46 (1981): 817–828.

37. F.Q. Nuttall et al., "Effect of Protein Ingestion on the Glucose and Insulin Response to a Stan-dardized Oral Glucose Load," *Diabetes Care* 7 (1984): 465–470.

38. I.H. Anderson et al., "Incomplete Absorption of the Carbohydrate in All-Purpose Wheat Flour," *New England Journal of Medicine* 304 (1981): 891–892.

39. D.E. Bowman, "Amylase Inhibitor of Navy Beans," *Science* 102 (1945): 358–359.

40. R.L. Rea et al., "Lectins in Foods and Their Relation to Starch Digestibility," *Nutrition Research* 5 (1985): 919–929.

41. H.F. Hintz et al., "Toxicity of Red Kidney Beans (*Phaseolus vulgaris*) in the Rat," *Journal of Nutrition* 93 (1967): 77–86.

42. J.H. Yoon et al., "The Effect of Phytic Acid on In Vitro Rate of Starch Digestibility and Blood Glucose Response," *The American Journal of Clinical Nutrition* 38 (1983): 835–842.

43. M.L. Kakade and R.J. Evans, "Growth Inhibition of Rats Fed Raw Navy Beans (*Phaseolus vulgaris*)," *Journal of Nutrition* 90 (1961): 191–198.

44. W. Puls and U. Keup, "Influence of an Alpha-Amylase Inhibitor (BAY d 7791) on Blood Glucose, Serum Insulin and NEFA in Starch Loading Tests in Rats, Dogs and Man," *Diabetologia* 9 (1973): 97–101.

45. I. Hillebrand et al., "The Effect of the Alpha-Glucosidase Inhibitor Bay g 5421 (Acarbose) on Meal Stimulated Elevations of Circulating Glucose, Insulin and Triglyceride Levels in Man," *Research in Experimental Medicine* 175 (1979): 81–86.

46. P. Snow and K. O'Dea, "Factors Affecting the Rate of Hydrolysis in Starch in Food," *American Journal of Clinical Nutrition* 34 (1981): 2721–2727.

47. Yoon et al., "The Effects of Phytic Acid on In Vitro Rate of Starch Digestibility and Blood Glucose Response."

48. P. Collings et al., "Effect of Cooking on Serum Glucose and Insulin Responses to Starch," *British Medical Journal* 282 (1981): 1032.

49. T.M.S. Wolever et al., "Glycemic Response to Pasta: Effect of Food Form, Cooking and Protein Enrichment," *Diabetes Care* 9 (1986): 401–404.

50. T.M.S. Wolever et al., "Comparison of Regular and Parboiled Rices: Explanation of Discrepancies between Reported Glycemic Responses to Rice," *Nutrition Research* 6 (1986): 349–357.

51. D. Jenkins et al., "Effect of Processing on Digestibility and the Blood Glucose Response: A Study of Lentils," *American Journal of Clinical Nutrition* 36 (1982): 1093–1101.

52. Jenkins et al., "Effect of Processing on Digestibility and the Blood Glucose Response: A Study of Lentils."

53. K. O'Dea et al., "Physical Factors Influencing Postprandial Glucose and Insulin Responses to Starch," *American Journal of Clinical Nutrition* 33 (1980): 760–765.

54. G. Collier and K. O'Dea, "Effects of Physical Form of Carbohydrate on the Postprandial Glucose, Insulin and Gastric Inhibitory Polypeptide Response in Type 2 Diabetes," *American Journal of Clinical Nutrition* 36 (1982): 10–14.

55. Wolever, "Glycemic Response to Pasta: Effect of Food Form, Cooking and Protein Enrichment."

56. W. James et al., "Calcium Binding by Dietary Fibre," *Lancet* 1 (1978): 638–639.

57. D. Jenkins et al., "Diabetic Glucose Control, Lipids, and Trace Elements on Long Term Guar," *British Medical Journal* 1 (1980): 1353–1354.

58. J. Anderson et al., "Mineral and Vitamin Status of High-Fiber Diets: Long-Term Studies of Diabetic Patients," *Diabetes Care* 3 (1980): 38–40.

59. A.N. Lindsay et al., "High-Carbohydrate, High-Fiber Diet in Children with Type I Diabetes Mellitus," *Diabetes Care* 7 (1984): 63–67.

60. J. Baumer et al., "Effects of Dietary Fibre and Exercise in Mid-Morning Diabetic Control: A Controlled Trial," *Archives of Disease in Childhood* 57 (1982): 905–909.

61. A.L. Kinmouth et al., "Whole Foods and Increased Dietary Fibre Improve Blood Glucose Control in Diabetic Children," *Archives of Disease in Childhood* 57 (1982): 187–194.

62. C. Kuhl et al., "Guar Gum and Glycemic Control of Pregnant Insulin-Independent Diabetic Patients," *Diabetes Care* 6 (1983): 152–154.

63. D. Ney et al., "Decreased Insulin Requirement and Improved Control of Diabetes in Pregnant Women Given a High-Carbohydrate, High-Fiber, Low-Fat Diet," *Diabetes Care* 5 (1982): 529–533.

64. James et al., "Calcium Binding by Dietary Fibre."

65. B. Canivet et al., "Fibre, Diabetes, and Risk of Bezoar," *Lancet* 2 (1980): 529–533.

66. L. Story et al., "Adherence to High-Carbohydrate, High-Fiber Diets: Long-Term Studies of Non-Obese Diabetic Men," *Journal of the American Dietetic Association* 85 (1985): 1105–1110.

67. D. Jenkins et al., "Unabsorbable Carbohydrates and Diabetes: Decreased Postprandial Hyperglycemia," *Lancet* 2 (1976): 172–174.

68. H. Vuorinen-Markkola et al., "Guar Gum in Insulin-Dependent Diabetes: Effects on Glycemic Control and Serum Lipoproteins," *American Journal of Clinical Nutrition* 56 (1980): 1056–1060.

69. J. Anderson, "The Role of Dietary Carbohydrate and Fiber in the Control of Diabetes," *Advances in Internal Medicine* 26 (1980): 67–96.

70. Jenkins et al., "Unabsorbable Carbohydrates and Diabetes: Decreased Postprandial Hyperglycemia."

71. Vuorinen-Markkola et al., "Guar Gum in Insulin-Dependent Diabetes: Effects on Glycemic Control and Serum Lipoproteins."

72. D.J.A. Jenkins et al. "Glycemic Response to Wheat Products: Reduced Response to Pasta but No Effect of Fiber," *Diabetes Care* 6 (1983): 155–159.

73. L. Tinker and M. Wheeler, "Fiber Metabolism and Use in Diabetes Therapy," in *Handbook of Diabetes Medical Nutrition Therapy*, ed. M.A. Powers (Gaithersburg, MD: Aspen Publishers, Inc., 1996), 405.

74. American Diabetes Association, "American Diabetes Association Position Statement: Nutrition Recommendations and Principles for People with Diabetes Mellitus."

75. Tinker and Wheeler, "Fiber Metabolism and Use in Diabetes Therapy."

76. R. Wolever and D. Jenkins, "The Use of the Glycemic Index in Predicting the Blood Glucose Response to Mixed Meals," *American Journal of Clinical Nutrition* 43 (1986): 167–172.

77. D. Jenkins et al., "Glycemic Index of Foods: A Physiological Basis for Carbohydrate Exchange," *American Journal of Clinical Nutrition* 34 (1981): 362–366.

78. D. Jenkins et al., "Exceptionally Low Blood Glucose Response to Dried Beans: Comparison with Other Carbohydrate Foods," *British Medical Journal* 281 (1980): 578–580.

79. T.M.S. Wolever et al., "Determinants of Diet Glycemic Index Calculated Retrospectively from Diet Records of 342 Individuals with Non–insulin-dependent Diabetes Mellitus," *American Journal of Clinical Nutrition* 9 (1994): 1265–1269.

80. J.C.B. Miller, "Importance of Glycemic Index in Diabetes," *American Journal of Clinical Nutrition* 59 (suppl.) (1994): 7475–7525.

81. P.B. Geil, "Complex and Simple Carbohydrates in Diabetes Therapy," in *Handbook of Diabetes Medical Nutrition Therapy*, ed. M.A. Powers (Gaithersburg, MD: Aspen Publishers, 1996), 312.

82. Expert Panel on Detection, Evaluation, and Treatment of High Blood Cholesterol in Adults, "Summary of the Second Report of the National Cholesterol Education Program (NCEP) Expert Panel on Detection, Evaluation, Treatment of High Blood Cholesterol in Adults (Adult Treatment Panel II)," *Journal of the American Medical Association* 269 (1993): 3015–3023.

83. O'Dea, "Physical Factors Influencing Post-Prandial Glucose, Insulin and Gastric Inhibitory Polypeptide Response in Type 2 Diabetes."

84. D. Jenkins et al., "Diabetic Diets, High Carbohydrate Combined with High Fiber," *American Journal of Clinical Nutrition* 33 (1980): 1729–1733.

85. S. Wong et al., "Factors Affecting the Rate of Hydrolysis of Starch in Legume," *American Journal of Clinical Nutrition* 42 (1985): 38–43.

86. G. Collier and K. O'Dea, "The Effect of Co-ingestion of Fat on the Glucose, Insulin, and Gastric Inhibitory Polypeptide Responses to Carbohydrate and Protein," *American Journal of Clinical Nutrition* 37 (1983): 941–944.

87. G. Collier and K. O'Dea, "The Effect of Co-ingestion of Fat on the Metabolic Responses to Slowly and Rapidly Absorbed Carbohydrates," *Diabetologia* 26 (1984): 50–54.

88. G. Collier et al., "Concurrent Ingestion of Fat and Reduction in Starch Content Impairs Carbohydrate Tolerance to Subsequent Meals," *American Journal of Clinical Nutrition* 45 (1987): 963–969.

89. E. Ferrannini et al., "Effect of Fatty Acids on Glucose Production and Utilization in Man," *Journal of Clinical Investigation* 72 (1983): 1737–1747.

90. B. Brackenridge, "Carbohydrate Counting for Diabetes Therapy," in *Handbook of Diabetes Medical Nutrition Therapy*, ed. M.A. Powers (Gaithersburg, MD: Aspen Publishers, 1996), 262–263.

91. H. Munro and J. Allison, *Mammalian Protein Metabolism*. Vol. 1 (New York: Academic Press, 1964), 162–170.

92. F.Q. Nuttal and M.C. Gannon, "Plasma Glucose and Insulin Response to Macronutrients in Nondiabetic and NIDDM Subjects," *Diabetes Care* 14 (1991): 824–834.

93. M.J. Oexmann, *Total Available Glucose, Diabetic Food System* (Charleston, SC: Medical University of South Carolina Printing Service, 1987).

94. Joint FAO/WHO Expert Committee on Food Additives, *Evaluation of Certain Food Additives and Contaminants, 37th Report,* Report no. 806, (Geneva: 1991).

95. American Diabetes Association, "Position Statement: Nutrition Recommendations and Principles for People with Diabetes Mellitus."

96. American Dietetic Association, "Position Statement: Use of Nutritive and Non-nutritive Sweeteners," *Journal of the American Dietetic Association* 93, no. 7 (1993): 816–820.

97. L. D. Steginck, "Aspartame Metabolism in Humans: Acute Dosing Studies," in *Aspartame: Physiology and Biochemistry*, eds. L.D. Steginck and L.J. Filer, Jr. (New York: Marcel Dekker, Inc., 1984), 509–554.

98. J.K. Nehrling et al., "Aspartame Use by Persons with Diabetes," *Diabetes Care* 8 (1985): 415–417.

99. W.C. Monte, "Aspartame: Methanol and the Public Health," *Journal of Applied Nutrition* 36 (1984): 42–54.

100. Nehrling et al., "Aspartame Use by Persons with Diabetes."

101. "Aspartame: Commissioner's Final Decision," *Federal Register* 46 (July 24, 1981): 38283.

102. "Saccharin and Its Salts," *Federal Register* 42 (December 9, 1977): 62209.

103. A.S. Morrison and J.E. Buring, "Artificial Sweeteners and Cancer of the Lower Urinary Tract," *New England Journal of Medicine* 302 (1980): 537–541.

104. Council on Scientific Affairs, "Saccharin—Review of Safety Issues," *Journal of the American Medical Association* 254 (1985): 2622.

105. American Diabetes Association, "Position Statement: Nutrition Recommendations and Principles for People with Diabetes Mellitus."

106. American Dietetic Association, "Position Statement: Use of Nutritive and Non-nutritive Sweeteners."

107. M.E. Hendrick, "Alitame," in *Alternative Sweeteners*, eds. L. O'Brien Nabors and R.C. Gelardi (New York: Marcel Dekker, Inc., 1991).

108. B.A. Bopp and P. Price, "Cyclamate," in *Alternative Sweeteners*, ed. L. O'Brien and R.C. Gelardi (New York: Marcel Dekker, Inc., 1991).

109. B.A. Bopp et al., "Toxicological Aspects of Cyclamate and Cyclohexylamine," *CRC Critical Reviews in Toxicology* 16 (1986): 213–306.

110. Bopp, "Cyclamate."

111. R. Newsome, "Sugar Substitutes," in *Low-Calorie Foods Handbook,* ed. A.M. Altschul (New York: Marcel Dekker, Inc., 1993), 139–170.

112. L. O'Brien and W.T. Miller, "Cyclamate—A Toxicological Review," *Comment on Toxicology* 3, no. 4 (1989): 307.

113. McNeil Specialty Products Company, *Sucralose: An Introduction to a New Low-Calorie Sweetener* (New Brunswick, NJ, 1994).

114. N. Mezitis et al., "Glycemic Response to Sucralose, a Novel Sweetener, in Subjects with Diabetes Mellitus," *Diabetes* 43, no. 5 (1994): S261A.

115. W.H. Bower, "The Effects of Sucralose on Coronal and Root-Surface Caries," *Journal of Dental Research* 69, no. 8 (1990): 1485–1487.

116. H.S. Warshaw, "Alternative Sweeteners—Past, Present and Potential," *Diabetes Spectrum* 3, no. 5 (1990): 335.

117. D.J. Walsh and D.J. O'Sullivan, "Effect of Moderate Alcohol Intake on Control of Diabetes," *Diabetes* 23 (1974): 440–442.

118. M.J. Franz, "Diabetes Mellitus: Consideration in the Development of Guidelines for the Occasional Use of Alcohol," *Journal of the American Dietetic Association* 83 (1983): 148–149.

119. R. Menze et al., "Effect of Moderate Ethanol Ingestion on Overnight Diabetes Control and Hormone Secretion in Type 1 Diabetic Patients," *Diabetologia* 34 (1991): A188.

120. American Diabetes Association, "Technical Review: Nutrition Principles for the Management of Diabetes and Related Complications," *Diabetes Care* 17, no. 5 (1994): 490.

121. K.D. Kulkarni, "Adjusting Nutrition Therapy for Special Situations," in *Handbook of Diabetes Medical Nutrition Therapy*, ed. M.A. Powers (Gaithersburg, MD: Aspen Publishers, Inc., 1996), 437–442.

122. M.J. Franz, "Exercise Benefits and Guidelines for Persons with Diabetes," in *Handbook of Diabetes Medical Nutrition Therapy*, ed. M.A. Powers (Gaithersburg, MD: Aspen Publishers, Inc., 1996), 107–129.

123. L. Jovanovic and C.M. Peterson, "The Clinical Utility of Glycosylated Hemoglobin," *American Journal of Medicine* 70 (1981): 331–338.

124. H.F. Bunn, "Nonenzymatic Glycosylation of Protein: Relevance to Diabetes," *American Journal of Medicine* 70 (1981): 325.

125. L. Jovanovic and C.M. Peterson, "Hemoglobin A1c—The Key to Diabetic Control," *Laboratory Medicine for the Practicing Physician* (July–August, 1978): 11.

126. C.M. Peterson and R.L. Jones, "Glycosylation Reactions and Reversible Sequelae of Diabetes Mellitus," in *Diabetes Management in the 80's*, ed. C.M. Peterson (New York: Praeger Publishers, 1982), 12–25.

127. D.J. Jenkins et al., "Glycemic Index of Foods: A Physiological Basis for Carbohydrate Exchange," *American Journal of Clinical Nutrition* 34 (1981): 184–190.

128. J. Choppin et al., "Matching Food with Insulin," *Diabetes Professional* (Spring 1991): 1–14.

129. Choppin et al., "Matching Food with Insulin."

130. B. Brackenridge, "Carbohydrate Counting for Diabetes Nutrition Therapy."

131. M.J. Oexmann, *Total Available Glucose, Diabetic Food System* (Charleston, SC: Medical University of South Carolina Printing Service, 1987).

132. Munro and Allison, *Mammalian Protein Metabolism,* 162–264.

133. G. Lusk, *The Elements of the Science of Nutrition* (Philadelphia: W.B. Saunders Co., 1928), 206–209.

134. J.A.T. Pennington, *Bowes and Church's Food Values of Portions Commonly Used* (Philadephia: J.B. Lippincott, 1994).

135. Oexmann, *Total Available Glucose.*

136. Munro and Allison, *Mammalian Protein Metabolism,* 164.

137. The Diabetes Control and Complications Research Group, "The Effect of Intensive Treatment of Diabetes."

138. L.M. West, "Diet Therapy of Diabetes: An Analysis of Failure," *Annals of Internal Medicine* 79 (1973): 425–534.

139. The Diabetes Control and Complications Research Group, "The Effect of Intensive Treatment of Diabetes."

140. J.D. Watkins et al., "A Study of Diabetes Patients at Home," *American Journal of Public Health* 57 (1967): 452–459.

141. B.A. Broussard et al., "Reasons for Diabetic Diet Noncompliance among Cherokee Indians," *Journal of Nutrition Education* 14 (1982): 56–57.

142. E.A. Schlenk and L.K. Hart, "Relationship Between Health Locus of Control, Health Values and Social Support and Compliance of Persons with Diabetes Mellitus," *Diabetes Care* 7 (1984): 566–574.

143. L. Eckerling and M.B. Kohrs, "Research on Compliance with Diabetic Regimens: Applications to Practice," *Journal of the American Dietetic Association* 84 (1984): 805–809.

144. R.L. Wiensier et al., "Diet Therapy of Diabetes: Description of a Successful Methodologic Approach to Gaining Adherence," *Diabetes* 23 (1974): 639–673.

145. Jean Hassell and Eva Medved, "Group/Audiovisual Instruction for Patients with Diabetes," *Journal of the American Dietetic Association* 66 (1975): 465–470.

146. Gwen S. Tani and Jean H. Hankin, "A Self-Learning Unit for Patients with Diabetes," *Journal of the American Dietetic Association* 58 (1971): 331–335.

147. Stewart M. Dunn et al., "Development of the Diabetes Knowledge Scales: Forms DKNA, DKNB, and DKNC," *Diabetes Care* 7 (1984): 36–41.

148. K.L. Webb et al., "Dietary Compliance Among Insulin-Dependent Diabetics," *Journal of Chronic Disease* 37 (1984): 633–643.

149. P.H. Sonksen et al., "Home Monitoring of Blood Glucose," *Lancet* 1 (1978): 727–732.

150. S. Walford et al., "Self-Monitoring of Blood Glucose," *Lancet* 1 (1978): 732–735.

151. M. Cohen and P. Zimmet, "Self-Monitoring of Blood Glucose Levels in Non-Insulin-Dependent Diabetes Mellitus," *Medical Journal of Australia* 2 (1983): 377–381.

152. The Diabetes Control and Complications Research Group, "The Effect of Intensive Treatment of Diabetes."

153. L.A. Slowie, "Patient Learning—Segments from Case Histories," *Journal of the American Dietetic Association* 58 (1971): 563–567.

154. M. Boutaugh, A. Hall, and W. Davis, "An Examination of Diabetes Educational Diagnosis Assessment Forms," *Diabetes Educator* 7 (1982): 29–34; *Dunn et al.*, "Development of the Diabetes Knowledge Scales"; and George E. Hess and Wayne K. Davis, "The Validation of a Diabetes Patient Knowledge Test," *Diabetes Care* 6 (1983); 591–596.

155. Webb et al., "Dietary Compliance Among Insulin-Dependent Diabetics.

156. R.J. Shenkel et al., "Importance of 'Significant Other' in Predicting Cooperation with Diabetic Regimen," *International Journal of Psychiatry in Medicine* 15 (1985): 149–155.

157. L.S. Schwartz et al., "The Role of Recent Life Events and Social Support in the Control of Diabetes Mellitus," *General Hospital Psychiatry* 8 (1986): 212–216.

158. M.A. Bush, "Compliance, Education, and Diabetes Control," *Mount Sinai Journal of Medicine* 54 (1987): 221–227.

159. R.R. Wing et al., "Behavioral Self-Regulation in the Treatment of Patients with Diabetes Mellitus," *Psychological Bulletin* 99 (1986): 78–89.

160. D.K. McColloush et al., "Influence of Imaginative Teaching on Diet on Compliance and Metabolic Control in Insulin Dependent Diabetes," *British Medical Journal* 287 (1983): 1858–1861.

161. B. McNeal et al., "Comprehension Assessment of Diabetes Education Program Participants," *Diabetes Care* 7 (1984): 232–235.

162. S.R. Rapp et al., "Food Portion Size Estimation by Men with Type II Diabetes," *Journal of the American Dietetic Association* 86 (1986): 249–251.

163. D.V. Ary et al., "Patient Perspective on Factors Contributing to Nonadherence to Diabetes Regimens," *Diabetes Care* 9 (1986): 168–172.

164. K. Glanz, "Nutrition Education for Risk Factor Reduction and Patient Education: A Review," *Preventive Medicine* 14 (1985): 721–752.

165. B. Martinez, "Perfection/Imperfection," *Diabetes Spectrum* 8 (1995): 304–307.

Adherence Tool 6–1: One-Day Food Record (Monitoring Device)

Name_____

		No. of Exchanges	Type of Foods and Amount
Breakfast	Bread		
	Fruit		
	Milk		
	Meat		
	Fat		
Midmorning	Bread		
	Fruit		
	Milk		
	Meat		
	Fat		
Lunch	Bread		
	Fruit		
	Veg. A		
	Veg. B		
	Milk		
	Meat		
	Fat		
Midafternoon	Bread		
	Fruit		
	Milk		
	Meat		
	Fat		
Dinner	Bread		
	Fruit		
	Veg. A		
	Veg. B		
	Milk		
	Meat		
	Fat		
Bedtime	Bread		
	Fruit		
	Milk		
	Meat		
	Fat		

Adherence Tool 6–2: One-Week Check-Off System To Identify Morning Snacking Problems (Monitoring Device)

Monday
_____

Tuesday
_____

Wednesday
_____

Thursday
_____

Friday
_____

Saturday
_____

Sunday

+ = Had a snack
* = Avoided a snack

Adherence Tool 6–3: Graph of Breakfast TAG Values Based on Diet Records Completed between Visits (Monitoring Device)

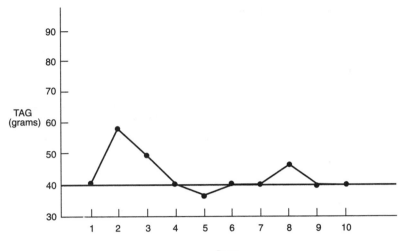

Adherence Tool 6–4: Graph of Blood Glucose and Glycosylated Hemoglobin Levels (Monitoring Device)

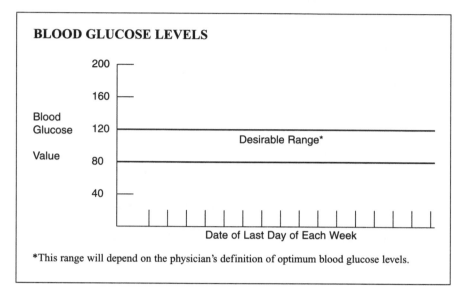

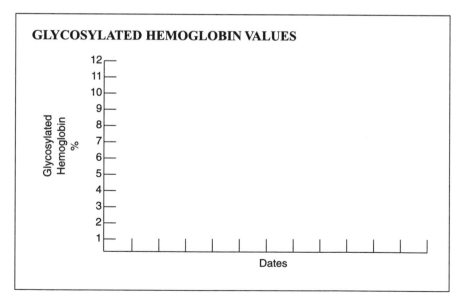

Adherence Tool 6–5: Monthly Check-Off System for Pre-Meal Insulin Injections (Monitoring Device)

ONE-MONTH

Sun.	Mon.	Tues.	Wed.	Thur.	Fri.	Sat.

Month of _____ 19 ____   If you have any questions, please call: _____

Adherence Tool 6–6: Individualized Exchanges for Meal Planning (Informational Device)

STARCH/BREAD LIST
Cereals/grains and pasta, ½ cup
    Grapenuts, ¼ cup
Starch vegetable
    Corn, ½ cup
    Potato, baked, 1 small (3 ounces)
Bread
    Whole wheat bread, 1 slice (1 ounce)

MEAT LIST
    Lean meats, 1 ounce
        Beef sirloin, 1 ounce
        Canned ham, 1 ounce
        Chicken, 1 ounce
        Tuna, 1 ounce
        Cottage cheese, ¼ cup

VEGETABLE LIST
    Cooked vegetables, ½ cup
    Raw vegetables, 1 cup

FRUIT LIST
    Apple, raw, 2 inches across, 1
    Banana (9 inches long), ½
    Pear, large, ½
    Raisins, 2 tablespoons
    Orange juice, ½ cup

MILK LIST
    1% milk, 1 cup

FAT LIST
    Margarine, 1 teaspoon
    Reduced-calorie mayonnaise, 1 tablespoon

Adherence Tool 6–7: Practice with Exchanges and Total Available Glucose (TAG) (Informational Device)

Determine the exchanges and TAG for each of the following foods:

	Exchanges	TAG
Corn, ½ cup		
Orange juice, 6 ounces		
Poached egg, 1		
Chicken, 3 ounces		
Pork chop, 2 ounces		
Tuna fish, ½ cup		
Green beans, ¾ cup		
Saltine crackers, 6		
Party crackers (Triscuits), 5		
Graham crackers, 3		
Skim milk, 8 ounces		
Whole milk, 8 ounces		
Peanut butter, 2 tablespoons		
Italian dressing, 1 tablespoon		
Wheat bread, 2 slices		
Mayonnaise, 1 tablespoon		
Grape juice, ⅔ cup		
Grapes, 15		
Watermelon, 1¼ cup		
Small olives, 10		
Stick pretzels, ¾ ounces		
Dry nonfat milk, ⅓ cup		
Baked beans, ½ cup		
French fries, 10 (3½ inches long)		
Muffin, 1, small plain		
Bacon, 2 slices		
American cheese, 1 ounce		
Bran Buds®, ½ cup		
Oatmeal, 1 cup		
Plain nonfat yogurt, 1 cup		
Sour cream, ½ cup		
Sherbert, ½ cup		

continues

Adherence Tool 6–7   (continued)

List the amount of carbohydrate, protein, fat, and kilocalories in the following exchange groups:

Exchange	Carbo- hydrate (grams)	Protein (grams)	Fat (grams)	Kilo- calories (grams)	TAG
Bread					
Milk (skim)					
Fat					
Vegetable					
Meat					
Fruit					

Adherence Tool 6–8:   Total Available Glucose (TAG) (Informational Device)

TAG = Carbohydrate (CHO) (g) + [Animal Protein (PRO) (g) × 0.58]

	CHO	+ PRO (0.58)	= TAG
1 Fruit Exchange	= 15 g	+ 0	= 15
1 Meat Exchange	= 0	+ 7 g (0.58)	= 4
1 Milk Exchange	= 12 g	+ 8 g (0.58)	= 17
1 Bread Exchange	= 15 g	+ 0	= 15
1 Vegetable Exchange	= 5 g	+ 0	= 5

The number that results from this formula can be used to determine what each of your meals might include.

Counting total available glucose (TAG) is a way of ensuring consistency in diet from day to day. We count carbohydrate because we know it tends to raise blood sugars. Animal proteins also raise blood sugar levels because they are eventually converted to carbohydrate by our bodies. Fat does not raise blood sugar levels because very little of it is converted to carbohydrate. We do try to keep fat intake low enough to prevent increases in weight and also consider the type of fat you eat to prevent coronary heart disease.

Adherence Tool 6–9:   Worksheet for Calculating Exchanges and Total Available Glucose (TAG) in a Recipe: Chocolate Cookies (Informational Device)

1¼ cups flour	1 egg
½ teaspoon baking soda	⅓ cup buttermilk
½ teaspoon salt	1 teaspoon vanilla
½ cup butter or margarine	2 ounces melted unsweetened chocolate
1 cup white sugar	½ cup chopped walnuts

Ingredients	Fruit	Veg	Bread	Meat	Fat	Milk	TAG
1¼ cups flour							
½ teaspoon baking soda							
½ teaspoon salt							
½ cup butter or margarine							
1 cup white sugar							
1 egg							
⅓ cup buttermilk							
1 teaspoon vanilla							
2 ounces melted chocolate							
½ cup walnuts							

Total Exchanges: Bread _____   Fruit _____

Meat _____   Vegetable _____

Fat_____   Milk _____

TAG _____

Exchanges per Serving _____

TAG per Serving _____

Directions: Indicate what portion of an exchange each ingredient contains. Divide by the number of servings for each ingredient to obtain total exchanges and exchanges per serving. Use Pennington* to calculate TAG for each ingredient and per serving.

*J.A.T. Pennington and H.N. Church, *Bowes and Church's Food Values of Portions Commonly Used*, copyright © 1995, Lippincott-Raven Publishers.

Adherence Tool 6–10:   Worksheet for Calculating Exchanges and Total Available Glucose (TAG) in a Recipe: Chicken Soup (Informational Device)

12 ounces cooked chicken (weigh
   after removing from bone)
$\frac{1}{3}$ cup rice, uncooked
$\frac{1}{2}$ cup diced celery
$\frac{1}{2}$ cup carrots, chopped

$\frac{1}{4}$ cup diced onion
$\frac{1}{2}$ teaspoon salt
$\frac{1}{8}$ teaspoon pepper
$\frac{1}{2}$ teaspoon celery salt
4 cups water

Ingredients	Fruit	Veg	Bread	Meat	Fat	Milk	TAG
12 ounces chicken							
$\frac{1}{3}$ cup rice, uncooked							
$\frac{1}{2}$ cup diced celery							
$\frac{1}{2}$ cup carrots, chopped							
$\frac{1}{4}$ cup diced onion							
$\frac{1}{2}$ teaspoon salt							
$\frac{1}{8}$ teaspoon pepper							
$\frac{1}{2}$ teaspoon celery salt							
4 cups water							

Total Exchanges: Bread _____   Fruit _____

Meat _____   Vegetable _____

Fat _____   Milk _____

TAG _____

Exchanges per Serving _____

TAG per Serving _____

Adherence Tool 6–11: Worksheet for Calculating Exchanges and Total Available Glucose (TAG) in a Recipe: Chicken Almond Oriental (Informational Device) (4–6 Servings)

Ingredients	Fruit	Veg	Bread	Meat	Fat	Milk	TAG
1 pound chicken breast without bone and skin							
1½ cups broccoli cut into 1″ pieces							
½ cup blanched almonds							
1 teaspoon cornstarch							
½ teaspoon sugar							
2 tablespoons soy sauce							
2 tablespoons dry sherry							
1 medium onion, cut into thin wedges							
½ cup water chestnuts, thinly sliced							
½ cup bamboo shoots							
Total Exchanges:							
Exchanges per Serving:							
TAG per Serving:							

Adherence Tool 6–12: Weighing and Measuring (Informational Device)

STANDARD:	Weight	Carbo-hydrate	Protein	Fat
Apple, raw, 1 medium, with skin (without core)	138 grams	21.1	0.3	0.5

ACTUAL:

Your apple weighs 200 grams (without core).

$$\frac{\text{Weight of Standards}}{\text{Carbohydrate (g) of Standard}} = \frac{\text{Weight of Actual}}{\text{Carbohydrate (g) in Actual}}$$

$$\frac{138}{21.1} = \frac{200}{X}$$

$$138X = 200 \times 21.1$$

$$X = \frac{200 \times 21.1}{138}$$

$$X = 30.6 \text{ g of Carbohydrate in your actual serving}$$

Adherence Tool 6–13: Total Available Glucose (TAG) for Mixed Food

1. Philly Sandwich

Carbo-hydrate	Protein	Fat
45 grams	28 grams	24 grams

2. How much of the 28 grams of protein is vegetable protein?
   How many bread exchanges are in 45 grams of carbohydrate?
   45/15 grams carbohydrate in each exchange = 3 bread exchanges.
   Protein = 3 grams in 1 bread exchange.
   $3 \times 3 = 9$ grams vegetable protein.

3. Subtract grams of vegetable protein from grams of total protein to get grams of animal protein.
   $28 - 9 = 19$ grams of animal protein

4. Use TAG formula:

TAG	= Carbohydrate grams + (Animal Protein $\times$ 0.58)
TAG	= 45 + (19 $\times$ 0.58 grams)
TAG	= 45 + 11.02
TAG	= 56.02 grams

Adherence Tool 6–14:   Calculating Total Available Glucose (TAG)

1. Look for food value in Pennington.*

$$\frac{\text{Standard Value:} \quad \text{3.5 oz. Meat}}{\text{25.2 g Protein}}$$

2. Determine (by weighing) your meat portion.

$$\frac{\text{2 oz. Meat}}{X}$$

3. Calculate the ratio and proportion.

$$\frac{3 \text{ oz.}}{25.2 \text{ grams Protein}} = \frac{2 \text{ oz.}}{X}$$

$$3X = 2 \times 25.2$$
$$3X = 50.4$$
$$X = 16.8 \text{ grams Protein}$$

4. Calculate TAG = grams Protein × 0.58

$$\text{TAG} = 16.8 \times 0.58$$
$$\text{TAG} = 9.74 \text{ grams}$$

5. Add this TAG to total Carbohydrate in rest of meal.

*Jean A.T. Pennington, *Bowes and Church's Food Values of Portions Commonly Used* (Philadelphia: J.B. Lippincott, 1994).

Adherence Tool 6–15: Your Favorite Meals: Are They Meeting Your Goals?

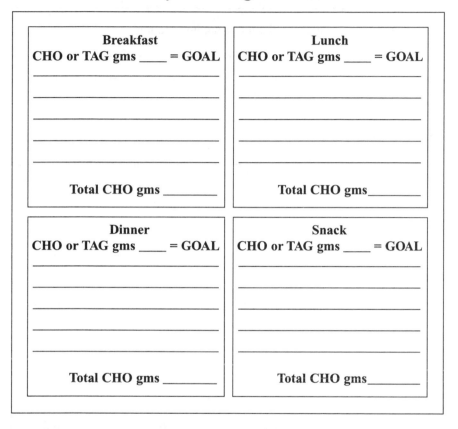

Breakfast
CHO or TAG gms _____ = GOAL

Total CHO gms _____

Lunch
CHO or TAG gms _____ = GOAL

Total CHO gms_____

Dinner
CHO or TAG gms _____ = GOAL

Total CHO gms _____

Snack
CHO or TAG gms _____ = GOAL

Total CHO gms_____

Adherence Tool 6–16:   Worksheet for Food Labeling (Informational Device)

1. Select a label and obtain the following information:

   Product name_____

   Serving size _____

   Number of servings per container_____

   Calories _____

   Protein (g) _____

   Carbohydrates (g) _____

   Fat (g) _____

   Ingredients_____

   _____

   _____

   _____

2. From the information listed above, calculate the exchanges and TAG contained in this product.

3. Use this product with other foods to create a balanced meal (breakfast, lunch, or dinner), using your meal pattern.

Exchange Lists for Meal Planning

STARCH LIST

Cereals, grains, pasta, breads, crackers, snacks, starchy vegetables, and cooked dried beans, peas, and lentils are starches. In general, one starch is:

- ½ cup of cereal, grain, pasta, or starchy vegetable
- 1 ounce of a bread product, such as 1 slice of bread
- ¾ to 1 ounce of most snack foods (Some snack foods may also have added fat.)

Nutrition Tips

1. Most starch choices are good sources of B vitamins.
2. Foods made from whole grains are good sources of fiber.
3. Dried beans and peas are a good source of protein and fiber.

Selection Tips

1. Choose starches made with little fat as often as you can.
2. Starchy vegetables prepared with fat count as one starch and one fat.
3. Bagels or muffins can be 2, 3, or 4 ounces in size, and can, therefore, count as 2, 3, or 4 starch choices. Check the size you eat.
4. Dried beans, peas, and lentils are also found on the Meat and Meat Substitutes list.

Source: The Exchange Lists are the basis of a meal-planning system designed by a committee of the American Diabetes Association and The American Dietetic Association. While designed primarily for people with diabetes and others who must follow special diets, the Exchange Lists are based on principles of good nutrition that apply to everyone. Reprinted with permission from The American Dietetic Association and the American Diabetes Association. Copyright © 1995, Chicago, Illinois.

5. Regular potato chips and tortilla chips are found on the Other Carbohydrates list.
6. Most of the serving sizes are measured after cooking.
7. Always check Nutrition Facts on the food label.

**One starch exchange equals 15 grams carbohydrate,
3 grams protein, 0–1 grams fat, and 80 calories.**

Bread

Bagel	½ (1 oz)
Bread, reduced-calorie	2 slices (1½ oz)
Bread, white, whole-wheat, pumpernickel, rye	1 slice (1 oz)
Bread sticks, crisp, 4 in long × ½ in.	2 (⅔ oz)
English muffin	½
Hot dog or hamburger bun	½ (1 oz)
Pita, 6 in across	½
Roll, plain, small	1 (1 oz)
Raisin bread, unfrosted	1 slice (1 oz)
Tortilla, corn, 6 in across	1
Tortilla, flour, 7–8 in across	1
Waffle, 4½-in square, reduced-fat	1

Cereals and Grains

Bran cereals	½ cup
Bulgur	½ cup
Cereals	½ cup
Cereals, unsweetened, ready-to-eat	¾ cup
Cornmeal (dry)	3 Tbsp
Couscous	⅓ cup
Flour (dry)	3 Tbsp
Granola, low-fat	¼ cup
Grape-Nuts	¼ cup
Grits	½ cup
Kasha	½ cup
Millet	¼ cup
Muesli	¼ cup
Oats	½ cup
Pasta	½ cup
Puffed cereal	1½ cups
Rice milk	½ cup
Rice, white or brown	⅓ cup
Shredded Wheat	½ cup

Sugar-frosted cereal . . . . ½ cup
Wheat germ. . . . . 3 Tbsp

Starchy Vegetables

Baked beans . . . . ⅓ cup
Corn. . . . . ½ cup
Corn on cob, medium . . . . 1 (5 oz)
Mixed vegetables with corn, peas, or pasta . . . . 1 cup
Peas, green . . . . ½ cup
Plaintain . . . . ½ cup
Potato, baked or boiled. . . . . 1 small (3 oz)
Potato, mashed . . . . ½ cup
Squash winter (acorn, butternut) . . . . 1 cup
Yam, sweet potato, plain . . . . ½ cup

Crackers and Snacks

Animal crackers. 8
Graham crackers, 2½-in square 3
Matzoh. . . . . ¾ oz
Melba toast. . . . . 4 slices
Oyster crackers 24
Popcorn (popped, no fat added or low-fat microwave) . . . . 3 cups
Pretzels. . . . . ¾ oz
Rice cakes, 4 in across. 2
Saltine-type crackers 6
Snack chips, fat-free (tortilla, potato). . . . . 15–20 (¾ oz)
Whole-wheat crackers, no fat added . . . . 2–5 (¾ oz)

Dried Beans, Peas, and Lentils
(Count as 1 starch exchange, plus 1 very lean meat exchange.)

Beans and peas (garbanzo, pinto, kidney, white, split, black-eyed) . . . . . . ½ cup
Lima beans. . . . . ⅔ cup
Lentils . . . . ½ cup
Miso* . . . . 3 Tbsp

Starchy Foods Prepared with Fat
(Count as 1 starch exchange, plus 1 fat exchange.)

Biscuit, 2½ in across 1

---

*400 mg or more sodium per exchange.

Chow mein noodles . . . . ½ cup
Corn bread, 2-in cube. . . . . 1 (2 oz)
Crackers, round butter type 6
Croutons . . . . 1 cup
French-fried potatoes . . . . 16–25 (3 oz)
Granola. . . . . ¼ cup
Muffin, small . . . . 1 (1½ oz)
Pancake, 4 in across. 2
Popcorn, microwave. . . . . 3 cups
Sandwich crackers, cheese or peanut butter filling. 3
Stuffing, bread (prepared). . . . . ⅓ cup
Taco shell, 6 in across 2
Waffle, 4½-in square 1
Whole-wheat crackers, fat added . . . . 4–6 (1 oz)

Some food you buy uncooked will weigh less after you cook it. Starches will often swell in cooking, so a small amount of uncooked starch will become a much larger amount of cooked food. The following table shows some of the changes.

Food (Starch Group)	Uncooked	Cooked
Oatmeal	3 Tbsp	½ cup
Cream of Wheat	2 Tbsp	½ cup
Grits	3 Tbsp	½ cup
Rice	2 Tbsp	⅓ cup
Spaghetti	¼ cup	½ cup
Noodles	⅓ cup	½ cup
Macaroni	¼ cup	½ cup
Dried beans	¼ cup	½ cup
Dried peas	¼ cup	½ cup
Lentils	3 Tbsp	½ cup

Common Measurements

3 tsp = 1 Tbsp	4 ounces = ½ cup
4 Tbsp = ¼ cup	8 ounces = 1 cup
5 ⅓ Tbsp = ⅓ cup	1 cup = ½ pint

FRUIT LIST

Fresh, frozen, canned, and dried fruits and fruit juices are on this list. In general, one fruit exchange is:

- 1 small to medium fresh fruit
- ½ cup of canned or fresh fruit or fruit juice
- ¼ cup dried fruit

Nutrition Tips

1. Fresh, frozen, and dried fruits have about 2 grams of fiber per choice. Fruit juices contain very little fiber.
2. Citrus fruits, berries, and melons are good sources of vitamin C.

Selection Tips

1. Count ½ cup cranberries or rhubarb sweetened with sugar substitutes as free foods.
2. Read the Nutrition Facts on the food label. If one serving has more than 15 grams of carbohydrate, you will need to adjust the size of the serving you eat or drink.
3. Portion sizes for canned fruits are for the fruit and a small amount of juice.
4. Whole fruit is more filling than fruit juice and may be a better choice.
5. Food labels for fruits may contain the words "no sugar added" or "unsweetened." This means that no sucrose (table sugar) has been added.
6. Generally, fruit canned in extra light syrup has the same amount of carbohydrate per serving as the "no sugar added" or the juice pack. All canned fruits on the fruit list are based on one of these three types of pack.

One fruit exchange equals 15 grams carbohydrate and 60 calories.
The weight includes skin, core, seeds, and rind.

Fruit

Apple, unpeeled, small	1 (4 oz)
Applesauce, unsweetened	½ cup
Apples, dried	4 rings
Apricots, fresh	4 whole (5½ oz)
Apricots, dried	8 halves
Apricots, canned	½ cup
Banana, small	1 (4 oz)
Blackberries	¾ cup
Blueberries	¾ cup
Cantaloupe, small	⅓ melon (11 oz) or 1 cup cubes
Cherries, sweet, canned	½ cup
Dates	3
Figs, fresh	1½ large or 2 medium (3½ oz)
Figs, dried	1½
Fruit cocktail	½ cup

Grapefruit, large . . . . ½ (11 oz)
Grapefruit sections, canned. . . . . ¾ cup
Grapes, small. . . . . 17 (3 oz)
Honeydew melon . . . . 1 slice (10 oz) or 1 cup cubes
Kiwi . . . . 1 (3½ oz)
Mandarin oranges, canned . . . . ¾ cup
Mango, small . . . . ½ fruit (5½ oz) or ½ cup
Nectarine, small. . . . . 1 (5 oz)
Orange, small . . . . 1 (6½ oz)
Papaya. . . . . ½ fruit (8 oz) or 1 cup cubes
Peach, medium, fresh. . . . . 1 (6 oz)
Peaches, canned . . . . ½ cup
Pear, large, fresh . . . . ½ (4 oz)
Pears, canned . . . . ½ cup
Pineapple, fresh . . . . ¾ cup
Pineapple, canned. . . . . ½ cup
Plums, small . . . . 2 (5 oz)
Plums, canned. . . . . ½ cup
Prunes, dried 3
Raisins . . . . 2 Tbsp
Raspberries. . . . . 1 cup
Strawberries . . . . 1¼ cup whole berries
Tangerines, small. . . . . 2 (8 oz)
Watermelon. . . . . 1 slice (13½ oz) or 1¼ cup cubes

Fruit Juice

Apple juice/cider . . . . ½ cup
Cranberry juice cocktail . . . . ⅓ cup
Cranberry juice cocktail, reduced-calorie. . . . . 1 cup
Fruit juice blends, 100% juice. . . . . ⅓ cup
Grape juice. . . . . ⅓ cup
Grapefruit juice . . . . ½ cup
Orange juice. . . . . ½ cup
Pineapple juice . . . . ½ cup
Prune juice . . . . ⅓ cup

MILK LIST

Different types of milk and milk products are on this list. Cheeses are on the Meat list and cream and other dairy fats are on the Fat list. Based on the amount of fat they contain, milks are divided into skim/very low-fat milk, low-fat milk, and whole milk. One choice of these includes:

	Carbohydrate (g)	Protein (g)	Fat (g)	Calories
Skim/very low-fat	12	8	0–3	90
Low-fat	12	8	5	120
Whole	12	8	8	150

Nutrition Tips

1. Milk and yogurt are good sources of calcium and protein. Check the food label.
2. The higher the fat content of milk and yogurt, the greater the amount of saturated fat and cholesterol. Choose lower-fat varieties.
3. For those who are lactose intolerant, look for lactose-reduced or lactose-free varieties of milk.

Selection Tips

1. One cup equals 8 fluid ounces or ½ pint.
2. Look for chocolate milk, frozen yogurt, and ice cream on the Other Carbohydrates list.
3. Nondairy creamers are on the Free Foods list.
4. Look for rice milk on the Starch list.
5. Look for soy milk on the Medium-Fat Meat list.

One milk exchange equals 12 grams carbohydrate and 8 grams protein.

Skim and Very Low-Fat Milk (0–3 grams fat per serving)

Skim milk . . . . 1 cup
1/2% milk . . . . 1 cup
1% milk . . . . 1 cup
Nonfat or low-fat buttermilk . . . . 1 cup
Evaporated skim milk . . . . ½ milk
Nonfat dry milk . . . . ⅓ cup dry
Plain nonfat yogurt . . . . ¾ cup
Nonfat or low-fat fruit-flavored yogurt sweetened
    with aspartame or with nonnutritive sweetener. . . . . 1 cup

Low-Fat Milk (5 grams fat per serving)

2% milk . . . . 1 cup
Plain low-fat yogurt . . . . ¾ cup
Sweet acidophilus milk . . . . 1 cup

Whole Milk (8 grams fat per serving)

Whole milk . . . . 1 cup
Evaporated whole milk . . . . ½ cup
Goat's milk . . . . 1 cup
Kefir . . . . 1 cup

OTHER CARBOHYDRATES LIST

You can substitute food choices from this list for a starch, fruit, or milk choice on your meal plan. Some choices will also count as one or more fat choices.

Nutrition Tips

1. These foods can be substituted in your meal plan, even though they contain added sugars or fat. However, they do not contain as many important vitamins and minerals as the choices on the Starch, Fruit, or Milk list.
2. When planning to include these foods in your meal, be sure to include foods from all the lists to eat a balanced meal.

Selection Tips

1. Because many of these foods are concentrated sources of carbohydrate and fat, the portion sizes are often very small.
2. Always check Nutrition Facts on the label. It will be your most accurate source of information.
3. Many fat-free or reduced-fat products made with fat replacers contain carbohydrate. When eaten in large amounts, they may need to be counted. Talk with your dietitian to determine how to count these in your meal plan.
4. Look for fat-free salad dressings in smaller amounts on the Free Foods list.

One exchange equals 15 grams carbohydrate,
or 1 starch, or 1 fruit, or 1 milk.

Food	Serving Size	Exchanges per Serving
Angel food cake, unfrosted	¹/₁₂ cake	2 carbohydrates
Brownie, small unfrosted	2-in square	1 carbohydrate, 1 fat
Cake, unfrosted	2-in square	1 carbohydrate, 1 fat
Cake frosted	2-in square	2 carbohydrates, 1 fat
Cookie, fat-free	2 small	1 carbohydrate
Cookie or sandwich cookie with creme filling	2 small	1 carbohydrate, 1 fat
Cupcake, frosted	1 small	2 carbohydrates, 1 fat
Cranberry sauce, jellied	¹/₄ cup	2 carbohydrates
Doughnut, plain cake	1 medium (1½ oz)	1½ carbohydrates, 2 fats
Doughnut, glazed	3¾ in across (2 oz)	2 carbohydrates, 2 fats
Fruit juice bars, frozen, 100% juice	1 bar (3 oz)	1 carbohydrate
Fruit snacks, chewy (pureed fruit concentrate)	1 roll (¾ oz)	1 carbohydrate
Fruit spreads, 100% fruit	1 Tbsp	1 carbohydrate
Gelatin, regular	½ cup	1 carbohydrate
Gingersnaps	3	1 carbohydrate
Granola bar	1 bar	1 carbohydrate, 1 fat
Granola bar, fat-free	1 bar	2 carbohydrates
Hummus	¹/₃ cup	1 carbohydrate, 1 fat
Ice cream	½ cup	1 carbohydrate, 2 fats
Ice cream, light	½ cup	1 carbohydrate, 1 fat
Ice cream, fat-free, no sugar added	½ cup	1 carbohydrate
Jam or jelly, regular	1 Tbsp	1 carbohydrate
Milk, chocolate, whole	1 cup	2 carbohydrates, 1 fat
Pie, fruit, 2 crusts	¹/₆ pie	3 carbohydrates, 2 fats
Pie, pumpkin or custard	¹/₈ pie	1 carbohydrate, 2 fats
Potato chips	12–18 (1 oz)	1 carbohydrate, 2 fats
Pudding, regular (made with low-fat milk)	½ cup	2 carbohydrates
Pudding, sugar-free (made with low-fat milk)	½ cup	1 carbohydrate
Salad dressing, fat-free*	¹/₄ cup	1 carbohydrate
Sherbert, sorbet	½ cup	2 carbohydrates
Spaghetti or pasta sauce, canned*	½ cup	1 carbohydrate, 1 fat

*400 mg or more sodium per exchange.

Sweet roll or danish . . . . 1 (2½ oz) . . . . 2½ carbohydrates, 2 fats
Syrup, light. . . . . 2 Tbsp . . . . 1 carbohydrate
Syrup, regular. . . . . 1 Tbsp . . . . 1 carbohydrate
Syrup, regular. . . . . ¼ cup . . . . 4 carbohydrates
Tortilla chips. . . . . 6–12 (1 oz). . . . . . . 1 carbohydrate, 2 fats
Yogurt, frozen, low-fat,
    fat-free . . . . ⅓ cup . . . . 1 carbohydrate, 0–1 fat
Yogurt, frozen, fat-free,
    no sugar added . . . . ½ cup . . . . 1 carbohydrate
Yogurt, low-fat with fruit . . . . . 1 cup . . . . 3 carbohydrates, 0–1 fat
Vanilla wafers. . . . . 5. . . . . 1 carbohydrate, 1 fat

VEGETABLE LIST

Vegetables that contain small amounts of carbohydrates and calories are on this list. Vegetables contain important nutrients. Try to eat at least two or three vegetable choices each day. In general, one vegetable exchange is:

- ½ cup of cooked vegetables or vegetable juice
- 1 cup of raw vegetables

If you eat one to two vegetable choices at a meal or snack, you do not have to count the calories or carbohydrates because they contain small amounts of these nutrients.

Nutrition Tips

1. Fresh and frozen vegetables have less added salt than canned vegetables. Drain and rinse canned vegetables if you want to remove some salt.
2. Choose more dark green and dark yellow vegetables, such as spinach, broccoli, romaine, carrots, chilies, and peppers.
3. Broccoli, brussels sprouts, cauliflower, greens, pepper, spinach, and tomatoes are good sources of vitamin C.
4. Vegetables contain 1 to 4 grams of fiber per serving.

Selection Tips

1. A 1-cup portion of broccoli is a portion about the size of a light bulb.
2. Tomato sauce is different from spaghetti sauce, which is on the Other Carbohydrates list.
3. Canned vegetables and juices are available without added salt.

4. If you eat more than 4 cups of raw vegetables or 2 cups of cooked vegetables at one meal, count them as 1 carbohydrate choice.
5. Starchy vegetables such as corn, peas, winter squash, and potatoes that contain larger amounts of calories and carbohydrates are on the Starch list.

**One vegetable exchange equals 5 grams carbohydrate,
2 grams protein, 0 grams fat, and 25 calories.**

Vegetables

Artichoke
Artichoke hearts
Asparagus
Beans (green, wax, Italian)
Bean sprouts
Beets
Broccoli
Brussels sprouts
Cabbage
Carrots
Cauliflower
Celery
Cucumber
Eggplant
Green onions or scallions
Greens (collard, kale, mustard, turnip)
Kohlrabi
Leeks
Mixed vegetables (without corn, peas, or pasta)

Mushrooms
Okra
Onions
Pea pods
Peppers (all varieties)
Radishes
Salad greens (endive, escarole, lettuce, romaine, spinach)
Sauerkraut*
Spinach
Summer squash
Tomato
Tomatoes, canned
Tomato sauce*
Tomato/vegetable juice*
Turnips
Water chestnuts
Watercress
Zucchini

MEAT AND MEAT SUBSTITUTES LIST

Meat and meat substitutes that contain both protein and fat are on this list. In general, one meat exchange is:

- 1 oz meat, fish, poultry, or cheese
- ½ cup dried beans

Based on the amount of fat they contain, meats are divided into very lean, lean, medium-fat, and high-fat lists. This is done so you can see which ones contain the least amount of fat. One ounce (one exchange) of each of these includes:

---

*400 mg or more sodium per exchange.

	Carbohydrate (g)	Protein (g)	Fat (g)	Calories
Very Lean	0	7	0–1	35
Lean	0	7	3	35
Medium-fat	0	7	5	75
High-fat	0	7	8	100

Nutrition Tips

1. Choose very lean and lean meat choices whenever possible. Items from the high-fat group are high in saturated fat, cholesterol, and calories and can raise blood cholesterol levels.
2. Meats do not have any fiber.
3. Dried beans, peas, and lentils are good sources of fiber.
4. Some processed meats, seafood, and soy products may contain carbohydrate when consumed in large amounts. Check the Nutrition Facts on the label to see if the amount is close to 15 grams. If so, count it as a carbohydrate choice as well as a meat choice.

Selection Tips

1. Weigh meat after cooking and removing bones and fat. Four ounces of raw meat is equal to 3 ounces of cooked meat. Some examples of meat portions are:
   - 1 ounce cheese = 1 meat choice and is about the size of a 1-inch cube
   - 2 ounces meat = 2 meat choices, such as
     - 1 small chicken leg or thigh
     - ½ cup cottage cheese or tuna
   - 3 ounces meat = 3 meat choices and is about the size of a deck of cards, such as
     - 1 medium pork chop
     - 1 small hamburger
     - ½ of a whole chicken breast
     - 1 unbreaded fish fillet
2. Limit your choices from the high-fat group to three times per week or less.
3. Most grocery stores stock Select and Choice grades of meat. Select grades of meat are the leanest meats. Choice grades contain a moderate amount of fat, and Prime cuts of meat have the highest amount of fat. Restaurants usually serve Prime cuts of meat.
4. "Hamburger" may contain added seasoning and fat, but ground beef does not.

5. Read labels to find products that are low in fat and cholesterol (5 grams or less of fat per serving).
6. Dried beans, peas, and lentils are also found on the Starch list.
7. Peanut butter, in smaller amounts, is also found on the Fat list.
8. Bacon, in smaller amounts, is also found on the Fat list.

Meal Planning Tips

1. Bake, roast, broil, grill, poach, steam, or boil these foods rather than frying.
2. Place meat on a rack so the fat will drain off during cooking.
3. Use a nonstick spray and a nonstick pan to brown or fry foods.
4. Trim off visible fat before or after cooking.
5. If you add flour, bread crumbs, coating mixes, fat, or marinades when cooking, ask your dietitian how to count it in your meal plan.

Very Lean Meat and Substitutes List

One exchange equals 0 grams carbohydrate, 7 grams protein, 0–1 grams fat, and 35 calories.

One very lean meat exchange is equal to one of the following items.

Poultry: Chicken or turkey (white meat, no skin), Cornish hen (no skin) . . . . 1 oz
Fish: Fresh or frozen cod, flounder, haddock, halibut, trout; tuna (fresh or canned in water) . . . . 1 oz
Shellfish: Clams, crab, lobster, scallops, shrimp, imitation shellfish . . . . . . 1 oz
Game: Duck or pheasant (no skin), venison, buffalo, ostrich . . . . 1 oz
Cheese with 1 gram or less of fat per ounce:
    Nonfat or low-fat cottage cheese. . . . . ¼ cup
    Fat-free cheese . . . . 1 oz
Other: Processed sandwich meats with 1 gram or less fat per ounce, such as deli thin, shaved meats, chipped beef,* turkey ham . . . . 1 oz
    Egg whites. 2
    Egg substitutes, plain . . . . ¼ cup
    Hot dogs with 1 gram or less fat per ounce* . . . . 1 oz
    Kidney (high in cholesterol) . . . . 1 oz
    Sausage with 1 gram or less fat per ounce. . . . . 1 oz

Count as one very lean meat and one starch exchange:
Dried beans, peas, lentils (cooked) . . . . ½ cup

---

*400 mg or more sodium per exchange.

Lean Meat and Substitutes List

**One exchange equals 0 grams carbohydrate, 7 grams protein,
3 grams fat, and 55 calories.**

One lean meat exchange is equal to any one of the following items:

Beef: USDA Select or Choice grades of lean beef trimmed of fat,
    such as round, sirloin, and flank steak; tenderloin; roast
    (rib, chuck, rump); steak (T-bone, porterhouse, cubed), ground round . . . 1 oz
Pork: Lean pork, such as fresh ham; canned, cured, or
    boiled ham; Canadian bacon*; tenderloin, center loin chop . . . . 1 oz
Lamb: Roast, chop, leg . . . . 1 oz
Veal: Lean chop, roast . . . . 1 oz
Poultry: Chicken, turkey (dark meat, no skin), chicken white meat
    (with skin), domestic duck or goose (well-drained of fat, no skin) . . . . . . 1 oz
Fish:
    Herring (uncreamed or smoked) . . . . 1 oz
    Oysters. . . . . 6 medium
    Salmon (fresh or canned), catfish . . . . 1 oz
    Sardines (canned). . . . . 2 medium
    Tuna (canned in oil, drained). . . . . 1 oz
Game: Goose (no skin), rabbit . . . . 1 oz
Cheese:
    4.5%-fat cottage cheese . . . . ¼ cup
    Grated Parmesan . . . . 2 Tbsp
    Cheeses with 3 grams or less fat per ounce . . . . 1 oz
Other:
Hot dogs with 3 grams or less fat per ounce* . . . . 1½ oz
Processed sandwich meat with 3 grams or less fat per ounce,
    such as turkey pastrami or kielbasa . . . . 1 oz
Liver, heart (high in cholesterol) . . . . 1 oz

Medium-Fat Meat and Substitutes List

**One exchange equals 0 grams carbohydrate, 7 grams protein,
5 grams fat, and 75 calories.**

One medium-fat meat exchange is equal to any one of the following items:

Beef: Most beef products fall into this category (ground beef,
    meatloaf, corned beef, short ribs, Prime grades of meat trimmed of fat,
    such as prime rib) . . . . 1 oz

---

*400 mg or more sodium per exchange.

Pork: Top loin, chop, Boston butt, cutlet . . . . 1 oz
Lamb: Rib roast, ground . . . . 1 oz
Veal: Cutlet (ground or cubed, unbreaded) . . . . 1 oz
Poultry: Chicken dark meat (with skin), ground turkey or ground chicken, fried
    chicken (with skin) . . . . 1 oz
Fish: Any fried fish product. . . . . 1 oz
Cheese with 5 grams or less fat per ounce:
    Feta. . . . . 1 oz
    Mozzarella . . . . 1 oz
    Ricotta . . . . ¼ cup (2 oz)
Other:
    Egg (high in cholesterol, limit to 3 per week) 1
    Sausage with 5 grams or less fat per ounce . . . . 1 oz
    Soy milk. . . . . 1 cup
    Tempeh . . . . ¼ cup
    Tofu . . . . 4 oz or ½ cup

High-Fat Meat and Substitutes List

**One exchange equals 0 grams carbohydrate, 7 grams protein,
8 grams fat, and 100 calories.**

Remember these items are high in saturated fat, cholesterol, and calories and may raise blood cholesterol levels if eaten on a regular basis. One high-fat meat exchange is equal to any one of the following items:

Pork: Spareribs, ground pork, pork sausage. . . . . 1 oz
Cheese: All regular cheeses, such as American,* cheddar,
    Monterey Jack, Swiss . . . . 1 oz
Other: Processed sandwich meats with 8 grams or less fat per ounce, such as
    bologna, pimento loaf, salami . . . . 1 oz
Sausage, such as bratwurst, Italian, knockwurst, Polish, smoked . . . . 1 oz
Hot dog (turkey or chicken)* 1 (10/lb)
Bacon . . . . 3 slices (20 slices/lb)

Count as one high-fat meat plus one fat exchange:

Hot dog (beef, pork, or combination)* 1 (10/lb)
Peanut butter (contains unsaturated fat). . . . . 2 Tbsp

---

*400 mg or more sodium per exchange.

FAT LIST

Fats are divided into three groups, based on the main type of fat they contain: monounsaturated, polyunsaturated, and saturated. Small amounts of monounsaturated and polyunsaturated fats in the foods we eat are linked with good health benefits. Saturated fats are linked with heart disease and cancer. In general, one fat exchange is:

- 1 teaspoon of regular margarine or vegetable oil
- 1 tablespoon of regular salad dressings

Nutrition Tips

1. All fats are high in calories. Limit serving sizes for good nutrition and health.
2. Nuts and seeds contain small amounts of fiber, protein, and magnesium.
3. If blood pressure is a concern, choose fats in the unsalted form to help lower sodium intake, such as unsalted peanuts.

Selection Tips

1. Check the Nutrition Facts on food labels for serving sizes. One fat exchange is based on a serving size containing 5 grams of fat.
2. When selecting regular margarine, choose those with liquid vegetable oil as the first ingredient. Soft margarines are not as saturated as stick margarines. Soft margarines are healthier choices. Avoid those listing hydrogenated or partially hydrogenated fat as the first ingredient.
3. When selecting low-fat margarines, look for liquid vegetable oil as the second ingredient. Water is usually the first ingredient.
4. When used in smaller amounts, bacon and peanut butter are counted as fat choices. When used in larger amounts, they are counted as high-fat meat choices.
5. Fat-free salad dressings are on the Other Carbohydrates list and the Free Foods list.
6. See the Free Foods list for nondairy coffee creamers, whipped topping, and fat-free products, such as margarines, salad dressings, mayonnaise, sour cream, cream cheese, and nonstick cooking spray.

Monounsaturated Fats List

One fat exchange equals 5 grams fat and 45 calories.

Avocado, medium . . . . ⅛ (1 oz)
Oil (canola, olive, peanut) . . . . 1 tsp

Olives: ripe (black) . . . . 8 large
    green, stuffed* . . . . 10 large
Nuts:
    almonds, cashews. . . . . 6 nuts
    mixed (50% peanuts) . . . . 6 nuts
    peanuts. . . . . 10 nuts
    pecans. . . . . 4 halves
Peanut butter, smooth or crunchy . . . . 2 tsp
Sesame seeds . . . . 1 Tbsp
Tahini paste . . . . 2 tsp

Polyunsaturated Fats List

One fat exchange equals 5 grams fat and 45 calories.

Margarine: stick, tub, or squeeze . . . . 1 tsp
    lower-fat (30% to 50% vegetable oil). . . . . 1 Tbsp
Mayonnaise: regular. . . . . 1 tsp
    reduced-fat . . . . 1 Tbsp
Nuts: walnuts, English . . . . 4 halves
Oil (corn, safflower, soybean). . . . . 1 tsp
Salad dressing: regular* . . . . 1 Tbsp
    reduced-fat . . . . 2 Tbsp
Miracle Whip Salad Dressing®: regular . . . . 2 tsp
    reduced-fat . . . . 1 Tbsp
Seeds: pumpkin, sunflower . . . . 1 Tbsp

Saturated Fats List**

One fat exchange equals 5 grams fat and 45 calories.

Bacon, cooked . . . . 1 slice (20 slices/lb)
Bacon, grease. . . . . 1 tsp
Butter: stick . . . . 1 tsp
    whipped . . . . 1 tsp
    reduced-fat . . . . 1 Tbsp
Chitterlings, boiled. . . . . 2 Tbsp (½ oz)
Coconut, sweetened, shredded. . . . . 2 Tbsp
Cream, half and half . . . . 2 Tbsp

---

*400 mg or more sodium per exchange.
**Saturated fats can raise blood cholesterol levels.

Cream cheese: regular . . . . 1 Tbsp (½ oz)
    reduced-fat . . . . 2 Tbsp (1 oz)
Fatback or salt pork, see below[†]
Shortening or lard . . . . 1 tsp
Sour cream: regular. . . . . 2 Tbsp
    reduced-fat . . . . 3 Tbsp

FREE FOODS LIST

A free food is any food or drink that contains less than 20 calories or less than 5 grams of carbohydrate per serving. Foods with a serving size listed should be limited to three servings per day. Be sure to spread them out throughout the day. If you eat all three servings at one time, it could affect your blood glucose level. Foods listed without a serving size can be eaten as often as you like.

Fat-Free or Reduced-Fat Foods

Cream cheese, fat-free. . . . . 1 Tbsp
Creamers, nondairy, liquid . . . . 1 Tbsp
Creamers, nondairy, powdered . . . . 2 tsp
Mayonnaise, fat-free . . . . 1 Tbsp
Mayonnaise, reduced-fat . . . . 1 tsp
Margarine, fat-free . . . . 4 Tbsp
Margarine, reduced-fat. . . . . 1 tsp
Miracle Whip®, nonfat . . . . 1 Tbsp
Miracle Whip®, reduced-fat . . . . 1 tsp
Nonstick cooking spray
Salad dressing, fat-free . . . . 1 Tbsp
Salad dressing, fat-free, Italian . . . . 2 Tbsp
Salsa . . . . ¼ cup
Sour cream, fat-free, reduced-fat. . . . . 1 Tbsp
Whipped topping, regular or light . . . . 2 Tbsp

Sugar-Free or Low-Sugar Foods

Candy, hard, sugar-free . . . . 1 candy
Gelatin dessert, sugar-free
Gelatin, unflavored

[†]Use a piece 1 in × 1 in × ¼ in if you plan to eat fatback cooked with vegetables. Use a piece 2 in × 1 in × ½ in when eating only the vegetables with the fatback removed.

Gum, sugar-free
Jam or jelly, low-sugar or light . . . . 2 tsp
Sugar substitutes[†]
Syrup, sugar-free . . . . 2 Tbsp

Drinks

Bouillon, broth, consommé*
Bouillon or broth, low-sodium
Carbonated or mineral water
Cocoa powder, unsweetened . . . . 1 Tbsp
Coffee
Club soda
Diet soft drinks, sugar-free
Drink mixes, sugar-free
Tea
Tonic water, sugar-free

Condiments

Catsup . . . . 1 Tbsp
Horseradish
Lemon juice
Lime juice
Mustard
Pickles, dill* . . . . 1½ large
Soy sauce, regular or light*
Taco sauce . . . . 1 Tbsp
Vinegar

Seasonings

Be careful with seasonings that contain sodium or are salts, such as garlic or celery salt, and lemon pepper.

---

*400 mg or more sodium per choice.

[†]Sugar substitutes, alternatives, or replacements that are approved by the Food and Drug Administration (FDA) are safe to use. Common brand names include: Equal® (aspartame); Sprinkle® (saccharin); Sweet One® (acesulfame K); Sweet-10® (saccharin); Sugar Twin® (saccharin); Sweet 'n Low® (saccharin).

Flavoring extracts
Garlic
Herbs, fresh or dried
Pimiento
Spices
Tabasco® or hot pepper sauce
Wine, used in cooking
Worcestershire sauce

COMBINATION FOODS LIST

Many of the foods we eat are mixed together in various combinations. These combination foods do not fit into any one exchange list. Often it is hard to tell what is in a casserole dish or prepared food item. This is a list of exchanges for some typical combination foods. This list will help you fit these foods into your meal plan. Ask your dietitian for information about any other combination foods you would like to eat.

Food Entrees	Serving Size	Exchanges per Serving
Tuna noodle casserole, lasagna, spaghetti with meatballs, chili with beans, macaroni and cheese**	1 cup (8 oz)	2 carbohydrates, 2 medium-fat meats
Chow mein (without noodles or rice)	2 cups (16 oz)	1 carbohydrate, 2 lean meats
Pizza, cheese, thin crust**	¼ of 10 in (5 oz)	2 carbohydrates, 2 medium-fat meats, 1 fat
Pizza, meat topping, thin crust**	¼ of 10 in (5 oz)	2 carbohydrates, 2 medium-fat meats, 2 fats
Pot pie*	1 (7 oz)	2 carbohydrates,1 medium-fat meat, 4 fats

Frozen Entrees

Salisbury steak with gravy, mashed potato*	1 (11 oz)	2 carbohydrates, 3 medium-fat meats, 3–4 fats

---

* 400 mg or more sodium per choice.
** 400 mg or more of sodium per exchange.

Turkey with gravy,
    mashed potato, dressing**. . 1 (11 oz). . . . . 2 carbohydrates, 2 medium-fat
                                                               meats, 2 fats
Entree with less than
    300 calories* . . . . 1 (8 oz). . . . . 2 carbohydrates, 3 lean meats

Soups

Bean*. 1 cup. . . . . 1 carbohydrate, 1 very lean meat
Cream (made with water)* . . . . 1 cup (8 oz) . . . . 1 carbohydrate, 1 fat
Split pea (made with water)* . . ½ cup (4 oz) . . . . 1 carbohydrate
Tomato (made with water)* . . . 1 cup (8 oz) . . . . 1 carbohydrate
Vegetable beef, chicken noodle,
    or other broth-type* . . . . 1 cup (8 oz) . . . . 1 carbohydrate

FAST FOODS LIST

Food	Serving Size	Exchanges per Serving
Burritos with beef** . . . . . . 2.		4 carbohydrates, 2 medium-fat meats, 2 fats
Chicken nuggets**. . . . . 6.		1 carbohydrate, 2 medium-fat meats, 1 fat
Chicken breast and wing, breaded and fried**. . . . . 1 each.		1 carbohydrate, 4 medium-fat meats, 2 fats
Fish sandwich/tartar sauce**. . . . . 1.		3 carbohydrates, 1 medium-fat meat, 3 fats
French fries, thin . . . . 20–25.		2 carbohydrates, 2 fats
Hamburger, regular . . . . 1.		2 carbohydrates, 2 medium-fat meats
Hamburger, large** . . . . 1.		2 carbohydrates, 3 medium-fat meats, 1 fat
Hot dog with bun**. . . . . . . 1.		1 carbohydrate, 1 high-fat meat, 1 fat
Individual pan pizza**. . . . . 1.		5 carbohydrates, 3 medium-fat meats, 3 fats
Soft-serve cone . . . . 1 medium.		2 carbohydrates, 1 fat
Submarine sandwich** . . . . 1 sub (6 in.) . . .		3 carbohydrates, 1 vegetable, 2 medium-fat meats, 1 fat
Taco, hard shell* . . . . 1 (6 oz).		2 carbohydrates, 2 medium-fat meats, 2 fats
Taco, soft shell*. . . . . 1 (3 oz).		1 carbohydrate, 1 medium-fat meat, 1 fat

* 400 mg or more sodium per exchange.
** 400 mg or more of sodium per serving.
Note: Ask your fast-food restaurant for nutrition information about your favorite fast foods.

Ethnic Food Exchanges

Food	Serving	Food Exchange
Mexican Foods		
Burrito, bean	1 small	2 starch
	1 large	1 medium-fat meat, 3 starch, 2 fat
Burrito, meat (beef)	1 small	1 starch, 1 medium-fat meat
	1 large	2½ starch, 3 medium-fat meat, 1 fat
Chili	1 cup	2 starch, 2 medium-fat meat, 1 fat
Chili sauce	2 tsp	⅓ fruit
Corn chips	1 oz (1 cup)	1 starch, 2 fat
Enchilada: meat or cheese	1 small (6″ tortilla)	1 medium-fat meat
Refried beans	½ cup	1 starch, 1 medium-fat meat
Spanish rice	1 cup	2 starch, 1 fat
Spanish sauce	½ cup	⅓ fruit, 1 fat
Tamale with sauce	1	1 starch, 1 medium-fat meat
Tortilla/taco shell	6″ diameter	1 starch
Taco (meat, cheese, lettuce, tomato)	1	1 starch, 2 medium-fat meat
Tostada		
with refried beans	1 small	2 starch
with meat	1 small	1 starch, 1 high-fat meat

Source: Data from *McCance and Widdowson's The Composition of Foods* by A.A. Paul and D.A. Southgate, Elsevier Science Publishing Company, Inc., © 1985 and *Food Values of Portions Commonly Used* by J.A.T. Pennington and H.N. Church, Harper & Row Publishers, Copyright © 1985.

Food	Serving	Food Exchange
Chinese Foods		
Egg flower, soup	1 cup	½ medium-fat meat
Fried rice		
(rice, meat, eggs, onions)	1 cup	1½ starch, ½ medium-fat meat
Fortune cookies	1	½ starch or ½ fruit
Egg roll	1	½ starch, 1 vegetable
Chow mein	1 cup	1 starch, 1 medium-fat meat, 1 vegetable
Sukiyaki	1 cup	3 medium-fat meat, 1 fat
Tofu	2 oz	½ medium-fat meat
Chop suey	1 cup	2 medium-fat meat, 1 vegetable
Pepper steak	1 cup	1 starch, 3 medium-fat meat, 1 vegetable
Chow mein noodles	½ cup	1 starch, 1 fat
Egg foo young	1	1 vegetable, 2 medium-fat meat, 2 fat
East Indian Foods		
Alu Mattar		
(curried potatoes and peas)	1 cup	1 vegetable, 1½ starch, 3 fat
Alu Paratha	6″ diameter	2½ starch, 6 fat
(flat whole wheat bread with spiced potato filling)		
Chana Dal (curried chick peas)	½ cup	2 medium-fat meat
Kheema do Pyaza	1 cup	2 vegetable, 3 lean meat, 3 fat
(curried ground lamb with onions)		
Kofta	3 balls (approx. 1½″ diameter)	3 high-fat meat, 4 fat
Machli aur tomatar		
(curried halibut)	3 oz fish	½ vegetable, 3 lean meat, 1½ fat
Masala dosai (crepe-like pancake with spiced potato filling)	1	2 starch, 4 fat
Chicken curry	3 oz chicken	½ vegetable, 3 lean meat, 2 fat
Samosas	1 large or 3 small (potato filling)	1 starch, 2 fat
(deep-fried filled pastries)	1 large or 3 small (lamb filling)	1 starch, ½ lean meat, 2½ fat

Food	Serving	Food Exchange
Italian Foods		
Vermicelli soup	1 cup	1 starch
Minestrone soup	1 cup	1 starch, 1 fat
Pasta, cooked	½ cup	1 medium-fat meat
Italian ham (Prosciutto)	1 oz	1 medium-fat meat
Meatballs	1 oz	1 medium-fat meat
Chicken cacciatore	3 oz chicken with sauce	3 lean meat, 1 vegetable, 1 fat
Eggplant parmesan	1 cup	2 medium-fat meat, 2 vegetable, 1 starch, 1½ fat
Veal parmesan	1 cutlet (4 oz)	1 starch, 4 medium-fat meat, 1 vegetable, 1 fat
Italian spaghetti	1 cup	2 starch, 2 vegetable, 2 medium-fat meat
Lasagna	1 (3″ × 4″) serving	1 starch, 1 vegetable, 2½ medium-fat meat
Manicotti	1 shell	1½ starch, 1 vegetable, 3 medium-fat meat, 2 fat
Pizza with cheese, sausage, pepperoni	¼ of 16 oz pizza	2 starch, 1 vegetable, 2 medium-fat meat, 1 fat
Ravioli		2 starch, 1 vegetable,
with cheese	1 cup	1 medium-fat meat, 1 fat
with beef	1 cup	2 starch, 1 vegetable, 1 medium-fat meat, 1 fat
Jewish Foods		
Bagel	½	1 starch
Bialy	1	1 starch
Challah	1 slice	1 starch
Matzo, 6″ diameter	1	1 starch
Matzo, crackers	7 (1½″ square each)	1 starch
Potato latkes (calculate the fat used in cooking)	½ cup	1 starch
Kippered herring	1 oz	1 lean meat
Pickle herring	1 oz	1 lean meat
Smoked salmon (lox)	1 oz	1 lean meat
Corned beef	1 oz	1 high-fat meat
Chopped liver	1 oz	1 high-fat meat

CHAPTER 7

Nutrition Counseling in Treatment of Renal Disease

CHAPTER OBJECTIVES

1. Identify factors that lead to inappropriate eating behaviors associated with protein-modified regimens.

2. Identify specific nutrients that should be emphasized in assessing a baseline eating pattern before providing dietary instruction.

3. Identify strategies to treat inappropriate eating behaviors associated with low-protein patterns.

4. Generate strategies to facilitate problem solving for clients who are following a protein-modified eating pattern.

5. Recommend dietary adherence tools for clients on protein-modified eating patterns.

This chapter guides the nutrition counselor who is working on potential prevention of dialysis or predialysis therapy for the person diagnosed with chronic renal insufficiency. Current facts and theories are discussed as researched by some of the foremost nephrologists in the world. The focus of this chapter is on the outpatient in a predialysis state.

THEORIES AND FACTS ABOUT NUTRITION AND CHRONIC RENAL FAILURE

Many nephrologists recommend low-protein diets as a means of halting deterioration of renal function. Protein restriction and control of blood pressure delay the progression of renal disease in laboratory animals.[1-3] Most studies in humans[4–10] have suggested that a restriction of dietary protein is beneficial, especially in patients with advanced renal disease,[11,12] but some of these studies were inconclusive because of deficiencies in their design or because changes in renal function were assessed only by measurements of serum creatinine, which may be affected by diet.

In 1978 Ibels and colleagues theorized that hyperphosphatemia was responsible for renal function deterioration,[13] and in 1982 Brenner and colleagues developed the glomerular hyperfiltration theory.[14] The Brenner hypothesis suggests that a low-protein diet halts the progression of chronic renal insufficiency in two ways: (1) by preventing the increase in glomerular plasma flow and (2) by preventing high capillary pressures. Accompanying proteinuria and structural alterations of epithelial cells seem to be less severe when predialysis persons are placed on low-protein diets. In the absence of a low-protein diet, glomerular hyperfiltration continues.[15,16] As the function of sclerosing glomeruli is lost, less severely affected glomeruli undergo further compensatory hyperfiltration with subsequent injury. This process favors progression of kidney damage and eventual total loss of glomerular and renal function.

To provide data beyond the above studies, the National Institutes of Health funded the Modification of Diet in Renal Disease (MDRD) Study that included two randomized, multicenter trials involving a total of 840 patients with various chronic renal diseases. It tested two hypotheses: (1) that two interventions—a reduction in dietary protein and phosphorus intake and the maintenance of blood pressure at a level below that usually recommended[17]—retard the progression of renal disease; and (2) that these interventions are safe and acceptable to patients for long-term use.[18–20]

In the MDRD Study, clients with moderate renal insufficiency experienced a slower decline in renal function four months after the introduction of the low-protein diet when compared with clients on a moderate-protein diet. This suggests the small benefit of low-protein diet in slowing the progression of renal disease in patients with moderate renal insufficiency. Among clients with more severe renal insufficiency, a very-low-protein diet, as compared with a low-protein diet, did not significantly slow the progression of renal disease.[21] Following the MDRD study, a moderately reduced protein intake has been recommended for clients with diabetes and pre-end stage disease. The American Diabetes Association recommends that clients with diabetic nephropathy restrict intake to ~0.8 grams of protein per kilogram body weight per day.[22] For clients with pre-end stage renal disease, the Renal Dietitians Dietetic Practice Group of the American Dietetic Association prescribes 0.6 to 0.8 grams of protein per kilogram body weight per day.[23]

The principle of reducing dietary protein and maximizing the biological quality of protein intake in predialysis clients has been generally accepted for decades.

These measures increase the efficiency with which nitrogen is used for synthesis and reduce the ingested quantities of total nitrogen, nonprotein nitrogen, potassium, phosphorus, and sulfur. This results in a reduction of the requirements for excretion of urea, uric acid, potassium, phosphate, sulfate, and acid and decreases the tendency of such persons to develop azotemia, acidosis, hyperkalemia, and hyperphosphatemia with their consequences.

The levels of dietary protein recommended for persons suffering from chronic renal failure to maintain nitrogen balance are controversial. Unlike persons with normal renal function, a person with renal insufficiency requires more protein because of the altered metabolism associated with uremia, which may promote protein catabolism. Most obvious are proteinuria and occult gastrointestinal bleeding. These problems increase protein requirements not only because blood proteins may not be completely reabsorbed, but also because they cannot be resynthesized with complete efficiency. Hormonal disturbances such as hyperglucagonemia and carbohydrate intolerance in uremic persons may increase protein requirements.[24,25] On the other hand, the reduced rates of excretion of nonurea urinary nitrogen components mentioned above reduce nitrogen requirements. Even though urea nitrogen reutilization is questioned, nitrogen balance can be maintained in some uremic persons on very low intakes.[26]

The estimated safe allowance for protein intake in persons without proteinuria or occult blood loss has been controversial. The many studies that have addressed this issue were reviewed by the Joint Food and Agriculture Organization/World Health Organization Expert Committee on energy and protein requirements, which recommended 0.60 gram of protein per kilogram of body weight to maintain positive nitrogen balance.[27]

The consensus among nephrologists seems to be that 0.57 gram per kilogram of protein (40 grams per 70 kilograms), predominantly of high biological value, is adequate to maintain nitrogen balance in the absence of substantial proteinuria or occult blood loss.[28] Researchers have found that nitrogen balance in persons with chronic renal failure can be maintained by giving 0.55 to 0.60 gram of protein per kilogram per day and a minimum of 35 kilocalories per kilogram per day.[29] In this study, positive nitrogen balance depended directly on caloric intake. Use of protein in uremia also depends, in part, on the biological value of protein. The literature indicates a range for intake of protein of high biological value from 70 to 75 percent.[30]

The role of serum phosphate in the progression of renal disease is also controversial.[31,32] Walser has found excellent clinical results with dietary phosphorus restrictions in persons with modest protein restrictions (40 grams).[33] Phosphorus was reduced by restricting intake of milk, milk products, cheese, cola beverages, and instant powdered beverages to bring the level of phosphorus down to approximately 600 milligrams, approximately one-half the usual daily intake. The

MDRD Study also describes a phosphorus restriction as a part of the dietary prescription.[34]

Early in the course of renal failure, intestinal calcium absorption is reduced before serum vitamin D levels fall.[35] Later vitamin D deficiency further aggravates this problem. Both azotemia and acidosis independently increase renal excretion of calcium.[36] Calcium balance is usually negative in uremic persons unless calcium supplementation is prescribed.[37]

Nutritionists should be aware of sodium, potassium, and acid-base balance. Persons with renal insufficiency suffer from uremic acidosis, a condition caused by accumulation of phosphate, sulfate, and organic acids, impaired ammonia excretion, and renal bicarbonate wastage. The degree of renal bicarbonate wastage is variable; therefore, the requirement for sodium bicarbonate also varies—from 0 to 14 milliequivalents per kilogram of body weight.

Decreasing dietary protein results in some improvement in acidosis because the major source of acid in acid-ash diets is dietary protein (particularly its sulfur content). Treating acidosis is important for several reasons:

- prevention of dissolution of bone salt
- reduction in symptoms associated with decreased pH (which usually are not apparent until serum bicarbonate is 16 millimoles or lower)
- prevention of the protein catabolic effect of acidosis (An alkaline-ash diet, comprised mostly of fruits and vegetables, may help but is rather monotonous.)

Persons with chronic uremia differ markedly from normal persons in their ability to vary renal excretion of sodium. They excrete a large, relatively fixed fraction of filtered sodium.

Various techniques have been developed to determine an optimal level of dietary sodium in a given client. Generally the sodium bicarbonate requirement should be assessed first, because it affects the level of sodium chloride to be given. Ideally 24-hour sodium output should be determined first. Providing an amount of sodium chloride equal to this quantity (in milliequivalents) minus the sodium bicarbonate intake will then maintain sodium balance.

Diuretics are indicated in most cases of moderate or severe renal failure.[38] When the diuretic is administered chronically, the same extracellular fluid volume may be maintained with higher salt intake, making the diet less difficult to follow.

Potassium balance in the chronic uremic client is less of a problem than sodium balance. However, hyperkalemia is quite common in more advanced stages of renal disease. Modest reductions in high-potassium foods such as tomatoes, bananas, potatoes, and oranges can be effective. A small number of persons with renal failure may exhibit a tendency toward hypokalemia. Increasing foods high in potassium and or potassium supplements is recommended for these individuals.

A few clients may develop hyponatremia, especially those whose intake of sodium is severely restricted or those with congestive heart failure. Water intake must be restricted to correct and prevent hyponatremia.

Vitamin and mineral levels must be assessed in the chronically uremic client. Supplements of B vitamins and vitamin C are indicated. Serum levels of vitamin A and of retinol-binding protein are commonly elevated.[39] Because these substances are normally cleared by the kidney, vitamin A should not be given. Uremic persons have low concentrations of zinc in their plasma leucocytes and hair, so supplementation is recommended.[40]

In summary, the client with chronic renal failure requires careful, consistent nutrition monitoring through blood and urine values. Low-protein, low-phosphorus diets require semimonthly to monthly nutritional monitoring.

RESEARCH ON ADHERENCE TO EATING PATTERNS IN TREATMENT OF RENAL DISEASE

Treatment for chronic renal failure involves major adjustments and stress for clients. Although compliance with renal diets can be easily monitored with laboratory tests, many physiological factors can modify the results of these tests. For persons who are losing weight because calorie intake on low-protein diets tends to be low, loss of muscle mass may contribute to urinary nitrogen, which is used as a marker for dietary compliance. There is much to learn about urinary nitrogen and the possible effect of chronic renal disease on that biological marker. In many cases, very compliant persons whose intake by self-report may look excellent are classified as noncompliant on analysis of urinary nitrogen. Researchers have found that food diaries underestimate dietary intake for a variety of reasons. In one study, subjects believed they were consuming a diet containing 0.6 grams of protein per kilogram of standard body weight based on their food record calculations, but estimated protein intake indicated they consumed approximately 0.8 grams of protein per kilogram of standard body weight.[41] Subject errors in calculating the protein content of food and/or discrepancies between protein values on the patient education materials and computerized database accounted for part of this discrepancy. Researchers in this study note that educating subjects on how to classify foods for protein content and calculate protein intake might have narrowed the difference between self-report records and the biological marker (urinary nitrogen). Nutritionists and physicians should be aware that discrepancies between urinary nitrogen excretion and reported protein intake may reflect factors other than willful noncompliance.

When patients with renal disease were asked which parts of a diet intervention program were most helpful, they indicated self-monitoring and dietitian support.[42] Clients who were satisfied with a low-protein eating pattern at the final visit in the MDRD Study had mean protein intakes closer to their assigned protein goals.[43]

The MDRD Study focused on behavioral dietary interventions and analyzed the factors that contributed to dietary adherence.[44] The dietary program emphasized appropriate food choices that promoted healthful, long-term eating patterns rather than food restrictions. Adherers indicated more favorable attitudes about their eating patterns and perceived themselves as more successful than nonadherers. More frequent telephone contacts were made with nonadherers. Dietitians made telephone calls to solve problems, reinforce strategies discussed during the visit, and provide contact between monthly visits. Results of this study indicate that adherence to low-protein eating patterns requires social support and assistance for replacing energy lost by decrease in protein intake. Adherence did not seem to require ongoing provision of guidelines for reducing protein intake. Adherent patients reported that the eating pattern did not interfere with their ability to socialize. Providing patients with protein-modified products and recipes and samples of products was beneficial in promoting adherence. The frequency of self-monitoring increased with those who were adherent. As many as 51 percent of adherent clients self-monitored on an average of six to seven days per week throughout the two-year period of this study.

INAPPROPRIATE EATING BEHAVIORS

The person with chronic renal insufficiency who is seen as an outpatient requires a great deal of assistance in dietary adherence. The MDRD Study showed that visits during months 1 through 4 lasted for a mean of 183 ± 1 to $116 + 41$ minutes.[45] The regimen for a predialysis client is extremely complicated and requires extra time and assistance from the dietitian. The exchange lists alone can be overwhelming for many clients who have followed other diets in the past. The MDRD Study used protein counting as a means of streamlining the renal diet.[46] A low-calorie diet in principle contrasts directly with the renal diet, so a person who has followed low-calorie diets in the past may find it difficult to readjust to the new principles of the renal diet. For example, on a low-calorie diet, fat and pure carbohydrate foods are discouraged, but on a low-protein diet they are encouraged. With reduction in protein, an increase in calories through fat and carbohydrate is essential. Weight maintenance is important.

A family member who is diabetic may influence a renal client to avoid foods high in simple sugars. The renal client may have difficulty accepting the idea that simple sugars are necessary on a low-protein diet to maintain adequate caloric intake.

Like clients on other restricted eating patterns, clients who have difficulties adhering to low-protein diets must struggle with social pressures that are multiplied by the large number of restrictions. Clients may drop out of social affairs to avoid the embarrassment of having to explain their health problems. "Everything in my life has changed!" is a common remark. Old eating habits are replaced by a constant preoccupation with restriction. The tradition of enjoying all food is replaced by a feeling that meals are never spontaneous but always associated with don'ts. For clients with a protein restriction, eating can become only a means of existence instead of a means of recreation.

On a protein- and phosphorus-restricted diet, usual foods may be replaced by low-protein and low-phosphorus foods that are less moist, have an aftertaste, and are lower in fiber (due to the phosphorus restriction). The result is less enjoyment in taste and texture sensations, and frequently an initial side effect is constipation because of the reduction in fiber. These negative associations with the protein-restricted diet can lead to inappropriate eating behaviors.

ASSESSMENT OF EATING BEHAVIORS

Early assessment of the client with chronic renal insufficiency is crucial to dietary success. Identification of potential problems is important. Because many of these clients suffer from uremic symptoms, signs of depression may be more frequent than in the normal population. Prior to instruction on an involved eating pattern, some clients may require psychological counseling. It is important to look for predictors of adherence, especially in clients for whom the dietary and medication regimens are very complicated. Along with the diet, there are many medications that must be taken daily (for example, multivitamins, calcium, iron, blood pressure regulators).

Identifying the support of others is crucial. Support from a spouse or significant other may signal excellent future adherence. Lack of support may signal poor adherence.

The assessment of the person with renal insufficiency also requires close attention to personal indicators. For example, before instituting a low-protein eating regimen, counselors should identify past dietary behaviors. Has the patient tried without success to follow a low-sodium diet? Good past performance is an indicator of future success with a new eating pattern. Initial assessment might include eliciting a list of reasons the client wants to follow the new eating pattern and take medications. Later, when commitment wanes, a review of the reasons and circumstances in the client's life that have altered commitment can improve adherence.

The nutrition counselor should provide an opportunity for the client to try out behaviors before actually starting a regimen. For example, holding a special event for clients centered around a holiday buffet can give them an opportunity to try some foods they might like to serve during the holiday season. Vegetable fettuccine made with low-protein pasta and nondairy creamer along with black forest cake prepared with low-protein flour and without eggs are examples of festive, low-protein dishes clients may wish to serve.

Careful, detailed assessments of dietary intake should include the protein content of the diet along with other baseline information on dietary phosphorus, potassium, sodium, calcium, and magnesium. Intake assessment might include several diet records (three a month for three months) and diet recalls (once a month for three months). In addition, a food frequency or diet history may be valuable. The questionnaire in Adherence Tool 7–1 can provide valuable information on past eating habits. Once the client is placed on the new eating pattern, Adherence Tool 7–2 might be used to monitor intake.

An assessment of medication-taking habits is also important. Many renal clients have taken blood pressure medications. Potential problems with taking medications at certain times of day may be apparent from a description of past habits.

Before providing information about a new eating pattern, the counselor should assess the client's knowledge of diets. What information does the client presently have concerning dietary exchange patterns? What impact will these patterns have on learning a new dietary exchange list? What basic principles taught in relation to past diets may no longer be true? For example, a client who has followed low-calorie diets in the past may have difficulty switching to a totally new exchange list in which foods are categorized based on protein content rather than calories. The idea of limiting high-carbohydrate, high-fat foods is no longer valid. It is extremely difficult to assure a client that on a low-protein diet it is not only good but mandatory to eat high-carbohydrate, high-fat foods on a daily basis for adequate caloric intake.

Assessment of adherence to a low-protein regimen may involve medication counting, review of urine urea nitrogens, a corresponding estimated protein intake,* and a review of laboratory serum and urine values. Adherence Tool 7–3 includes a worksheet to help calculate percent adherence to medications. Adherence Tool 7–4 is an accompanying list of adherence rates at each visit that serves as a monitoring device for clients and clinicians. Graphs can also be used to track diet adherence (Adherence Tool 7–5). It is extremely important to track serum and urine laboratory values for clients on low-protein eating patterns. The laboratory data can help determine how well the client is adhering to diet and medication. Adherence Tool 7–6 includes space for recording laboratory values and corresponding normal ranges for each chemistry value.

---

*Equation: 6.25 × [Urine Urea Nitrogen + (0.31 × Standard Body Weight) + Urine Protein] = Estimated Protein Intake (grams per kilogram).

If urine protein is greater than 5, add it into this equation. If it is less than 5, set urine protein equal to 0. Standard body weight is rounded to the nearest 10.

TREATMENT STRATEGIES

Problems with low-protein eating patterns fall into the three categories mentioned for other diets: lack of knowledge, forgetfulness, and lack of commitment. As with all dietary regimens, lack of knowledge can be easily remedied. Cueing devices can provide help when forgetting is a problem. Lack of commitment is the most difficult problem to solve.

Strategies To Deal with Lack of Knowledge

Before dealing with problems involving lack of knowledge, counselors have at their disposal large quantities of information to present to the client in a variety of ways. The most potent strategy to solve lack of knowledge is tailoring. The ideal situation for tailoring allows for an individual dietary pattern and an individualized exchange list for each person. The pattern shows exchanges with amounts tailored to each client's preferred eating style, such as X ounces or grams of meat, X servings of vegetables, X servings of fruits, X servings of milk, and so on. The tailored exchange list includes only foods the client eats; all others are eliminated from the list. **The tailored list is preferred over one general list for the following reasons:**

- **A tailored list can be very short and thus less cumbersome.** Fewer items mean less work for the person learning the list.
- **It allows for much greater detail.** With fewer items, more information can be included for each item, such as protein, phosphorus, and calories, automatically giving the person using the list more information about the eating pattern.
- **It stimulates learning because it can create a feeling of ownership.**

Along with individualizing exchanges, individualized menu planning with active client participation can be an aid to later adherence. The MDRD Study used protein counting as a method of facilitating dietary adherence. When other nutrients or calories required monitoring, the nutrition counselor specified changes in certain foods which were favorites for the client.

Once counselors have presented individualized crucial information to each client, they must stage changes in eating habits to coincide with the recommended dietary components. Counselors should avoid creating the impression that they are the "experts" and in sole control. Too often, counselors present forms, lists, and other documents in a way that leaves clients feeling totally removed from the process of change. Clients begin to regard themselves as unwilling objects to be moved, shaped, and molded by the counselors. The goal during the sessions should be to shape the eating patterns with clients as they continue to follow the dietary prescription.

Researchers in the MDRD Study found that the need to provide knowledge decreased over time,[47] and the behavioral skills discussed below increased.

Staging or setting priorities for the components of a diet with several restrictions, all of which clients must follow as a package, can be difficult. Staging allows clients to solve one problem at a time while continuing to follow all restrictions to the best of their ability. Once again, clients must be very actively involved in the developmental process. In choosing which problems to work on first, counselors should consider several factors:

- Which problem, if solved, will allow the most success? Initial success can be very important to continued improvement in dietary adherence.
- Which problem is the most difficult and inhibiting from the standpoint of dietary adherence? The counselor and client may need to deal first with a very large problem that precludes following the diet. A client who refuses to comply with any recommendations may need to be seen by a psychologist or psychiatrist before any instruction on a dietary regimen.
- Which problems will be moderately difficult to solve? Once the client feels he or she is in an action stage ready for change, the nutrition counselor should focus on the easiest problems to solve, then rank the more difficult problems and discuss each separately. The ultimate choice should be a product of client-counselor teamwork.

In dealing with a client on a low-protein eating pattern, staging learning can be very important. Counselors should begin by focusing on selecting appropriate amounts of food from an exchange group high in protein, choosing a group less preferred by the client so that cutting back is not impossible. The counselor should try to ensure success. The area listed as most difficult should be the last. Staging makes it possible to use *attribution* to facilitate adherence to a more difficult problem. For example, the counselor might say, "You have done so well in eating the required amounts of food in the milk category (Attribution). You should eventually do well in cutting back on meat." Staging may also take the form of menu planning initially to provide direct guidance in dietary adherence. As time passes, the client will become comfortable assuming personal responsibility for menu planning.

Lack of knowledge can often be the major problem in a variety of issues. One of clients' most commonly voiced concerns is social eating, which includes eating at friends' homes and in restaurants. Tracking adherence to diets and medications shows major decreases in group adherence rates during holidays such as Hanukkah and Christmas and during vacation periods. These times involve accelerated social eating. Initial assistance in this area can be informational. Counselors can involve clients by asking them to plan a menu (Adherence Tool 7–7). Adherence Tools 7–8 and 7–9 provide practice in learning exchanges and modifying recipes, and listing favorite low-protein foods. During the holidays, counselors can help clients adhere to the eating pattern by giving information as shown in Adherence Tool 7–10. This tool was designed to allow a client who has used up all exchanges for breakfast, lunch, and dinner to select foods spontaneously at a late-night party. It shows many "free" items in terms of protein content, allows a few lower-protein foods, and says "stop" to many high-protein foods. Adherence Tool 7–11 is a birthday card that includes a recipe for a low-protein birthday cake. When signed by all clinical staff, the card becomes an important reminder and aid in following the new eating pattern at a difficult time.

Restaurant eating can be very difficult for clients following a low-protein eating pattern. It is important to provide adequate information so clients can follow the diet when eating out. A file of menus for the client's favorite restaurant is extremely valuable. Counselors can ask clients to plan a day's menu that includes eating out. It is helpful to call the restaurant before; use a menu and elicit as much information as possible on serving sizes. By giving clients enough information, counselors can make restaurant eating much less difficult.

Eating at home when following restricted-protein eating patterns can be easier if the client has access to low-protein products that provide added calories. Adherence Tool 7–12 provides space to identify low-protein products along with company names. These products make it possible to include a greater amount of some high-protein foods. For example, by eating rice, which has minimal protein content, more protein can come from meat products rather than regular bread products.

Lack of knowledge may be evidenced by the lack of ability to identify circumstances preceding and following a behavior. For example, if snacking in the evening seems to be a behavior that pushes protein intake over the recommended amount, examining events leading to that behavior may help determine how to modify it. The chain of events might be as follows: Eat dinner, wash dishes, watch TV (*antecedents*), eat snack of cheese and crackers (*behavior*), tell myself how bad I've been, feel depressed, eat a peanut butter sandwich (*consequences*).

Identifying the ABCs of behavior (antecedents, behavior, and consequences) makes a variety of solutions available. First, the counselor can determine how important regular, as opposed to low-protein, crackers are. It is very easy to suggest low-protein crackers and jelly as an alternative to regular crackers and cheese. If this change is too drastic, a compromise might be a mixture of mayonnaise and very small amounts of cheese (0.2 ounces), mixed and microwaved, on low-protein crackers. The positive self-reinforcement that replaces the negative reinforcement indicated in the above chain will probably make the additional peanut butter sandwich less tempting. By saying, "This is great! I can eat this snack without increasing my protein intake significantly," the client can eliminate the feelings of depression and subsequent eating.

The more self-management through self-reinforcement a counselor can help the client achieve, the greater the likelihood of dietary success.

Strategies To Deal with Forgetfulness

Cueing devices can be very helpful in avoiding problems of forgetting. A note on the refrigerator saying, "Eat rice with margarine today" may help keep protein low and calories high. Placing hard candy in jars throughout the house can cue the client to eat adequate calories without added protein.

Forgetting is often a problem in dealing with medication. Pill boxes with sections for each day's doses (morning, noon, evening, and before bed) are useful. If placed in visible areas, such as the kitchen table or counter, they can serve as prompts to taking medication (see Adherence Tool 7–13).

During vacation times, a postcard (Adherence Tool 7–14) with cues to remind the client to take medications during the trip can help avoid poor adherence. Calendars (Adherence Tool 7–15) can help document times when clients forget to take medication. Recording the amount of medication taken at each time of day can help clients see when they miss medications, and the recording may be a cue to improve adherence.

Strategies To Deal with Lack of Commitment

On a low-protein regimen with many restrictions, almost every client inevitably faces periods when commitment wanes. The degree is directly related to the number of adherence predictors identified during the initial assessment. Counselors should watch persons prone to depression for periods of decreased commitment to diet and adherence to medication. Lack of support or constant negative reinforcement by a spouse or significant other may set the stage for more frequent and longer periods of decreased commitment. Clients who have tried in vain to follow an eating pattern in the past will probably experience periods of poor adherence to the low-protein eating pattern.

The first indication of reduced commitment may be a comment such as, "I'm tired of taking medications and following this strict diet." Assuming the counselor has provided enough information about the diet and the medication regimen and has offered cueing devices that the client is using, this comment indicates the following:

- More dietary information will probably only aggravate the situation. The client is not looking for more information at this point.
- Failing to remember to take the medication and follow the diet is not the major problem. Offering more cueing devices will only make the client angry because, as a counselor, you are not listening to what the client is saying.

At this point, the skills of communication discussed in Chapter 2 become very important. The counselor may either alienate the client by giving short, uninsightful answers such as "You just need to eliminate meat products," or, more positively, retrieve a potential nonadherer and improve adherence at the same time. The dialogue that follows illustrates one way to approach the person who lacks commitment:

> *Client:* "I'm really tired of following this diet and taking all those medications."
> *Nutrition Counselor:* "When you say you are 'tired,' what specifically do you mean?"
> *Client:* "I have lost the desire to fight. I look at my pill dispenser and notice that I should take a noon dose of blood pressure medication, but I don't have the desire to do it. So I don't. I have started eating a second serving of meat at night."
> *Nutrition Counselor:* "You were so committed when we started. I remember you listed several reasons for wanting to do well. I have the list here: (1) "I don't want my disease to get worse." (2) "I want to feel better." (3) "I want to succeed."
> *Client*: "Yes, I remember, but many things have changed since then. I lost my job. My husband was laid off. It is hard to succeed or even see a reason to succeed if your future looks so bleak. We have so many financial problems that the diet and taking my medications have taken a back seat."

In many cases, lack of commitment may mean that other stressful life events have taken priority over adhering to an eating pattern or medication regimen. One of the most positive aspects in maintaining adherence to the low-protein regimen is that in the predialysis client it can result in uremic symptoms that are less severe. During life events when the stress factor is temporary, a short time of reducing dietary and medication requirements until life events stabilize may be necessary. For example, if a client is going through a divorce, the counselor can help the client identify the most difficult time period and arrange a way of decreasing monitoring during that time, or set up a contract (Adherence Tool 7–16). The client can agree to monitor medication and dietary intake for one meal with a calendar every other week and try to do well without monitoring during the other weeks.

In some cases a client may adhere poorly to diet for a few days when eating at home is impossible. Once again, a contract (Adherence Tool 7–17) can avoid monumental indiscretions and create controlled ones. Instead of following a pattern of 0.8 grams per kilogram of protein, for a time the diet might be 0.9 grams per kilogram of protein. This process of relaxing the rules can help in times of crisis and serve as a way of staging back to the original prescription—from 0.9 grams per kilogram of protein to 0.85 grams per kilogram and finally back to 0.8 grams per kilogram. The contract written during this period should clearly indicate the times during which the rules will be relaxed and state exactly what relaxing the rules will change. The contract should make it very clear that the rules will be relaxed only while the client is recovering from an experience that precludes following the diet. The counselor should stress that the ultimate goal is to follow the diet 100 percent of the time.

At certain points, constructive confrontation may be necessary:

> *Nutrition Counselor:* "I've enjoyed working with you over the past few weeks and I really thought you were making progress. (Personal and Relationship Statements) As I review your urine urea nitrogen levels, it is evident that you have not been following your low-protein eating pattern. Your diet records also show an increase in protein intake." (Description of Behavior)
>
> *Client:* "I really want to do well, but particularly during breaks at work I just can't resist."
>
> *Nutrition Counselor:* "I am confused when you say you want to do well but your behavior during breaks shows that you actually do the opposite. There seem to be two messages. (Description of Feelings and Interpretation of Client's Situation) Do you understand what I mean?"
>
> *Client:* "Yes." (Understanding Response)
>
> *Nutrition Counselor:* "How do you feel about what I am saying?" (Perception Check)
>
> *Client:* "I am giving a mixed message. You are right, but it is so hard to say 'No' to my friends."
>
> *Nutrition Counselor:* "You seem to feel confused. You want to follow the diet, but the urgings of friends during breaks push you into eating more protein that you would like. (Interpretive Response) Can we come up with a solution?" (Constructive Feedback) or "Look at how far you have come. You began eating 90 grams of protein and now you are down to 45 grams." (This is constructive feedback for this person who who has slipped into a contemplation stage. Note that no advice is given.)

For the client with little support from a spouse or significant other and who is in the action phase (wanting to change), several alternatives are valuable. One is to identify another support person—a friend, daughter, sister, brother, cousin, or someone on a similar diet who is doing well. A second alternative is to train the spouse to give positive reinforcement. For example, the counselor can provide many examples of positive reinforcement during a counseling session when a husband and wife are present. A third alternative is to help clients with self-reinforcement. Counselors can ask clients to record thoughts about eating and help the client turn negative to positive thoughts during the next counseling session.

For example, a client might say, "I ate the cottage cheese and I know it is increasing my protein intake beyond what is recommended. I might as well give up." A more positive way to approach the situation is to say, "I ate more protein at this meal than I should have but tonight at supper I can keep the amount of protein down by eating a small lettuce salad, toasted low-protein bread and margarine, 7-Up, low-protein jello, and two low-protein cookies. I don't have to go over my protein allowance just because I have a problem with one meal." Adherence Tool 7–18 is a form on which to record both positive and negative monologues.

In summary, major problems with adherence to new eating patterns and supplementary medications involve information regarding the protein content of foods and means of applying this knowledge to specific situations. Cueing devices can be helpful in altering events to take medications and follow low-protein eating patterns. The most difficult problem involving lack of commitment might be approached with strategies such as self-monitoring, contracting, reinforcement, and positive thinking.

Review of Chapter 7
(Answers in Appendix H)

1. List four factors associated with inappropiate eating behaviors when following a protein-modified eating pattern:

   a. _____

   b. _____

   c. _____

   d. _____

2. Identify five possible nutrients that should be identified as to baseline intake:

   a. _____

   b. _____

   c. _____

   d. _____

   e. _____

3. List four strategies to treat inappropiate eating behaviors associated with protein-modified patterns:

   a. _____

   b. _____

   c. _____

   d. _____

4. The following is an exercise to help in applying the ideas just discussed:

John is a 31-year-old minister who eats all of his meals at home except for a few social gatherings. His major problem is his wife's reluctance to help him modify his diet because she feels there are too many restrictions. Explain what you would do, and why, to change the wife's feelings about the diet. (Don't presume the significant other's behavior will change.)

_____

_____

_____

_____

_____

_____

_____

_____

_____

_____

_____

NOTES

1. S. Klahr et al., "Role of Dietary Factors in the Progression of Chronic Renal Disease," *Kidney International* 24 (1983): 579–587.

2. B.M. Brenner, "Hemodynamically Mediated Glomerular Injury and the Progressive Nature of Kidney Disease," *Kidney International* 23 (1983): 647–655.

3. W.F. Keane et al., "Angiotensin Converting Enzyme Inhibitors and Progressive Renal Insufficiency: Current Experience and Future Directions," *Annals of Internal Medicine* 111 (1989): 503–516.

4. W.E. Mitch et al., "The Effect of a Keto Acid-Amino Acid Supplement to a Restricted Diet on the Progression of Chronic Renal Failure," *New England Journal of Medicine* 311 (1984): 623–629.

5. J.B. Rosman et al., "Prospective Randomized Trial of Early Dietary Protein Restriction in Chronic Renal Failure," *Lancet* 2 (1984): 1291–1296.

6. L.G. Hunsicker, "Studies of Therapy of Progressive Renal Failure in Humans," *Seminars in Nephrology* 9 (1989): 380–394.

7. B.U. Ihle et al., "The Effect of Protein Restriction on the Progression of Renal Insufficiency," *New England Journal of Medicine* 321 (1989): 1773–1777.

8. A.S. Levey et al., "Assessing the Progression of Renal Disease in Clinical Studies: Effects of Duration of Follow-Up and Regression to the Mean: Modification of Diet in Renal Disease (MDRD) Study Group," *Journal of the American Society of Nephrology* 1 (1991): 1087–1094.

9. D. Fouque et al., "Controlled Low Protein Diets in Chronic Renal Insufficiency: Meta-Analysis," *British Medical Journal* 304 (1992): 216–220.

10. M. Walser et al., "A Crossover Comparison of Progression of Chronic Renal Failure: Ketoacids versus Amino Acids," *Kidney International* 43 (1993): 933–939.

11. Mitch et al., "The Effect of a Keto Acid-Amino Acid Supplement."

12. Walser et al., "A Crossover Comparison of Progression of Chronic Renal Failure."

13. L.S. Ibels et al., "Preservation of Function in Experimental Renal Disease by Dietary Phosphate Restriction," *New England Journal of Medicine* 298 (1978): 122–126.

14. B.M. Brenner et al., "Dietary Protein Intake and the Progressive Nature of Kidney Disease," *New England Journal of Medicine* 307 (1982): 652–659.

15. T.H. Hostetter et al., "Hyperfiltration in Remnant Nephrons: A Potentially Adverse Response to Renal Ablation," *American Journal of Physiology* 241 (1981): F83–F93.

16. J.L. Olson et al., "Altered Glomerular Permeability and Progressive Sclerosis Following Ablation of Renal Mass," *Kidney International* 22 (1982): 112–126.

17. "The Fifth Report of the Joint National Committee on Detection, Evaluation, and Treatment of High Blood Pressure," *Archives of Internal Medicine* 153 (1993):154–183.

18. S. Klahr, "The Modification of Diet in Renal Disease Study," *New England Journal of Medicine* 320 (1989): 864–866.

19. G.J. Beck et al., "Design and Statistical Issues of the Modification of Diet in Renal Disease Trial: The Modification of Diet in Renal Disease Study Group," *Controlled Clinical Trials* 12 (1991): 566–586.

20. "The Modification of Diet in Renal Disease Study: Design, Methods, and Results from the Feasibility Study," *American Journal of Kidney Disease* 20 (1992): 18–33.

21. S. Klahr et al., "The Effects of Dietary Protein Restriction and Blood-Pressure Control on the Progression of Chronic Renal Disease," *New England Journal of Medicine* 330 (1994): 877–884.

22. American Diabetes Association, "Nutrition Recommendations and Principles for People with Diabetes Mellitus," *Diabetes Care* 17 (1994): 519–522.

23. Renal Dietitians Dietetic Practice Group of the American Dietetic Association, *National Renal Diet: Professional Guide* (The American Dietetic Association, Chicago, IL, 1993), 6.

24. G.L. Bilbrey et al., "Hyperglucagonemia of Renal Failure," *Journal of Clinical Investigation* 53 (1974): 841–847.

25. R.A. DeFronzo and A. Alvestrand, "Glucose Intolerance in Uremia: Site and Mechanism," *American Journal of Clinical Nutrition* 33 (1980): 1438–1445.

26. C. Giordano et al., "Urea Index and Nitrogen Balance in Uremic Patients on Minimal Nitrogen Intakes," *Clinical Nephrology* 3 (1975): 168–171.

27. World Health Organization, *Energy and Protein Requirements, Report of a Joint FAO/WHO/UNU Expert Consultation,* Technical Report Series 724 (Geneva: 1985), 206.

28. J.D. Kopple, "Nutritional Therapy in Kidney Failure," *Nutrition Review* 39 (1981): 193–206.

29. J.D. Kopple et al., "Energy Expenditure in Chronic Renal Failure and Hemodialysis Patients" (Abstract), *American Journal of Nephrology* (1983): 50A.

30. S.R. Acchiardo et al., "Does Low Protein Diet Halt the Progression of Renal Insufficiency?" *Clinical Nephrology* 25 (1986): 289–294.

31. Ibels et al., "Preservation of Function in Experimental Renal Disease by Dietary Phosphate Restriction."

32. R.C. Tomford et al., "Effect of Thyroparathyroidectomy and Parathyroidectomy on Renal Function and Nephrotic Syndrome in Rat Nephrotoxic Serum Nephritis," *Journal of Clinical Investigation* 68 (1981): 655–664.

33. M. Walser, "Nutrition in Renal Failure," *Annals of the Review of Nutrition* 3 (1983): 133–134.

34. Klahr, "The Effects of Dietary Protein Restriction and Blood Pressure Control on the Progression of Chronic Renal Disease," 879.

35. J.W. Coburn et al., "Intestinal Absorption of Calcium, Magnesium and Phosphorus in Chronic Renal Insufficiency," in *Calcium Metabolism in Renal Failure and Nephrolithiasis,* ed. D.S. David (New York: John Wiley & Sons, 1977), 77–109.

36. C.C. Marone et al., "Acidosis and Renal Calcium Excretion in Experimental Chronic Renal Failure," *Nephron* 28 (1981): 294–296.

37. Coburn, "Intestinal Absorption of Calcium, Magnesium and Phosphorus in Chronic Renal Insufficiency," 402.

38. G.T. Wollam et al., "Diuretic Potency of Combined Hydrochlorothiazide and Furosemide Therapy in Patients with Azotemia," *American Journal of Medicine* 72 (1982): 929–938.

39. F.R. Smith and D.S. Goodman, "The Effects of Disease in Liver, Thyroid and Kidneys on Transport of Vitamin A in Human Plasma," *Journal of Clinical Investigation* 50 (1971): 2426–2436.

40. S. Mahajan et al., "Zinc Metabolism and Taste Acuity in Renal Transplant Recipients," (Abstract), *Clinical Research* 30 (1982): 246A.

41. L.G. Snetselaar et al., "Protein Calculation from Food Diaries of Adult Humans Underestimates Values Determined Using a Biological Marker," *Journal of Nutrition* 125 (1995): 2333–2340.

42. B.P. Gillis, et al., "Nutrition Intervention Program of the Modification of Diet in Renal Disease Study: A Self-Management Approach," *Journal of the American Dietetic Association* 95 (1995): 1288–1294.

43. T. Coyne et al., "Dietary Satisfaction Correlated with Adherence in the Modification of Diet in Renal Disease Study," *Journal of the American Dietetic Association* 95 (1995): 1301–1306.

44. N.C. Milas et al., "Factors Associated with Adherence to the Dietary Protein Intervention in the Modification of Diet in Renal Disease Study," *Journal of the American Dietetic Association* 95 (1995): 1295–1300.

45. T.A. Dolecek et al., "Registered Dietitian Time Requirements in the Modification of Diet in Renal Disease Study," *Journal of the American Dietetic Association* 95 (1995): 1307–1312.

46. Milas, "Factors Associated with Adherence to the Dietary Protein Intervention in the Modification of Diet in Renal Disease Study," 1296.

47. Gillis, "Nutrition Intervention Program of the Modification of Diet in Renal Disease Study: A Self-Management Approach," 1288.

Adherence Tool 7–1: Client Questionnaire for Protein-Restricted Eating Patterns (Monitoring Device)

Name: _____

Address: _____

Sex: M____ F____

Birthdate: _____

Home Phone: _____

Office Phone: _____

Doctor's name: _____

Anthropometry:

Elbow Breadth ____

Frame Size ____

Standard Body Weight ____ (Use Metropolitan Life Insurance Tables)

WEIGHT HISTORY

1. Your present weight _____ height _____

2. Describe your present weight (check one).

____ Very overweight

____ Slightly overweight

____ About average

____ Average

____ Slightly underweight

3. Are you dissatisfied with the way you look at this weight? (check one)

____ Completely satisfied

____ Satisfied

____ Neutral

____ Dissatisfied

____ Very dissatisfied

continues

Adherence Tool 7–1   continued

4. What do you do for physical exercise and how often do you do it?

ACTIVITY	FREQUENCY
(for example, swimming, jogging, and dancing)	(daily, weekly, monthly)

_____

_____

_____

_____

PAST DIETS

(If you have never followed a special diet, skip to question 12.)

5. Have you followed a low-protein diet in the past? _____ If "yes," what was the number of grams of protein eaten per day? _____ When did you start this diet? _____ Are you still following it? _____

6. How would you describe your ability to follow the diet? (check one)

____ Excellent

____ Good

____ Fair

____ Poor

7. What were or are the attitudes of the following people about your attempts to follow the low-protein diet? (Place an _X_ in the appropriate box.)

	Negative (They disapprove or are resentful.)	_Indifferent_ (They don't care or don't help.)	_Positive_ (They encourage me and are understanding.)
Husband			
Wife			
Children			
Parents			
Employer			
Friends			

8. Did or do these attitudes affect your ability to follow the low-protein diet?____. If "yes," please describe: _____

_____

_____

_____

_____

9. What other diets have you followed in the past or are you currently following? (Check as many as apply.)

____ High-calorie   ____ Diabetic

____ Low-cholesterol, low-fat   ____ Low-potassium

____ Low-calorie   ____ High-potassium

____ Low-salt   ____ Low-phosphorus

____ Other

10. What special products did you use or are you currently using?

____ Low-protein products

____ Low-salt products

____ Sugar-free products

____ Other _____

11. Have you had a major mood change while or after following a special diet? Indicate any mood changes on the following checklist.

Mood	No Change	A Little Change	Moderate Change	A Lot of Change	Extreme Change
A. Depressed, sad, feeling down, unhappy, the blues					
B. Anxious, nervous, restless, or uptight all the time					
C. Physically weak					
D. Elated or happy					

continues

Adherence Tool 7–1   continued

Mood	No Change	A Little Change	Moderate Change	A Lot of Change	Extreme Change
E. Easily irritated, annoyed, or angry					
F. Fatigued, worn out, tired all the time					
G. A lack of self-confidence					

MEDICAL HISTORY

12. What was the date of your last physical exam? _____

13. Other than your kidney disease, do you currently have other medical problems?

14. What medications or drugs do you take regularly?

_____

_____

_____

_____

15. List any medications, drugs, or food to which you are allergic:

_____

_____

_____

16. List any hospitalizations or operations. Indicate how old you were at each hospital admission.

    Age   Reason for hospitalization

_____

_____

_____

_____

17. List any serious illnesses you have had that have not required hospitalization. Indicate how old you were during each illness.

    Age   Illness

_____

_____

_____

_____

_____

18. How much alcohol do you usually drink per week? _____ ounces

19. List any psychiatric contact, individual counseling, or marital counseling that you have had or are now having.

    Age   Reason for contact and type of therapy

_____

_____

_____

_____

_____

20. List any recurring symptoms you are currently experiencing, vomiting, diarrhea, constipation, weak feeling, etc.

_____

_____

_____

_____

_____

SOCIAL HISTORY

21. Circle the last year of school attended:

    1 2 3 4 5 6 7 8   9 10 11 12   1 2 3 4   MA/MS   PhD/MD

        grade school   high school   college

continues

Adherence Tool 7–1   continued

22. Describe your present occupation: _____

_____

_____

(If self-employed, skip to question 24.)

23. How long have you worked for your present employer? _____

24. Present marital status (check one):

    ___ Single   ___ Widowed

    ___ Engaged   ___ Separated

    ___ Married   ___ Divorced

25. Describe spouse's occupation: _____

_____

_____

_____

26. Who lives at home with you?

_____

_____

_____

_____

FAMILY HISTORY

27. Is your father living? Yes _____ No _____
    Father's age now, or age at and cause of death: _____

_____ _____

_____

28. Is your mother living? Yes _____ No _____
    Mother's age now, or age at and cause of death: _____

_____

_____

29. Please add any additional information you feel may be relevant to your dietary success. This includes interactions with your family and friends that might sabotage your ability to follow a low-protein diet and additional family or social history that you feel might help us understand problems you will encounter with eating low-protein meals.

_____

_____

_____

_____

Adherence Tool 7–2: Daily Record of Foods Containing Protein (Monitoring Device)

Time	Protein-Containing Food	Amount	Source

Adherence Tool 7–3: Calculating Adherence (Monitoring Device)

Last visit date _____

Last visit number _____

Start counting for next visit adherence on   (date)

                              _____
                              (AM, PM, or bedtime dose)

Number of days since last visit _____

Number of prescribed pills per day _____

   a. Number of pills issued since last visit _____

   b. Returned by client this visit _____

   c. Left at home or accidentally destroyed_____

   d. Not taken ($b + c$) _____

   e. Subject has taken since last visit ($a - d$) _____

   f. Should have taken _____

   g. Percent adherence to nearest whole number_____
      ($a/f \times 100$)

   h. Number of days missed ($f - e$) / number of pills_____

Since your last visit, have you stopped taking your medicine for any reason? _____

_____

Since your last visit, have you changed the dose of medicine for any reason? _____

_____

Adherence Tool 7–4: Record of Adherence Percentages (Monitoring Device)

Medication:_____

Dosage: _____

Date	Percent Adherence

Adherence Tool 7–5: Graph of Protein Intake (Monitoring Device)

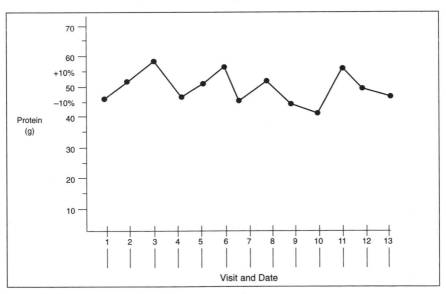

Adherence Tool 7–6: Laboratory Data
(Monitoring Device)

Name: _____

Hospital Number: _____

Diagnosis: _____

Visit: _____ Date: _____	Normal Values						
Serum Values							
Total Protein							
Albumin							
Transferrin							
Urea nitrogen appearance (UNA)							
Creatinine							
Sodium							
Potassium							
Chloride							
Bicarbonate							
Calcium							
Phosphorus							
Magnesium							
Iron							
Glucose							
White Blood Cells							
Hemoglobin							
Hematocrit							
Urine Values							
Protein							
Creatinine							
Phosphorus							
pH							
Glucose							

Adherence Tool 7–7: Client Diet Basics and One-Day Menu (Informational Device)

My diet should contain _____ grams of protein per day.
Examples of foods containing all essential amino acids:

Meats	Fish	Milk
Poultry	Eggs	Cheese

Examples of foods lacking one or more essential amino acids:

Breads	Fruits	Cereals
Vegetables	Gelatin	

Essential amino acids are:

Histidine	Threonine
Isoleucine	Tryptophan
Leucine	Valine
Lysine	

Plan one day's menu using protein-containing foods:

Breakfast	Lunch	Dinner	Snacks

Adherence Tool 7–8:   Exchange Practice for Your Low-Protein Eating Pattern (Informational Device)

Please write in the amount of protein coming from the food in the list and its exchange amount.

Food	Amount of Protein	Amount of Phosphorus	Exchange*
¼ cup corn			
½ cup ice cream			
8 ounces grape juice			
1 ounce hard candy			
4 saltine crackers			
⅛ of or 7″ of apple pie			
¾ cup applesauce			
¼ cup mashed potatotes			
28 grams lean roast beef			
28 grams lean ham			
56 grams frankfurters			
28 grams cheddar cheese			
¼ cup yogurt			

*Only the amount of protein may be important if exchanges are unnecessary.

Adherence Tool 7–9:   Recipe Modifications for Your Low-Protein Diet (Informational Device)

Title of Recipe: _____

Ingredients	Amount	Grams of Protein	Milligrams of Phosphorus	Calories

Total Protein _____ grams

Animal Protein _____ grams

Total Phosphorus _____ milligrams

Calories _____

Exchanges _____

_____

_____

Adherence Tool 7–10: Holiday Eating (Informational Device)

Christmas Goodies That Are "Go"	Use Caution with These	Stop!
Candy Canes	Raw Vegetables:	Sour Cream Dips
Lollipops	Carrot Sticks (not more	Chocolate Candies
Cut Rock (Prim Rose	than 4[3″] sticks)	Fudge
brand)	Celery sticks (not more	Meat and Cheese Appetizers
Mint Filled Straws (Prim	than 3[3″] sticks)	and Snacks
Rose brand)	Broccoli (not more than	Nuts
Holiday Mints (Brachs)	1 florette)	Peanut Brittle
Yule Mints (Brachs)	Cherry Tomato (not	Cheese Spreads
Christmas Jellies (Brachs)	more than 1 small)	Ice Cream
Cinnamon Santas (Brachs)	Radishes (not more than	Munchies: Pretzels, Crack-
Starlight Mints (Brachs)	5 small)	ers, Popcorn, Melba
Jelly Wreaths and Trees	Mushrooms (not more	Toast, Bread Sticks,
(Brachs)	than 2 tablespoons)	Potato Chips (over ¼
Ribbon Candy (Brachs)	Fruits:	cup), Cheese Curls, Corn
Pastel Mints (Richardson)	Kumquat, raw (not more	Chips
Gumdrops (Brachs)	than 1 average)	
Lifesavers	Apple, raw (not more	
Hard Candy	than ½ large)	
Spice Drop Candy (Sweets	Cranberry-Orange Relish	
and Treats Candy Shop)	(not more than ¼ cup)	
Christmas Gummy Bear	Pear, raw with skin (not	
(Sweets and Treats)	more than ½ medium)	
Mini Fruit Balls (Sweets	Pineapple, raw, cubed	
and Treats)	(not more than ¼ cup)	
Rock Candy (Sweets and	Potato Chips (not more than	
Treats)	¼ cup)	
Fruit Flavored Ices (Baskin	Mayonnaise Dips (not more	
Robbins)	than 1 tablespoon)	
Orange Ice (Sealtest)	Salad Dressing Dips (i.e.,	
Carbonated Beverages	Miracle Whip) (not more	
Apple Juice, Apple Cider	than 2 tablespoons)	
Cranberry Juice		
Wine		
Whiskey (mixed with water)		
Candied Apricots, Cherries,		
Citron, Lemons, Oranges		

Courtesy of Lisa Brooks and Dru Mueller.

Adherence Tool 7–11: Birthday Card (Informational Device)

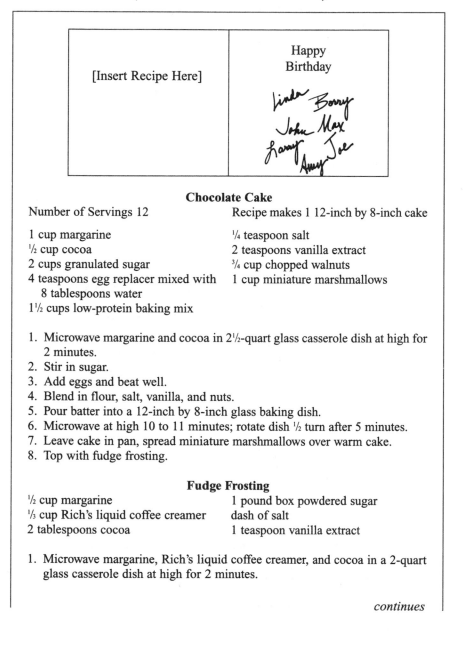

[Insert Recipe Here]	Happy Birthday

Chocolate Cake

Number of Servings 12   Recipe makes 1 12-inch by 8-inch cake

1 cup margarine
½ cup cocoa
2 cups granulated sugar
4 teaspoons egg replacer mixed with
    8 tablespoons water
1½ cups low-protein baking mix

¼ teaspoon salt
2 teaspoons vanilla extract
¾ cup chopped walnuts
1 cup miniature marshmallows

1. Microwave margarine and cocoa in 2½-quart glass casserole dish at high for 2 minutes.
2. Stir in sugar.
3. Add eggs and beat well.
4. Blend in flour, salt, vanilla, and nuts.
5. Pour batter into a 12-inch by 8-inch glass baking dish.
6. Microwave at high 10 to 11 minutes; rotate dish ½ turn after 5 minutes.
7. Leave cake in pan, spread miniature marshmallows over warm cake.
8. Top with fudge frosting.

Fudge Frosting

½ cup margarine
⅓ cup Rich's liquid coffee creamer
2 tablespoons cocoa

1 pound box powdered sugar
dash of salt
1 teaspoon vanilla extract

1. Microwave margarine, Rich's liquid coffee creamer, and cocoa in a 2-quart glass casserole dish at high for 2 minutes.

continues

Adherence Tool 7–11   continued

2. Stir in sugar, salt, and vanilla.
3. Spread on warm cake.

Note: Do not freeze.

Protein	3.4 grams	Serving Size: 1/12 cake
HBV* Protein	0.3 gram	Serving Weight: 130 grams
LBV** Protein	3.1 grams	
Calories	625	
Phosphorus	104 milligrams	

 *HBV = High biological value
**LBV = Low biological value

Adherence Tool 7–12: Low-Protein Foods for Your Diet (Informational Device)

Item Description	Company

Adherence Tool 7–13: Pill Box (Cueing Device)

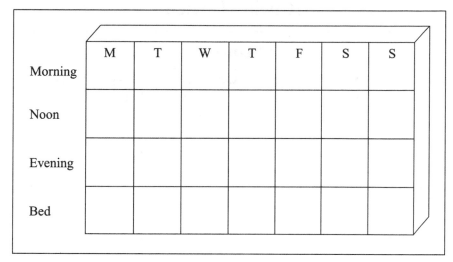

	M	T	W	T	F	S	S
Morning							
Noon							
Evening							
Bed							

Adherence Tool 7–14: Vacation Postcard (Cueing Device)

Your travel checklist. Have you done the following?

Yes No

☐ ☐ Temporarily cancelled the newspaper

☐ ☐ Put a stop on mail delivery

☐ ☐ Locked all doors and windows

☐ ☐ Counted your medication pills and added ones in case you stay longer than planned

☐ ☐ Obtained a medication letter for customs clearance if traveling abroad

☐ ☐ Checked and fueled your car, if driving

☐ ☐ Left your destination phone number with a friend

☐ ☐ Confirmed all reservations

Adherence Tool 7–15: Calendars
(Cueing Device)

ONE-MONTH

Sun.	Mon.	Tues.	Wed.	Thur.	Fri.	Sat.

Month of _____ 19 ____   If you have any questions, please call: _____

ONE-WEEK

NAME: _____

ATTN:_____   THANK YOU!

Adherence Tool 7–16: Reinstituting Commitment, Contract I (Behavioral Device)

During the week of January 2 (January 2–9) I agree to limit my monitoring of medication to every other day. For all other weeks in the month of January, I will monitor daily. I will record the exact amount of medication I take at breakfast, lunch, and dinner on the calendar provided. Each evening, I will allow myself to watch TV, call my friend, or read a book if I have been successful in recording for that week. If I fail to achieve this goal on designated weeks (all of those other than the week of January 2), I will not allow myself to engage in any of these behaviors. I will not reinforce during the week of January 2.

I understand that this break in my monitoring will be only temporary. Once life is back to normal (following the week of January 2), I will return to my old routine on January 10.

Client _____

Spouse/Parent/Friend _____

Nutrition Counselor _____

Physician_____

Adherence Tool 7–17: Reinstituting Commitment, Contract II (Behavioral Device)

During the week of Feburary 3 (February 3–9) I agree to limit my dietary intake to the new and temporary exchange list (0.9 grams per kilogram of protein per day) provided by my dietitian. Each day that I successfully follow this exchange pattern, I will reward myself by reading a book, going shopping, or visiting my cousin. If I do not follow the diet on a day, I will not allow myself to engage in any of these behaviors.

I recognize that this change in diet is temporary. On February 10, I will return to an intermediate dietary exchange pattern (0.85 grams per kilogram of protein per day). On February 17, I will return to my old exchange pattern (0.8 grams per kilogram of protein per day).

Client _____

Spouse/Parent/Friend _____

Nutrition Counselor _____

Physician_____

Adherence Tool 7–18: Reinstituting Commitment, Record of Monologues (Monitoring Device)

Time	Food Eaten	Thoughts

CHAPTER 8

Nutrition Counseling in Treatment of Hypertension

CHAPTER OBJECTIVES

1. Identify factors that lead to inappropriate eating behaviors associated with sodium-modified regimens.

2. Identify important steps in the assessment of a baseline diet for clients following a sodium-modified eating pattern.

3. Identify strategies to treat inappropriate eating behaviors associated with sodium-modified patterns.

4. Generate strategies to use in facilitating problem solving for clients who are following sodium-modified patterns.

5. Recommend dietary adherence tools for clients on sodium-modified eating patterns.

THEORIES AND FACTS ABOUT NUTRITION AND HYPERTENSION

The *Fifth Report of the Joint National Committee on Detection, Evaluation, and Treatment of High Blood Pressure* states that the goal of treating patients with hypertension is to prevent morbidity and mortality associated with high blood pressure and to control blood pressure by the least intrusive means possible.[1] The committee states that lifestyle modifications including weight reduction, increased physical activity, and moderation of dietary sodium and alcohol intake are definitive or adjunctive therapy for hypertension.[2,3] These lifestyle factors form the basis for intervention strategies that have shown promise in the prevention of high blood pressure.[4-7] However, their capacity to reduce morbidity or mortality in those with elevated blood pressure is not conclusively documented. In spite of this lack of conclusive evidence, lifestyle modifications offer multiple benefits at little cost and with minimal risk. Even when lifestyle modifications are not adequate in themselves to control hypertension, they may reduce the number and doses of antihypertensive medications needed to manage the condition.[8] Researchers have found that lifestyle modifications are helpful in the large proportion of hypertensive patients who have additional risk factors for premature cardiovascular disease, especially dyslipidemias or diabetes.[9] The Joint National Committee states that clinicians should vigorously encourage their patients to adopt these lifestyle modifications. The Joint National Committee also recommends the classification scheme in Table 8–1 for blood pressure levels.

Table 8–1 Classification of Blood Pressure for Adults Age 18 Years and Older*

Category	Systolic (mm Hg)	Diastolic (mm Hg)
Normal†	<130	<85
High normal	130–139	85–89
Hypertension**		
STAGE 1 (Mild)	140–159	90–99
STAGE 2 (Moderate)	160–179	100–109
STAGE 3 (Severe)	180–209	110–119
STAGE 4 (Very Severe)	≥210	≥120

*Not taking antihypertensive drugs and not acutely ill. When systolic and diastolic pressures fall into different categories, the higher category should be selected to classify the individual's blood pressure status. For instance, 160/92 mm Hg should be classified as Stage 2, and 180/120 mm Hg should be classified as Stage 4. Isolated systolic hypertension (ISH) is defined as SBP ≥ 140 mm Hg and DBP <90 mm Hg and staged appropriately (e.g., 170/85 mm Hg is defined as Stage 2 ISH).

†Optimal blood pressure with respect to cardiovascular risk is SBP <120 mm Hg and DBP <80 mm Hg. However, unusually low readings should be evaluated for clinical significance.

**Based on the average of two or more readings taken at each of two or more visits following an initial screening.

Note: In addition to classifying stages of hypertension based on average blood pressure levels, the clinician should specify presence or absence of target-organ disease and additional risk factors. For example, a patient with diabetes and a blood pressure of 142/94 mm Hg plus left ventricular hypertrophy should be classified as "Stage 1 hypertension with target-organ disease (left ventricular hypertrophy) and with another major risk factor (diabetes)." This specificity is important for risk classification and management.

Source: Reprinted from the National High Blood Pressure Education Program; National Institutes of Health; National Heart, Lung, and Blood Institute, *The Fifth Report of the Joint National Committee on Detection, Evaluation, and Treatment of High Blood Pressure*, 1994.

Research on Weight Control and Hypertension

A compelling body of evidence relates obesity to hypertension.[10–13] Many studies in epidemiology have shown the relationship of body weight and arterial pressure in both hypertensive and normotensive persons.[14–19] In smaller studies, body weight and blood pressure have also been correlated in children and adolescents.[20,21] In adults, relative body weight, body weight change over time, and skinfold thickness have been directly related to blood pressure levels and to subsequent rate of development of hypertension.[22] In addition, the risk of normotensive persons later becoming hypertensive is related to the degree of obesity. Several additional studies have documented the importance of weight gain in subsequent development of hypertension.[23–26]

Additional evidence indicates that truncal or abdominal fat deposition may be important to hypertension. The deposition of excess fat in this upper body region correlates with hypertension, dyslipidemia, diabetes, and increased coronary heart disease mortality.[27]

Researchers have provided a variety of evidence that weight reduction induced by calorie restriction lowers blood pressure. Experimental starvation studies have shown falls in systolic pressure from 104 mm Hg (millimeters of mercury) to 93 mm Hg and diastolic pressures from 70 mm Hg to 63 mm Hg. All subjects were normotensive. With refeeding, blood pressure values returned to prestarvation levels.[28]

Research correlating changes in blood pressure in hypertensive persons with changes in weight began in the 1920s. Rose found that weight reduction resulted in lower pressures,[29] and later many researchers reported reduced blood pressure with weight loss.[30–37]

In the Chicago Coronary Prevention Evaluation Program, a considerable decrease in body weight was associated with decreases in pressure, heart rate, and serum cholesterol.[38] A later Israeli study indicated that most obese hypertensive persons achieved normal pressure when they lost only half of their excess weight, even though they remained very obese.[39] Achieving ideal body weight was not crucial to reducing blood pressure, and the pressure fall persisted as long as the decreased body weight was maintained. Researchers in the Dusseldorf Obesity study found that, for hypertensive persons not receiving antihypertensive medication over four and one-half years, the pressure fall was greatest in those who lost 12 kilograms.[40] In another study, the decrease in blood pressure in subjects who lost weight was associated with contraction of plasma volume and a decline in cardiac output, which in turn was related to slower heart rate and decreases in plasma cholesterol, uric acid, and blood glucose.[41]

Weight reduction reduces blood pressure in a large proportion of hypertensive individuals who are more than 10 percent above ideal weight.[42] A reduction in blood pressure usually occurs early during a weight-loss program, often with weight loss as small as 10 pounds.[43]

Basic conclusions from these studies follow:

- Elevated blood pressure correlates with increased body mass.
- Decreases in blood pressure result when weight is reduced.
- With weight loss, cardiovascular morbidity and mortality will decrease even if pressure does not. For persons on antihypertensive drugs the number and/or dosage of these agents may be reduced with decreases in blood pressure following weight loss.

The 1994 Joint National Committee on Detection, Evaluation, and Treatment of High Blood Pressure issued the following recommendations about weight control and hypertension:

- All hypertensive patients who are above their ideal weight should initially be placed on an individualized, monitored weight-reduction program involving caloric restriction and increased caloric expenditure by regular physical activity.
- In overweight patients with stage 1 hypertension, an attempt to control blood pressure with weight loss and other lifestyle modifications should be tried for at least three to six months prior to initiating pharmacologic therapy. If pharmacologic therapy is needed, patients should continue to pursue vigorously the weight-loss program.[44]

Research on Dietary Sodium Restriction and Hypertension

A second nonpharmacological method for controlling high blood pressure is restricting dietary sodium. Epidemiologic observations and clinical trials support an association between dietary sodium intake and blood pressure. Based on linear regression analysis within populations, a 100 mmol (millimole) per day lower average sodium intake was associated with a 2.2 mm Hg lower systolic blood pressure (SBP) in 10,000 people,[45] and a 5 to 10 mm Hg lower SBP in multiple other studies involving 47,000 participants.[46] Furthermore, a 100 mmol per day lower sodium intake was associated with a 9 mm Hg decrease in the rise of SBP in persons between the ages of 25 and 55 years.[47]

Multiple therapeutic trials document a reduction of blood pressure in response to reduced sodium intake. In short-term trials, moderate sodium restriction in hypertensive individuals on average reduces SBP by 4.9 mm Hg and diastolic blood pressure (DBP) by 2.6 mm Hg.[48] In trials involving people aged 50 to 59 and lasting five weeks or longer, a 50 mmol per day reduction of sodium intake was associated with an average of 7 mm Hg reduction in SBP in hypertensive persons and a 5 mm Hg reduction in normotensive people.[49]

Individuals vary in their blood pressure response to changes in dietary sodium.[50] African Americans, older people, and patients with hypertension are more sensitive to changes in dietary sodium.[51,52]

The 1994 Joint National Committee on Detection, Evaluation and Treatment of High Blood Pressure issued the following recommendations about sodium restriction and hypertension.

- Because the average American consumes more than 150 mmol of sodium per day, moderate dietary sodium reduction to a level of less than 100 mmol per day (less than 6 grams of table salt or less than 2.3 grams of sodium per day) is recommended.
- For patients with stage 1 hypertension, the above degree of restriction may result in controlled blood pressure.
- For patients needing drug therapy, dietary sodium restriction may decrease the medication requirements.[53]

Research on Alcohol and Hypertension

A third important nonpharmacological method of helping to lower blood pressure is reduction in alcohol consumption. Epidemiological surveys have shown that consuming more than 60 to 80 grams (1½ to 2 ounces) of alcohol per day is associated with a significantly higher prevalence of hypertension.[54-57] In one study, 51.5 percent of clients who consumed more than 80 grams of alcohol per day had hypertension (blood pressure greater than 140/90 mm Hg) on admission to a hospital.[58] Following elimination of alcohol, systolic and diastolic pressures decreased; only 9 percent remained hypertensive. Those who abstained from alcohol over time remained normotensive; most of those who reverted back to drinking also reverted to previous elevated levels of blood pressure.

Although these studies point to the importance of abstinence from the standpoint of hypertension, almost all epidemiological evidence has shown lower morbidity and mortality from coronary heart disease in people who consume one to two ounces of ethanol per day compared with those who do not drink.[59,60]

The 1994 Joint National Committee on Detection, Evaluation and Treatment of High Blood Pressure issued the following recommendations about alcohol and hypertension:

- Persons with hypertension who drink alcohol-containing beverages should be counseled to limit their daily intake to 1 ounce of ethanol (2 ounces of 100-proof whiskey, 8 ounces of wine, or 24 ounces of beer).
- Significant hypertension may develop during withdrawal from heavy alcohol consumption, but the pressor effect of alcohol withdrawal reverses a few days after alcohol consumption is reduced.[61,62]

Research on Potassium and Hypertension

A high dietary potassium intake may protect against developing hypertension,[63] and potassium deficiency may increase blood pressure and induce ventricular ectopy.[64] The Joint National Committee on Detection, Evaluation, and Treatment of High Blood Pressure recommends the following:

- Normal plasma concentrations of potassium should be maintained, preferably from food sources.
- If hypokalemia occurs during diuretic therapy, additional potassium may be needed either from potassium-containing salt substitutes, potassium supplements, or use of a potassium-sparing diuretic. Potassium chloride supplements and potassium-sparing diuretics must be used with caution in patients susceptible to hyperkalemia.[65]

Research on Calcium and Hypertension

In many but not all epidemiologic studies, there is an inverse association between dietary calcium and blood pressure. Calcium deficiency is associated with an increased prevalence of hypertension, and a low calcium intake may amplify the effects of a high sodium intake on blood pressure.[66] An increased calcium intake may lower blood pressure in some patients with hypertension. However, the overall effect is minimal, and there is no way to predict which patients will benefit.[67] Based on this evidence, there is currently no rationale for recommending calcium intakes in excess of the recommended daily allowance of 20 to 30 mmol (800 to 1200 mg) in an attempt to lower blood pressure.[68]

Research on Magnesium and Hypertension

Suggestive evidence of an association between lower dietary magnesium intake and higher blood pressures exists. However, the Joint National Committee on Detection, Evaluation, and Treatment of High Blood Pressure states that, given no convincing data, they do not recommend an increased magnesium intake in an effort to lower blood pressure.[69]

Summary of Research Findings

In conclusion, three methods of dietary treatment, weight control, sodium restriction, and alcohol restriction, are recommended for management of hypertension (Exhibit 8–1). Evidence is too meager to justify recommendations about other nutrients in relation to hypertension. The research behind recommendations

Exhibit 8–1 Lifestyle Modifications for Hypertension Control and/or Overall Cardiovascular Risk

---

- Lose weight if overweight.
- Limit alcohol intake to no more than 1 ounce of ethanol per day (24 ounces of beer, 8 ounces of wine, or 2 ounces of 100-proof whiskey).
- Exercise (aerobic) regularly.
- Reduce sodium intake to less than 100 mmol per day (<2.3 grams of sodium or <6 grams of sodium chloride).
- Maintain adequate dietary potassium, calcium, and magnesium intake.
- Stop smoking and reduce dietary saturated fat and cholesterol intake for overall cardiovascular health. Reducing fat intake also helps reduce caloric intake—important for control of weight and Type II diabetes.

Source: National High Blood Pressure Education Program; National Institutes of Health; National Heart, Lung, and Blood Institute, *The Fifth Report of the Joint National Committee on Detection, Evaluation, and Treatment of High Blood Pressure*, NIH Publication No. 93-1088 (Bethesda, Md: March 1994), 14.

---

for low-calorie, low-sodium diets adds strength to the overall objective of reducing high blood pressure. The following sections provide research on adherence to changes in eating patterns; examples of inappropriate eating behaviors; methods of assessing those behaviors; and strategies for dealing with lack of knowledge, forgetfulness, and lack of commitment to low-sodium methods of altering high blood pressure. Indeed, persons who are hypertensive at ideal body weight may require only the low-sodium diet to normalize blood pressure. Suggestions for weight-loss strategies are covered in Chapter 4.

RESEARCH ON ADHERENCE TO EATING PATTERNS IN TREATMENT OF HYPERTENSION

Steckel and Swain found contingency contracting effective in reducing weight in a hypertensive client population.[70] Further, a feasibility test for the Dietary Intervention Study of Hypertension showed that interventions for weight reduction and sodium-potassium modification among hypertensives can be relatively independent,[71] implying that a hypertension education program could be divided into these components or that these interventions could be used separately.

Monitoring of and feedback on urinary sodium levels resulted in successful sodium reductions in studies by Kaplan et al. and Nugent et al.[72,73] The simplification of urine sodium estimation procedures through use of overnight instead of

24-hour urine samples and immediate feedback by analysis using chloride titrator strips are important advances in the practicality of these monitoring techniques.

Hovell and colleagues stressed the importance of regular monitoring of both behavioral (pill counts) and physiological outcome (blood pressure) data to avoid accidentally blaming clients for inadequate therapeutic response.[74] Indeed, a client may be an excellent adherer but show little physiological response if treatment is inappropriate or inadequate. Evers and associates suggested that the primary cause of dietary noncompliance may be inadequate dietary counseling.[75] Nurses trained by the medical director, a physician, counseled 489 subjects, who received information on the causes and results of hypertension and the elimination of salt at the table and in cooking, and discussed lists of high-sodium foods and substitutes. The 12 subjects in the control group were treated by family physicians in their usual manner, which generally included advice to restrict salt usage but no intensive dietary counseling or extra assistance. The failure to note differences in the two groups in this study was attributed to a lack of nutrition counseling as described by Tillotson, Winston, and Hall and others.[76–78] Evers also stated that the counseling sessions involved only the client; yet family support has been found to be important in successful adherence to dietary regimens.[79]

A study in Finland showed favorable results when cooperation between physician and client improved.[80] Physicians began providing oral and written information on hypertension that emphasized the importance of adherence to treatment. Clients also received a blood pressure follow-up card on which the blood pressure reading and the precise time of the next appointment were recorded. Clients who missed their appointments were sent a new invitation.

Miller, Weinberger, and Cohen stressed the importance of clients' believing that the benefits of hypertensive treatment outweigh the adverse effects.[81] Many clients believe that taking medicine should make them feel better. Since hypertension is an asymptomatic illness, the client does not obtain symptom relief from the medication or diet.

Kerr found that in chronic health care situations such as hypertension, a belief in shared control or cooperation between clients and health care providers lays the groundwork for optimum treatment outcomes.[82] This finding suggests that other, internal and powerful characteristics may interact in the best interest of the client. Shared responsibility in control of hypertension may be critical to increasing adherence in the client with uncontrolled hypertension.

Schlundt et al. and Cohen described components of a structured behavior modification program: (1) self-monitoring of sodium and/or calorie intake, (2) nutrient and behavior goal setting, (3) structured problem solving, and (4) skill training.[83,84] Prevention of relapse should be addressed in the context of emotional, social, and environmental forces that impinge upon the individual's behavior. Elements in the relapse prevention program include (1) introducing the client to the concept of high-risk situations and assessing previous coping strategies; (2) including skill training and behavior rehearsal to increase the client's coping skills in response to negative emotions, interpersonal conflict, and social pressure; (3) enhancing motivation through an emphasis on the long-term consequences of engaging in prohibited behaviors; (4) teaching clients how to cope cognitively and behaviorally with slips; (5) tailoring the rules of a low-sodium, weight-loss eating pattern to the individual's unique situation; (6) teaching strategies for minimizing high-risk situations; and (7) teaching clients to seek and enhance the social support available for following an antihypertensive eating pattern. Schlundt and others also emphasized the importance of follow-up contact after completion of the initial program and recommended individual counseling, group meetings, telephone contact, and regular mail contact for at least the first three to six months—the time the majority of relapses occur.[85,86]

INAPPROPRIATE EATING BEHAVIORS

Diets modified in sodium content may be extremely difficult for most clients with whom nutrition counselors must deal. Salt is used as a flavoring agent in nearly every food. Altering such dietary habits means drastic changes for most clients.

Nutrition counselors frequently hear the complaint, "I really miss familiar flavors," or "Everything I eat tastes like sawdust." For unconscious salters (those who salt without tasting), the true flavors of foods may never have come through. They can gradually discover the natural flavors in foods through strategies suggested in this chapter.

The new eating pattern limits clients' food options because most commercial products are very high in sodium. With the trend toward prepackaged commercial meals and other products, clients on a low-sodium regimen are left with fewer choices. This limitation has led to many alterations in old eating habits. Clients not only must change what they usually eat but also must become accustomed to a new and foreign range of food flavors.

The food industry, in an effort to assist these persons, has developed a variety of low-salt products. However, these generate comments such as, "Do you expect me to eat this low-sodium soup? It's terrible." Another complaint is that some salt substitutes leave a bitter aftertaste. Objections to commercial low-sodium products constitute a recurring problem for nutrition counselors.

ASSESSMENT OF EATING BEHAVIORS

For clients who must follow a low-sodium diet, a baseline assessment is crucial. Such regimens require changes in many foods that individuals routinely and even unconsciously consume. Identifying when, where, with whom, and how much sodium is consumed can be of great benefit in helping to reduce salt intake patterns. The format in Exhibit 8–2 can be used to collect baseline data.

In collecting this information, the clients self-monitor their sodium intake. Before using the form, clients might be asked simply to observe their general behaviors involving sodium consumption (for example, salting before tasting). They might be given ideas on which basic foods are high in sodium.

During the baseline data collection, clients begin counting sodium intake occurrences, along with collecting related information indicated in the form. The following guidelines can be of help:

- The form must be portable and readily available for recording.
- Clients must be familiar enough with high-sodium foods to record all occurrences of the target behavior (sodium intake).
- Clients should record the data as the behaviors occur.
- Clients always should keep written records—memory is not adequate for baseline data collection.

During this period, some changes in behavior may occur automatically and make the nutrition counselors' job that much easier. Unfortunately, not all clients

Exhibit 8–2 Sodium Intake Information

| Food | Amount | | Time | Place | Who Present |
	In Cooking	At Table			

respond with behavior changes during this time, and some need guidance in the treatment phase. Counselors should emphasize to clients that treatment interventions should begin after, not before, the baseline data collection.

During data collection, clients will experience increasing awareness of and attention to sodium intake. For example, during a meal they may become conscious of salting food before tasting. Clients might elicit help from friends and family. There are many ways family members can delicately and supportively point out excessive use of sodium.

Clients should never allow recordkeeping to become a punishment, so counselors must help find ways to reinforce this function positively.

Clients should be aware of the importance of baseline data in identifying types of foods, amounts, and related factors—information that will improve their adherence to the dietary pattern. At this point, they might well ask, "How long should I keep baseline data?" The reply depends on the following factors:

- The data collection should continue for at least one week, since the intake of sodium occurs daily.
- It is best to gather data for two weeks if an initial review reveals large variations in sodium intake from one day to the next.
- Data should be recorded for a long enough time to provide a good estimate of when in a day the largest amounts of sodium are consumed.
- Data gathering can end when clients and counselors are satisfied that the records show the actual patterns and frequencies of sodium intake.

Clients may wonder when they have reached a stable baseline. Watson and Tharp provide the following guidelines:

- It is rare to get a stable baseline in less than one week. Data collection generally should run at least one "normal" week and should go beyond three or four weeks only rarely.
- The greater the variation from day to day, the longer it will take to get a stable baseline.
- Clients should be asked to be sure the period during which the data were gathered is representative of their usual lifestyle.[87]

In helping clients fill out the recording form, counselors should ask the following questions:

- Are the categories to be recorded defined specifically?
- Are sodium intakes and related factors recorded?
- Will the form always be present during times of food consumption?
- Is the format simple and not punishing or intimidating?
- Is it possible to reinforce the recordkeeping positively?

The sodium intake form in Exhibit 8–2 can identify a wealth of information related to eventual treatment. Assessment based on this form can lead to identification of causes of hypertension and of strategies to control blood pressure.

TREATMENT STRATEGIES

The treatment strategies that follow are organized around three topics—lack of knowledge, forgetfulness, and lack of commitment.

Strategies To Deal with Lack of Knowledge

Initially, providing adequate information for the client who wishes to follow a low-sodium diet is crucial. Before recommending treatment strategies, counselors should identify a general problem to solve. Along with the statement of that problem, inappropriate regular eating patterns should be identified. Clients should be asked to help discover possible solutions, and the counselors should provide expertise by drawing from the strategies described below.

Tailoring and staging strategies help focus the dietary pattern on the clients' special needs. Behavior change is necessary for social occasions and for the routine alterations in eating style that the regimen requires.

Most nutrition counselors provide lists of standard dos and don'ts for low-sodium eating patterns. These do not allow for individualizing eating patterns to meet each client's needs. The counselor should tailor the eating pattern to the client, first by carefully studying the baseline information. Attention must be paid not only to consumption of sodium but also to other factors associated with its intake. If the client has a favorite high-sodium food, the counselor can discuss how it might be incorporated to meet a 2,000-milligram sodium limit, cautioning that other foods containing sodium may have to be eliminated or reduced. Compromises as to the amount of the favorite foods allowed might be discussed as well. In tailoring, the counselor should point out which foods on the diet record qualify for the sodium-restricted eating pattern. Foods the client routinely eats and likes should be discussed, and the counselor should explain the reasons for full acceptance, curtailment, or elimination. Any and all positive aspects of the low-sodium eating pattern should be emphasized.

Staging the diet can be crucial in maintaining adherence over time. It is very tempting for counselors to hand clients a list of foods high in sodium and send them on their way complaining that they never will be able to follow the diet. In beginning the staging process there are two simple rules: (1) it can never begin too low and (2) the steps upward can never be too small. As the interviews progress, these rules should be individualized for each client. If the sessions move too slowly, the counselors can move up a step or discuss fewer steps. This type of staging helps clients feel that changes are easy and, therefore, that their chances for success are increased. Staging also can help in analysis of the component parts of these situations.

An alternative to this approach is to stage the dietary restrictions for sodium, with the client slowly adjusting to sets of restrictions. One way is to start with the group of foods easiest to begin using in low-sodium form, which enables the client to succeed with the initial food group. The baseline data can be used to prepare lists in consultation with the client.

Another strategy is to provide good substitutions for salt—other flavoring agents such as spices, herbs, fruit juices, etc.—as proposed in Table 8–2. Adherence Tool 8–1 provides a brief guide to low-sodium meal planning and space to practice applying the ideas. The average sodium content of all spices is less than 1 milligram per teaspoon. The spice highest in sodium is parsley flakes, which contain not quite 6 milligrams per teaspoon. In comparison, one gram of salt contains 2,300 milligrams of sodium.

The importance of reading labels carefully should be stressed, because some spices are prepared in combination with salt. Anyone on a low-sodium diet should avoid the spice-salt combination products. Table 8–3 indicates the sodium content of spices prepared without salt. Adherence Tool 8–2 provides estimates of the natural sodium content of foods.

Strategies To Deal with Forgetfulness

Calendars may serve as reminders to take blood pressure medications. For clients who must take medication, forgetting to take medications can result in increased blood pressure. The calendar in Adherence Tool 7–16 provides a means of checking on days or on times of day when patients find it most difficult to take medications. The calendar can also function as a cueing device to remind the client to take medication.

Adherence Tool 8–3 is a monitoring device that can be used to record when a client eats a high-sodium meal. If lunch has been targeted as a difficult meal, marking an X on days when lunch was high in sodium lets the counselor and the client know on what days the client needs special help in changing habits. The calendar helps remind the client, "I must watch Monday lunches." By planning ahead, the client may avoid slipping into old high-sodium eating habits.

Strategies To Deal with Lack of Commitment

Frequently model adherers to diet revert to old habits. They tire of always choosing low-sodium meals and decide to "live a little." In some cases, this lack of commitment is short-lived and may end after one or two days. Indeed, a client

Table 8–2 Chart of Spices That Can Substitute for Salt

Spice	Appetizer	Soup	Meat & Eggs	Fish & Poultry	Sauces	Vegetables	Salad & Dressing	Desserts
Allspice	Cocktail Meatballs	Pot au Feu	Hamsteak	Oyster Stew	Barbecue	Eggplant Creole	Cottage Cheese Dressing	Apple Tapioca Pudding
Basil	Cheese Stuffed Celery	Manhattan Clam Chowder	Ragout of Beef	Shrimp Creole	Spaghetti	Stewed Tomatoes	Russian Dressing	
Bay Leaf	Pickled Beets	Vegetable Soup	Lamb Stew	Simmered Chicken	Bordelaise	Boiled New Potatoes	Tomato Juice Dressing	
Caraway Seed	Mild Cheese Spreads		Sauerbraten		Beef à la Mode Sauce	Cabbage Wedges		
Cinnamon	Cranberry Juice	Fruit Soup	Pork Chops	Sweet and Sour Fish	Butter Sauce for Squash	Sweet Potato Croquettes	Stewed Fruit Salad	Chocolate Pudding
Cayenne	Deviled Eggs	Oyster Stew	Barbecued Beef	Poached Salmon Hollandaise	Bearnaise	Cooked Greens	Tuna Fish Salad	
Celery Salt and Seed	Ham Spread (Salt)	Cream of Celery (Seed)	Meat Loaf (Seed)	Chicken Croquettes (Salt)	Celery Sauce (Seed)	Cauliflower (Salt)	Cole Slaw (Seed)	
Chervil	Fish Dips	Cream Soup	Omelet	Chicken Saute	Vegetable Sauce	Peas Francaise	Caesar Salad	
Chili Powder	Seafood Cocktail Sauce	Pepper Pot	Chilli con Carne	Arroz con Pollo	Meat Gravy	Corn Mexicali	Chili French Dressing	
Cloves	Fruit Punch	Mulligatawney	Boiled Tongue	Baked Fish	Sauce Madeira	Candied Sweet Potatoes		Stewed Pears
Curry Powder	Curried Shrimp	Cream of Mushroom	Curry of Lamb	Chicken Hash	Orientale or Indienne	Creamed Vegetables	Curried Mayonnaise	
Dill Seed	Cottage Cheese	Split Pea	Grilled Lamb Steak	Drawn Butter for Shellfish	Dill Sauce for Fish or Chicken	Peas and Carrots	Sour Cream Dressing	
Garlic Salt or Powder	Clam Dip	Vegetable Soup	Roast Lamb	Bouillabaisse	Garlic Butter	Eggs and Tomato Casserole	Tomato and Cucumber Salad	
Ginger	Broiled Grapefruit	Bean Soup	Dust lightly over Steak	Roast Chicken	Cocktail	Buttered Beets	Cream Dressing for Ginger Pears	Stewed Dried Fruits

continues

Table 8-2 continued

Spice	Appetizer	Soup	Meat & Eggs	Fish & Poultry	Sauces	Vegetables	Salad & Dressing	Desserts
Mace	Quiche Lorraine	Petite Marmite	Veal Fricassee	Fish Stew	Creole	Succotash	Fruit Salad	Cottage Pudding
Marjoram	Fruit Punch Cup	Onion Soup	Roast Lamb	Salmon Loaf	Brown	Eggplant	Mixed Green Salad	
Mint	Fruit Cup	Sprinkle over Split Pea	Veal Roast	Cold Fish	Lamb	Green Peas	Cottage Cheese Salad	Ambrosia
Mustard Powdered Dry	Ham Spread	Lobster Bisque	Virginia Ham	Deviled Crab	Cream Sauce for Fish	Baked Beans	Egg Salad	Gingerbread Cookies
Nutmeg	Chopped Oysters	Cream DuBarry	Salisbury Steak Meat Loaf	Southern Fried Chicken	Mushroom	Glazed Carrots Broiled Tomatoes	Sweet Salad Dressing	Sprinkle over Vanilla Ice Cream
Onion Powder, Salt, Flakes, and Instant Minced Onion	Avocado Spread (Powder)	Consommés (Flakes)	(Instant Minced Onion)	Fried Shrimp (Salt)	Tomato (Powder)	(Salt)	Vinaigrette Dressing (Instant Minced Onion)	
Oregano	Sharp Cheese Spread	Beef Soup	Swiss Steak	Court Bouillon	Spaghetti	Boiled Onions	Sea Food	
Paprika	Creamed Seafood	Creamed Soup	Hungarian Goulash	Oven Fried Chicken	Paprika Cream	Baked Potato	Cole Slaw	
Parsley Flakes	Cheese Balls	Cream of Asparagus	Irish Lamb Stew	Broiled Mackerel	Chasseur	French Fried Potatoes	Tossed Green Salad	
Rosemary	Deviled Eggs	Mock Turtle	Lamb Loaf	Chicken à la King	Cheese	Sauteed Mushrooms	Meat Salad	
Sage	Cheese Spreads	Consommé	Cold Roast Beef	Poultry Stuffing	Duck	Brussels Sprouts	Herbed French Dressing	
Savory	Liver Paste	Lentil Soup	Scrambled Eggs	Chicken Loaf	Fish	Beets	Red Kidney Bean Salad	
Tarragon	Mushrooms à la Greque	Snap Bean Soup	Marinated Lamb or Beef	Lobster	Green	Buttered Broccoli	Chicken Salad	
Thyme	Artichokes	Clam Chowder	Use sparingly in Fricassees	Poultry Stuffing	Bordelaise	Lightly on Sauteed Mushrooms		Tomato Aspic

Source: Reprinted from *How To Stay on a Low-Calorie, Low-Sodium Diet* with permission of the American Spice Trade Association, © 1980.

Table 8–3 Sodium Content of Spices

Spice	Milligrams/ teaspoon	Spice	Milligrams/ teaspoon
Allspice	1.4	Nutmeg	0.2
Basil Leaves	0.4	Onion Powder	0.8
Bay Leaves	0.3	Oregano	0.3
Caraway Seed	0.4	Paprika	0.4
Cardamom Seed	0.2	Parsley Flakes	5.9
Celery Seed	4.1	Pepper, Black	0.2
Cinnamon	0.2	Pepper, Chili	0.2
Cloves	4.2	Pepper, Red	0.2
Coriander Seed	0.3	Pepper, White	0.2
Cumin Seed	2.6	Poppy Seed	0.2
Curry Powder	1.0	Rosemary Leaves	0.5
Dill Seed	0.2	Sage	0.1
Fennel Seed	1.9	Savory	0.3
Garlic Powder	0.1	Sesame Seed	0.6
Ginger	0.5	Tarragon	1.0
Mace	1.3	Thyme	1.2
Marjoram	1.3	Turmeric	0.2
Mustard Powder	0.1		

Source: Reprinted from *Low-Sodium Spice Tips* with permission of the American Spice Trade Association, © 1980.

who can limit indiscretions to a two-day period should be commended. But others may have difficulty working back to appropriate eating habits and need assistance in renewing commitment.

A common experience in following a low-sodium eating pattern is the plateau. Week after week, clients make excellent progress; then, suddenly, they stop—they enter the contemplation phase. Moving up through all the previous steps may have seemed so easy, but now a new step—the same size as all the rest—seems very difficult. The first step to facilitate the move from contemplation to action is to show the client progress. "Look at this graph of your sodium intake. See how far you have come." If action seems possible, move to small steps of change and provide constant reinforcement. The easiest way to continue to progress is to subdivide the difficult step. If this does not help, the counselor should try increasing reinforcement.

Many clients confide to practitioners that they are guilty of cheating—taking the reinforcers even though they have not achieved a particular step. In such cases, the counselor must redesign the staged schedule so clients can be reinforced at a level they find achievable.

Some clients complain that they are losing the willpower to follow the low-sodium diet. They may experience this in two ways: (1) if they cannot get started, counselors and clients may not have set the initial step low enough (this can be resolved by moving to a lower step); (2) if they have started but insist that they see no progress, smaller steps are necessary.

In changing eating behaviors, counselors must review with clients the *antecedent-behavior-consequence* sequence. **The counselors begin to identify antecedents (events that precede a behavior) by asking the clients to think about the following questions as they relate to an eating occurrence:**

- What were the physical circumstances? (i.e., was the client surrounded by large tables of food?)
- What was the social setting?
- What was the behavior of others?
- What did you think or say to yourself?[84]

The client should be asked to collect data on these antecedents.

One tactic in changing eating behaviors is to lengthen the chain of events before partaking of a desired item such as high-sodium cheese. By pausing before eating, immediate gratification is delayed and the behavior eventually may not occur at all. It also may be possible to interrupt the chain by identifying an early link; a discontinuance or prolonged pause at that point may prevent the inappropriate behavior. The events also may be scrambled so that the eventual behavior is never reached.

Social occasions can present special problems. Clients can begin to learn to cope with such situations by collecting data on what types of reinforcers lead them to eat high-sodium foods during social events. The same reinforcer that maintains an undesired eating behavior can be used to strengthen appropriate conduct. For example:

> *Client* (at a party): "Boy, do those salty chips look good. But I know that they aren't on my diet. Over here, though, are some fresh vegetables. They look just as good and are on my diet. I feel really good about myself after eating them and I haven't cheated on my diet."

A list of positive reinforcers may help clients maintain a low-sodium diet. Watson and Tharp provide a set of questions clients might be asked when making a list of positive reinforcers:

1. What kinds of low-sodium foods do you like to eat?
2. What are your major interests?

3. What are your hobbies?
4. What people do you like to be with?
5. What do you like to do with these people?
6. What do you do for fun, for enjoyment?
7. What do you do to relax?
8. What do you do to get away from it all?
9. What makes you feel good?
10. What would be a nice present to receive?
11. What kinds of things are important to you?
12. What would you buy if you had an extra five dollars? Ten dollars? Fifty dollars?
13. What behaviors do you perform every day?
14. Are there any behaviors that you usually perform instead of the target behavior?
15. What would you hate to lose?
16. Of the things you do every day, what would you hate to give up?[88]

Counselors can construct additional questions. Determining the best reinforcers will depend upon each individual client. Before choosing a reinforcer, counselors should consider how closely the consequence meets a client's needs and desires. The reinforcer must be manageable from the client's point of view and must be contingent on performance of the desired behavior—eating low-sodium foods. The reinforcer should be strong enough to help in changing behavior.

The next step in helping to alter behavior is to set up a contract (Exhibit 8–3) that should specify stages of the change in eating habits, kinds of reinforcers to be gained at each step, and self-agreement to make gaining those reinforcers contingent on changing eating behavior involving high-sodium foods.

Ideally, a contract should be written and signed and should specify each detail of dietary change. Each element of this intervention plan should be very specific. A plan—a written contract—will help clients in those inevitable moments of weakness.

Reinforcers should fall within the realm of possibility or be readily accessible. They also should be potent. For example, buying clothes is not a potent reinforcer if the client does not enjoy doing it. The clients should be told to use "intuition" or estimate potency. The counselors' own data, collected during intervention, can indicate whether the chosen reinforcer is sufficiently powerful. A desired eating behavior should be reinforced immediately after the client has performed it. The longer reinforcement is delayed, the less effective it will be.

In summary, treatment strategies for low-sodium eating patterns involve tailoring and staging with calendars as a means of dealing with forgetting. To deal with a lack of commitment, it is important to make a list of self-reinforcers, use contracting, and stage the steps toward a goal.

Exhibit 8–3 Contract for a Sodium-Modified Diet

I agree to carry out each of the following steps and supply each reinforcer listed as each step is achieved:

Steps	Reinforcer
1. Eliminate salting before tasting.	Read a new cookbook.
2. Slowly eat unsalted foods to allow detection of true flavors.	Buy a new scarf.
3. Add new spices to foods in place of salt.	Buy a new pair of shoes.

Signed: _____

Cosigned (nutrition counselor): _____

Date: _____

Review of Chapter 8
(Answers in Appendix H)

1. List four factors that lead to inappropriate eating behaviors associated with sodium-modified patterns.

    a. _____

    b. _____

    c. _____

    d. _____

2. Identify three important steps in the assessment of a baseline diet for clients following a low-sodium regimen.

    a. _____

    _____

    b. _____

    _____

    c. _____

    _____

3. List four strategies to use in treating problems associated with eating patterns low in sodium.

a. _____

_____

b. _____

_____

c. _____

_____

d. _____

_____

4. Mrs. B. is 40 years old and has just been placed on a low-sodium diet. She has collected baseline information. She says she has tried and failed to follow a low-sodium diet previously. She loves cheese and cold cuts. What other facts would be beneficial to know? Based on hypothetical answers to those facts, what strategies would you recommend to solve her problems with low-sodium eating patterns? Explain why you would use these strategies.

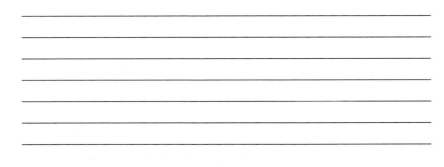

NOTES

1. National High Blood Pressure Education Program; National Institutes of Health; National Heart, Lung, and Blood Institute, *The Fifth Report of the Joint National Committee on Detection, Evaluation, and Treatment of High Blood Pressure*, NIH Publication No. 93-1088 (Bethesda, MD: March 1994), 11.

2. Treatment of Mild Hypertension Research Group, "The Treatment of Mild Hypertension Study: A Randomized, Placebo-Controlled Trial of a Nutritional-Hygenic Regimen along with Various Drug Monotherapies," *Archives of Internal Medicine* 151 (1991): 1413–1423.

3. S. Wassertheil-Smoller et al., "The Trial of Antihypertensive Interventions and Management (TAIM) Study: Adequate Weight Loss, Alone and Combined with Drug Therapy in the Treatment of Mild Hypertension," *Archives of Internal Medicine* 152 (1992): 131–136.

4. Trials of Hypertension Prevention Collaborative Research Group, "The Effects of Nonpharmacologic Interventions on Blood Pressure of Persons with High Normal Levels: Results of the Trials of Hypertension Prevention, Phase I," *Journal of the American Medical Association* 267 (1992): 1213–1220.

5. Hypertension Prevention Trial Research Group, "The Hypertension Prevention Trial: Three-Year Effects of Dietary Changes on Blood Pressure," *Archives of Internal Medicine* 150 (1990): 153–162.

6. Subcommittee on Nonpharmacologic Therapy of the 1984 Joint National Committee on Detection, Evaluation, and Treatment of High Blood Pressure, "Nonpharmacological Approaches to the Control of High Blood Pressure," *Hypertension* 8 (1986): 444–467.

7. R. Stamler et al., "Nutritional Therapy for High Blood Pressure: Final Report of a Four-Year Randomized Controlled Trial—The Hypertension Control Program," *Journal of the American Medical Association* 257 (1987): 1484–1491.

8. P. Little et al., "A Controlled Trial of a Low Sodium, Low Fat, High Fibre Diet in Treated Hypertensive Patients: Effect on Antihypertensive Drug Requirement in Clinical Practice," *Journal of Human Hypertension* 5 (1991): 175–181.

9. Working Group on Management of Patients with Hypertension and High Blood Cholesterol, "National Education Programs Working Group Report on the Management of Patients with Hypertension and High Blood Cholesterol," *Annals of Internal Medicine* 114 (1991): 224–237.

10. "Health Implications of Obesity: National Institutes of Health Consensus Development," *Annals of Internal Medicine* 103 (1985): 977–1077.

11. E.D. Frohlich et al., "The Problems of Obesity and Hypertension," *Hypertension* 5 (1983): Suppl. III-71–III-78.

12. L.B. Page et al., "Antecedents of Cardiovascular Disease of Six Solomon Island Societies," *Circulation* 49 (1974): 1132–1146.

13. B.N. Chiang et al., "Overweight and Hypertension," *Circulation* 39 (1969): 403–421.

14. I.A.M. Prior et al., "Sodium Intake and Blood Pressure in Two Polynesian Populations," *New England Journal of Medicine* 279 (1968): 515–520.

15. H.M. Whyte, "Body Build and Blood Pressure of Men in Australia and New Guinea," *Australian Journal of Experimental Biology and Medical Science* 41 (1963): 395–404.

16. G.V. Mann et al., "Cardiovascular Disease in the Masai," *Journal of Atherosclerosis Research* 4 (1964): 289–312.

17. C.R. Lowe, "Arterial Pressure, Physique and Occupation," *British Journal of Preventive and Social Medicine* 18 (1964): 115–124.

18. H.F. Epstein et al., "Prevalence of Chronic Disease and Distribution of Selected Physiological Variables in a Total Community, Tecumseh, Michigan," *American Journal of Epidemiology* 81 (1965): 307–323.

19. S. Padmavati and S. Gupta, "Blood Pressure Studies in Rural and Urban Groups in Delhi," *Circulation* 19 (1959): 395–405.

20. A.W. Voors et al., "Body Height and Body Mass as Determinants of Basal Blood Pressure in Children: The Bogalusa Heart Study," *American Journal of Epidemiology* 106 (1977): 101–108.

21. J.A. Morrison et al., "Studies of Blood Pressure in School Children (Ages 6–19) and Their Parents in an Integrated Suburban School District," *American Journal of Epidemiology* 111 (1980): 156–165.

22. W.B. Kannel et al., "Relation of Adiposity to Blood Pressure and Development of Hypertension: The Framingham Study," *Annals of Internal Medicine* 67 (1967): 48–59.

23. R.S. Paffenbarger et al., "Chronic Disease in Former College Students: VII. Characteristics in Youth Predisposing to Hypertension in Later Years," *American Journal of Epidemiology* 88 (1968): 25–32.

24. A. Oberman et al., "Trends in Systolic Blood Pressure in the Thousand Aviator Cohort over a Twenty-Four-Year Period," *Circulation* 36 (1967): 812–822.

25. A.L. Johnson et al., "Influence of Race, Sex and Weight on Blood Pressure Behavior in Young Adults," *American Journal of Cardiology* 35 (1975): 523–530.

26. S. Heyden et al., "Elevated Blood Pressure Levels in Adolescents, Evans County, GA: Seven-Year Follow-Up of 30 Patients and 30 Controls," *Journal of the American Medical Association* 209 (1969): 1683–1689.

27. J.P. Despres et al., "Regional Distribution of Body Fat, Plasma Lipoproteins, and Cardiovascular Disease," *Arteriosclerosis* 10 (1990): 497–511.

28. J. Bronzek et al., "Drastic Food Restriction," *Journal of the American Medical Association*, 137 (1948): 1569–1574.

29. R.H. Rose, "Weight Reduction and Its Remarkable Effect on High Blood Pressure," *New York Medical Journal* 115 (1922): 752–759.

30. M.F. Hovel, "The Experimental Evidence for Weight Loss Treatment of Essential Hypertension: A Critical Review," *American Journal of Public Health* 72 (1982): 359–368.

31. E. Reisin et al., "Effect of Weight Loss without Salt Restriction on the Reduction of Blood Pressure in Overweight Hypertensive Patients," *New England Journal of Medicine* 298 (1981): 1–10.

32. B. Fagerberg et al., "Blood Pressure Control during Weight Reduction in Obese Hypertensive Men: Separate Effects of Sodium and Energy Restriction," *British Medical Journal* 288 (1984): 11–14.

33. M.H. Maxwell et al., "Blood Pressure Changes in Obese Hypertensive Subjects during Rapid Weight Loss: Comparison of Restricted versus Unchanged Salt Intake," *Archives of Internal Medicine* 144 (1984): 1581–1584.

34. M.L. Tuck et al., "Reduction in Plasma Catecholamines and Blood Pressure during Weight Loss in Obese Subjects," *Acta Endocrinologica (Copenhagen)* 102 (1983): 252–257.

35. K.H. Stokholm et al., "Correlation between Initial Blood Pressure and Blood Pressure Decrease after Weight Loss," *International Journal of Obesity* 6 (1982): 307–312.

36. J. Stamler et al., "Prevention and Control of Hypertension by Nutritional-Hygienic Means," *Journal of the American Medical Association* 243 (1980): 1819–1823.

37. H.E. Eliaho et al., "Body Weight Reduction Necessary to Attain Normotension in the Overweight Hypertensive Patient," *International Journal of Obesity* (Supplement 1) (1981): 157–163.

38. J. Stamler et al., "Prevention and Control of Hypertension by Nutritional-Hygenic Means, *Journal of the American Medical Association* 243 (1980): 1819–1823.

39. Eliaho et al., "Body Weight Reduction Necessary To Attain Normotension in the Overweight Hypertensive Patient."

40. V. Jorgens et al., "Long-Term Effects of Weight Changes on Cardiovascular Risk Factors over 4.7 Years in 247 Obese Patients" (Abstract), Presented at the 4th International Congress of Obesity, New York, 1983, 68a.

41. E. Reison et al., "Cardiovascular Changes after Weight Reduction in Obesity Hypertension," *Annals of Internal Medicine* 98 (1983): 315–319.

42. H.G. Langford et al., "Effect of Drug and Diet Treatment of Mild Hypertension on Diastolic Blood Pressure," *Hypertension* 17 (1991): 210–217.

43. D.E. Schotte and A.J. Stunkard, "The Effects of Weight Reduction on Blood Pressure in 301 Obese Patients," *Archives of Internal Medicine* 150 (1990): 1701–1704.

44. National High Blood Pressure Education Program; National Institutes of Health; National Heart, Lung, and Blood Institute, *The Fifth Report of the Joint National Committee on Detection, Evaluation, and Treatment of High Blood Pressure,* 12.

45. Intersalt Cooperative Research Group, "Intersalt: An International Study of Electrolyte Excretion and Blood Pressure. Results for 24 Hour Urinary Sodium and Potassium Excretion," *British Medical Journal* 297 (1988): 319–328.

46. M.R. Law et al., "By How Much Does Dietary Salt Reduction Lower Blood Pressure? I—Analysis of Observational Data among Populations," *British Medical Journal* 302 (1991): 811–815.

47. Intersalt Cooperative Research Group, "Sodium, Potassium, Body Mass, Alcohol and Blood Pressure: The Intersalt Study," *Journal of Hypertension* 6, Supplement 4 (1988): S584–S586.

48. J.A. Cutler et al., "An Overview of Randomized Trials of Sodium Reduction and Blood Pressure," *Hypertension* 17, Supplement I (1991): I-27–I-33.

49. M.R. Law et al., "By How Much Does Dietary Salt Reduction Lower Blood Pressure? III— Analysis of Data from Trials of Salt Reduction," *British Medical Journal* 302 (1991): 819–824.

50. J. Sullivan, "Salt Sensitivity: Definition, Conception, Methodology, and Long-Term Issues," *Hypertension* 17, Supplement I (1991): I-61–I-68.

51. J.M. Flack et al., "Racial and Ethnic Modifiers of the Salt-Blood Pressure Response," *Hypertension* 17, Supplement I (1991): I-115–I-121.

52. D.E. Grobbee, "Methodology of Sodium Sensitivity Assessment: The Example of Age and Sex," *Hypertension* 17, Supplement I (1991): I-109–I-114.

53. National High Blood Pressure Education Program; National Institutes of Health; National Heart, Lung, and Blood Institute, *The Fifth Report of the Joint National Committee on Detection, Evaluation, and Treatment of High Blood Pressure,* 13.

54. World Hypertension League, "Alcohol and Hypertension—Implications for Management: A Consensus Statement by the World Hypertension League," *Journal of Human Hypertension* 5 (1991):1854–1856.

55. C.H. Hennekens, "Alcohol," in *Prevention of Coronary Heart Disease,* ed. N.N. Kaplan and J. Stamler (Philadelphia: W.B. Saunders, 1983), 130–138.

56. S.W. MacMahon et al., "Obesity, Alcohol Consumption and Blood Pressure in Australian Men and Women: The National Heart Foundation of Australia Risk Factor Prevalence Study," *Journal of Hypertension* 2 (1984): 85–91.

57. G.D. Friedman et al., "Alcohol, Tobacco and Hypertension," *Hypertension* 4, Supplement III (1982): III-43–III-150.

58. J.B. Saunders et al., "Alcohol-Induced Hypertension," *Lancet* 2 (1981): 653–656.

59. M.G. Marmot, "Alcohol and Coronary Heart Disease," *International Journal of Epidemiology* 13 (1984): 160–167.

60. T. Gordon and W.B. Kannel, "Drinking and Mortality: The Framingham Study," *American Journal of Epidemiology* 120 (1984): 97–107.

61. R. Maheswaran et al., "High Blood Pressure Due to Alcohol: A Rapidly Reversible Effect," *Hypertension* 17 (1991): 787–792.

62. National High Blood Pressure Education Program; National Institutes of Health; National Heart, Lung, and Blood Institute, *The Fifth Report of the Joint National Committee on Detection, Evaluation, and Treatment of High Blood Pressure,* 12.

63. Intersalt Cooperative Research Group, "Intersalt: An International Study of Electrolyte Excretion and Blood Pressure. Results for 24-Hour Urinary Sodium and Potassium Excretion," 319–328.

64. S.L. Linas, "The Role of Potassium in the Pathogenesis and Treatment of Hypertension," *Kidney International* 39 (1991): 771–786.

65. National High Blood Pressure Education Program; National Institutes of Health; National Heart, Lung, and Blood Institute, *The Fifth Report of the Joint National Committee on Detection, Evaluation, and Treatment of High Blood Pressure,* 13.

66. P. Hamet et al., "Interactions among Calcium, Sodium, and Alcohol Intake as Determinants of Blood Pressure," *Hypertension* 17, Supplement I (1991): I-150–I-154.

67. J.A. Cutler and E. Brittain, "Calcium and Blood Pressure: An Epidemiologic Perspective," *American Journal of Hypertension* 3 (1990): 137S–146S.

68. National High Blood Pressure Education Program; National Institutes of Health; National Heart, Lung, and Blood Institute, *The Fifth Report of the Joint National Committee on Detection, Evaluation, and Treatment of High Blood Pressure,* 14.

69. National High Blood Pressure Education Program; National Institutes of Health; National Heart, Lung, and Blood Institute, *The Fifth Report of the Joint National Committee on Detection, Evaluation, and Treatment of High Blood Pressure,* 14.

70. S.B. Steckel and M.A. Swain, "Contracting with Patients to Improve Compliance," *Hospitals* 51 (December 1977): 81–83.

71. R.R. Wing et al., "Dietary Approaches to the Reduction of Blood Pressure: Independence of Weight and Sodium/Potassium Interventions," *Preventive Medicine* 13 (1984): 233–244.

72. N.M. Kaplan et al., "Two Techniques to Improve Adherence to Dietary Sodium Restriction in the Treatment of Hypertension," *Archives of Internal Medicine* 142 (1982): 1638–1641.

73. C.A. Nugent et al., "Salt Restriction in Hypertensive Patients: Comparison of Advice, Education and Group Management," *Archives of Internal Medicine* 144 (1984): 1415–1417.

74. M.F. Hovel et al., "Experimental Analysis of Adherence Counseling Implications for Hypertension Management," 14 (1985): 648–654.

75. S.E. Evers et al., "Lack of Impact of Salt Restriction Advice on Hypertensive Patients," *Preventive Medicine* 16 (1987): 213–220.

76. J.L. Tillotson, M.C. Winston, and Y. Hall, "Critical Behaviors in the Dietary Management of Hypertension," *Journal of the American Dietetic Association* (1984): 290–293.

77. U.S. Department of Health and Human Services, "Report of the Working Group Critical Patient Behaviors in the Dietary Management of High Blood Pressure," NIH Publication No. 81-2269 (1981).

78. K. Glanz, "Compliance with Dietary Regimens: Its Magnitude, Measurement and Determinants," *Preventive Medicine* 9 (1980): 787–804.

79. Evers et al., "Lack of Impact of Salt Restriction Advice on Hypertensive Patients."

80. J. Takala, A. Leminen, and T. Telaranta, "Strategies for Improving Compliance in Hypertensive Patients," *Scandinavian Journal of Primary Health Care* 3 (1985): 233–238.

81. J.Z. Miller, M.H. Weinberger, and S.J. Cohen, "Advances in Non-Pharmacologic Treatment of Hypertension: A New Approach to the Problem of Effective Dietary Sodium Restriction, 1. Sodium in the Diet: Patient Compliance," *Indiana Medicine* (October 1985): 893–895.

82. J.A.C. Kerr, "Multidimensional Health Locus of Control Adherence and Lowered Diastolic Blood Pressure," *Heart and Lung* 15 (1986): 87–93.

83. D.G. Schlundt, E.C. McDonel, and H.G. Langford, "Compliance in Dietary Management of Hypertension," *Comprehensive Therapy* 11 (1985): 18–21.

84. S.J. Cohen, "Improving Patients' Compliance with Antihypertensive Regimens," *Comprehensive Therapy* 11 (1985): 18–21.

85. Schlundt, McDonel and Langford, "Compliance in Dietary Management."

86. M.G. Perri et al., "Maintaining Strategies for the Treatment of Obesity: An Evaluation of Relapse Prevention Training and Post-Treatment Contact by Mail and Telephone," *Journal of Consulting and Clinical Psychology* 52 (1984): 404–413.

87. D.L. Watson and R.G. Tharp, *Self-Directed Behavior: Self-Modification for Personal Adjustment* (Monterey, CA: Brooks/Cole Publishing, 1972), 85–89.

88. D.L. Watson and R.G. Tharp, *Self-Directed Behavior: Self-Modification for Personal Adjustment,* 108.

Adherence Tool 8–1: Spices for Low-Sodium Diets (Informational Device)

Spices for Use with Meats:

Dill seed for fish or chicken sauces
Garlic powder for bouillabaisse
Ginger for roast chicken
Mace for fish stew
Marjoram for salmon loaf
Mint for veal or lamb roast
Mustard for cream sauce on fish

Nutmeg for southern fried chicken
Oregano for Swiss steak
Rosemary for chicken à la king
Savory for chicken loaf
Tarragon for marinated beef
Thyme for clam chowder

Spices for Use with Vegetables:

Allspice for eggplant creole
Basil for stewed tomatoes
Bay leaf for boiled new potatoes
Caraway seed for cabbage wedges
Cinnamon for sweet potatoes
Celery seed for cauliflower
Chili powder for Mexican-style corn
Cloves for candied sweet potatoes
Curry for creamed vegetables
Dill seed for peas and carrots
Garlic for stewed tomatoes

Ginger for beets
Mace for succotash
Mint for green peas
Powdered dry mustard for baked beans
Nutmeg for glazed carrots
Rosemary for sauteed mushrooms
Sage for brussels sprouts
Savory for beets
Tarragon for broccoli
Thyme lightly on sauteed mushrooms

Plan menus for three meals. The menus should be low in sodium and should use the spices suggested above. Choose spices you think you and your family would enjoy.

Breakfast	Lunch	Dinner

Adherence Tool 8–2:   Estimated Natural Sodium Content of Foods (Informational Device)

A rough guide follows for the natural sodium content of foods that are grown or produced and processed without the addition of sodium.

8 oz. milk	=	120 mg. of sodium
1 oz. meat	=	25 mg. of sodium
1 egg	=	70 mg. of sodium
½ cup vegetable	=	9 mg. of sodium
½ cup fruit	=	2 mg. of sodium
1 slice of bread	=	5 mg. of sodium
1 teaspoon of fat	=	0 mg. of sodium

Source: Reprinted with permission from H.S. Mitchell et al., *Nutrition in Health and Disease,* p. 430, © 1976; Lippincott-Raven.

Adherence Tool 8–3:   Daily Food Record with Emphasis on Sodium Intake (Monitoring Device)

Time	Food Eaten	Amount	Low in Sodium*	Moderate in Sodium*	High in Sodium*

*Place an *X* in the column to indicate whether the food is high, moderate, or low in sodium.

CHAPTER 9

Nutrition Counseling for Cancer Risk Prevention

CHAPTER OBJECTIVES

1. Identify common inappropriate eating behaviors associated with following a fat-controlled eating pattern.

2. Identify how to assess problems associated with inappropriate eating patterns in following a fat-controlled regimen.

3. List strategies to overcome inappropriate eating behaviors associated with eating patterns controlled for fat.

Cancer is the second most common cause of death in Western societies. Because cancer is largely a disease of old age, as the population ages the number of cancer deaths increases. Most research in this area has been directed toward treatment and cure of cancers as they arise, a singularly unsuccessful policy. The prognosis of individuals with cancer of the lung, breast, large bowel, stomach, prostate, and pancreas is very discouraging. Successful approaches to diseases such as smallpox, rabies, plague, cholera, whooping cough, and diphtheria have focused on prevention rather than treatment.[1]

Approximately 40 percent of human cancers may have dietary causes.[2,3] Little is known about specific dietary factors responsible for cancer and dietary changes necessary for cancer prevention, but dietary evidence continues to accumulate.[4–7]

A variety of dietary factors have been associated with cancer. This chapter focuses on modifications in fat intake. Other approaches include an increase in fruits, vegetables, and grains to maximize fiber.

THEORIES AND FACTS ABOUT NUTRITION AND CANCER

Role of Dietary Fats in Cancer

Despite some inconsistencies in the data relating dietary fat to cancer causation, animal studies show an effect of dietary fat on carcinogenesis and suggest that dietary fat has a cancer-promoting role. International epidemiologic studies have suggested that differences in dietary fat intake may provide a meaningful key to prevention of cancer.

Animals fed a high-fat diet often have higher rates of carcinogen-induced cancers of the breast, colon, and pancreas than those fed low-fat diets.[8] Evidence of the positive connection between fat intake and cancer was shown in studies of experimental animals.[9] The combination of high fat and low dietary fiber is associated most highly with increased rates of cancers.[10]

The arguments and counterarguments based on human epidemiologic data are well summarized based on a 1990 symposium on the topic.[11-15] Studies of migrant populations have found that people who move to a country with a higher incidence of breast cancer than their native country tend to acquire the dietary habits of their new country of residence and may experience a cancer incidence that changes with the change in dietary fat.[16,17] Epidemiological studies show positive and negative associations for breast cancer and total fat consumption.[18-22] While methodological problems may have obscured a true risk association in the studies that have found negative associations,[23-25] these studies reinforce the need for cautious interpretation and additional study of diet and breast cancer risk.[26]

Substantial epidemiologic and animal evidence supports a relationship between dietary fat and the incidence of both breast cancer[27] and colon cancer.[28] Indeed, a comparison of populations indicates that death rates for cancers of the breast, colon, and prostate are directly proportional to estimated dietary fat intakes.[29,30] Other cancers that have been related to fat intake are those of the rectum,[31] ovaries,[32] and endometrium.[33] Considerable uncertainties remain to be resolved about these relationships. For example, the effects of different types of dietary fat (i.e., saturated versus unsaturated, animal versus plant origin) have not been separately analyzed in most human studies. In some human studies, low-fat and low polyunsaturated fatty acid (PUFA) (omega-6 acid) diets are associated with enhanced natural killer cytotoxicity for tumor cells in vitro, and effects are especially pronounced; however, the results are not entirely clear. The low-fat diets (25 percent or 30 percent of calories) did have such an effect; alterations in polyunsaturated to saturated fat ratio (P/S ratio) did not.[34,35] Thus, at present, the role of PUFA is not clear; several reports suggest that the data are mixed.[36,37] Investigators have studied the role of the omega-3 fish oils in animal models and have concluded that many effects operate through prostaglandin metabolism. Because the omega-3 and omega-6 fatty acids are metabolized to prostaglandins of different types and different activities, their effects may be quite different. The omega-3 fatty acids give rise to prostaglandins that appear to have lower biological activity than those formed from the omega-6 fatty acids, affecting not only natural killer cell activity, but other mediators such as the lymphokines, leukotrienes, and thromboxanes.[38] Although the mechanisms are not yet clear, immunosurveillance is thought to be involved.[39] Studies in humans are now being completed.

Table 9–1 summarizes several feasibility studies testing the hypothesis that low-fat diets are achievable among women living in various Western countries. The Women's Health Initiative is a study funded by The National Institutes of Health and designed to address the issue in a clinical trial design. It is an ongoing study with no outcome data reported at this time.[40]

In summary, the majority of the studies to date are strongly suggestive of the role for dietary fat in the etiology of some types of cancer. This chapter focuses on total fat intake as a possible means of modifying cancer incidence.

RESEARCH ON ADHERENCE TO EATING PATTERNS IN CANCER RISK PREVENTION

No systematic studies of the role of nutrition education in reducing cancer risk have been completed, although the National Cancer Institute has sponsored field trials for high-risk persons as well as the public. The Women's Health Initiative is one of the long-term clinical trials designed to look at the preventive effect of dietary fat intake with increases in fruits, vegetables, and grains. The Women's Intervention Nutrition Study (WINS) is designed to study a reduced fat diet (15 percent of calories from fat) with a different ratio of types of fat consumed and an increase in wheat fiber and its effect on tumor recurrence either with or without chemotherapeutic or antiestrogen therapy. Each of these clinical trials will provide evidence on the relationship between diet and cancer. The Polyps Prevention Trial is also designed to determine if diets low in fat and high in fiber affect polyp occurrence.

Planning nutrition education programs for reducing cancer risk involves many issues. Considerable controversy still exists about the extent to which dietary changes alone can reduce cancer morbidity. There is also much room for confusion about the specificity of cancers that are affected by certain nutrients in the diet. References to cancer in public health education may unnecessarily raise both the fears and the expectations of clients. Health professionals who are planning nutrition education on cancer risk must weigh the implications of the strategies and messages they plan to use.[41] Patterson and her colleagues have provided data from the Women's Health Initiative on low-fat diet practices of older women.[42] These practices can provide valuable information on planning nutrition programs.

Table 9–1 Characteristics of Selected Feasibility Studies for Reducing Dietary Fat

				Study			
		WHT[5-7]		Swedish Breast Cancer Study[8]		AHF Study[9]	
Characteristic	NAS[1-4]	Intervention Group	Control Group	Intervention Group	Control Group	Cancer	Cystic Disease
Group size		220					
Treatment	17			121 randomized, 63 completed (52%)		19 breast cancer	
Control	11			119 randomized, 106 completed (89%)		16 fibrocystic disease	
Diet assessment methods	4 DDR at baseline, 3 mo.	Baseline, 6, 12, 24 mo. SQFF, 24-hr. recall to compare to 4 DDR, fat score used to measure adherence		Diet histories (all) Food records (treatment only)		4DDR	
Study Duration, Months	3	12		24		3	
Calories							
Baseline	1840 (419)	7258 KJ (122)	7148 (168) KJ	7.7 MJ	8.2 MJ	1504	1743
3-month follow-up	1365 (291)						
% decrease	25%						
12-month follow-up		5460 (112)	6619 (158)				
% decrease		-24%	-7%				
24-month follow-up		5691	6675	6.8	7.6	1347 (3 mo.)	1344
% Decrease from baseline		-22%	-5%	-11.6%	-7.3%	-10.4%	22.8%
% Decrease from 12 months		+2%	+2%				
Fat, % Calories							
Baseline	38% (4.3)	39%	39%	36.9%	37.2%	33.5%	35.6%
?-months follow-up	23% (7.8)	22%					
% decrease	56%						

12-month follow-up	22%	37%	24.0	34.1	(3 mo.)20.7	21.4
% Decrease	-17%	-2%	-12.9%	-3.1%	-12.8%	-14.2%
24-month follow-up	23%	37%			22.6 g	15.5 g/day
% Decrease	+1%	0%				
Weight Loss, g/day						
Actual	31 g	40 g (3 mo.)	Not reported precisely, but intervention group decreased slightly (most in first year) then increased but not to baseline; but controls increased		66.33	59.3
Predicted from calorie deficit reported	65 g	53 g (3 mo.)	Should have decreased in both groups almost equally if reporting were equally erroneous		64.29	57.9

Notes: NAS = Nutrition Adjuvant Study DDR = Dietary Diary Record MJ = Millijoules
WHT = Women's Health Trial SQFF = Semiquantified Food Frequency
AHF = American Health Foundation KJ = Kilojoules

1. R.T. Chlebowski et al., "Breast Cancer Nutrition Adjuvant Study (NAS): Protocol Design and Initial Patient Adherence," *Breast Cancer Research Treatment* 10 (1987): 21.
2. I.M. Buzzard et al., "Diet Intervention Methods To Reduce Fat Intake: Nutrient and Food Group Composition of Self-Selected Low Fat Diets," *Journal of the American Dietetic Association* 90 (1990): 42.
3. R.T. Chlebowski et al., "Adjuvant Dietary Fat Intake Reduction in Postmenopausal Breast Cancer Patient Management," *Breast Cancer Research and Treatment* 20 (1991): 73–84.
4. R.T. Chlebowski et al., "The Nutrition Adjuvant Study Experience and Commentary," *Controlled Clinical Trials* 10 (1989): 368.
5. R.L. Prentice et al., "Aspects of the Rationale for the Women's Health Trial," *Journal of the National Cancer Institute* 80 (1988): 802.
6. R.L. Prentice and L. Sheppard, "Validity of International, Time Trend, and Migrant Studies of Dietary Factors and Disease Risk," *Preventive Medicine* 18 (1989): 167.
7. W. Insull et al., "Results of a Randomized Feasibility Study of a Low Fat Diet," *Archives of Internal Medicine* 150 (1990): 421.
8. E. Nordevang et al., "Dietary Intervention in Breast Cancer Patients: Effects on Dietary Habits and Nutrient Intake," *European Journal of Clinical Nutrition* 44 (1990): 681.
9. A.P. Boyar et al., "Recommendations for the Prevention of Chronic Disease: The Application for Breast Disease," *American Journal of Clinical Nutrition* 48 (1988): 896.

Source: Johanna Dwyer, Director, Frances Stern Nutrition Center, Box 783, New England Medical Center Hospital, 750 Washington Street, Boston, MA 02111.

This study showed that 69 percent of 7,419 women, aged 50 to 75 years, who responded to a food questionnaire rarely or never ate skin on chicken, 76 percent rarely or never ate fat on meat, 36 percent usually drank nonfat milk, 52 percent usually ate low-fat or fat-free mayonnaise, 59 percent ate low-fat chips/snacks, and 42 percent ate nonfat cheese. African American and Hispanic women of lower socioeconomic status reported significantly fewer low-fat practices than white women and women of higher socioeconomic status.[43]

Glanz stressed the importance of support from the family and health care providers.[44] Carson reported on a team approach to nutrition for persons with cancer, in which nutritionists helped clients solve a variety of diet-related problems and provided information or referral to other team members as necessary. Nutritionists also provided credible information and answered questions about unorthodox dietary practices. Carson's article gave case examples to illustrate these activities.[45] Campbell et al. taught systematic relaxation techniques to 22 persons with cancer in their homes in an effort to promote weight gain in underweight persons. Only 55 percent of these persons practiced the relaxation techniques regularly, but nutritional status and cancer performance status improved among the compliers.[46] This preliminary study suggested that for motivated persons, relaxation techniques may help with diet, pain control, and anxiety reduction.

Nutrition education for persons with cancer must be part of the comprehensive treatment program and account for individual needs and preferences. It will probably gain more attention as survival rates for various cancers increase in the years ahead.[47]

The discussion below is devoted to a diet recommended in a feasibility study and an ongoing clinical trial for the National Cancer Institute—The Women's Health Trial* and the Women's Health Initiative.** An example of how to apply

---

*The efforts of the following persons who developed the intervention component of the Women's Health Trial are acknowledged: Laura Coleman, MS, RD; Joanne Csaplar, MS, RD; Johanna Dwyer, DSc, RD; Carole Palmer, MEd, RD; and Molly Holland, MPH, RD. Many of the concepts discussed in this chapter were originally printed in materials designed by this group at Frances Stern Medical Center and New England Medical Center Hospitals with funding from the Nutrition Coordinating Unit, Tufts University School of Medicine, or the National Institutes of Health.

**The efforts of the following persons who developed the intervention component of the Women's Health Initiative are acknowledged: Beth Barrows, MS, RD; Carolyn Ehret, MS, RD; and Lesley Tinker, PhD, RD. Many of the concepts discussed in this chapter were originally printed in materials designed by this group at Fred Hutchison Cancer Research Center—Clinical Coordinating Center, 1124 Columbia Street, MP1002, Seattle, Washington 98104 with funding from the National Institutes of Health. All Adherence Tool materials are modifications of Women's Health Initiative concepts to fit this nutrition counseling text.

counseling skills to a specific low-fat diet for cancer prevention is provided in the following section.

INAPPROPRIATE EATING BEHAVIORS

For the client who has difficulty with simple math, adding up total grams of fat consumed in a day can be very difficult. For some, just finding the time to make the computations may be a problem. The low-fat diet may be very different from the client's traditional high-fat diet. For example, a client might state, "I miss fried meats, fried potatoes, gravy, and vegetables smothered with butter. I don't know how to avoid those favorite dishes."

ASSESSMENT OF EATING BEHAVIORS

Assessing intake of fat might require using several three-day diet records and a quantified food frequency. Initially, the Client Eating Questionnaire for clients following cholesterol- and fat-controlled eating patterns might be of value (Adherence Tool 4–1).

TREATMENT STRATEGIES

Treatment strategies can be divided into three categories: those dealing with lack of knowledge, forgetfulness, and lack of commitment.

Strategies To Deal with Lack of Knowledge

Three-day diet diaries can be used to identify problem areas. Once the counselor and client have mutually identified a problem area, the counselor can determine exactly where knowledge may be lacking. The following are examples of problem areas:

- using mathematical skills
- knowing what to look for on a label
- cooking high-fat, ethnic dishes in a low-fat manner
- eating in restaurants

Using Mathematical Skills

For the person who has problems using math skills, the counselor can identify exactly where problems are occurring (for example, whether the math calculations for certain meals like breakfast are easier while calculations for other meals may be more difficult because of the variations in foods). The counselor should praise the use of math skills at one meal and build upon those for a more difficult meal.

> *Client:* "I especially have trouble calculating grams of fat in meat at dinner."
> *Counselor:* "You have done an excellent job with breakfast. I'm glad you brought up this problem with dinner so that we can try to solve it."
> *Client:* "I'm no good at math. I can't handle this problem."
> *Counselor:* "You have proven that you can use math skills in more routine situations at breakfast. Let's use some of those same skills for the dinner meal. You have said meat is a major problem; let's try to calculate it."

Reading Labels

A second problem involves lack of knowledge of what to look for on a label. Sometimes examples are unclear or covered too quickly in a nutrition counseling session for the client to gain adequate understanding of how to apply the knowledge to all situations. In subsequent sessions, it is up to the counselor to assess a problem in this area and allow for enough rehearsal to transfer general information adequately to specific individual situations.

> *Client:* "I just don't know what to look for on food labels. It's so frustrating."
> *Counselor:* "Can you give me an example of a label that has been difficult to figure out?"
> *Client:* "Yes, this ingredient list says that there is no fat in this macaroni dish. But I have added margarine to the dry ingredients, so I know fat is included."
> *Counselor:* "The ingredient list will not include those items added to a product, only items in the box as you buy it. It is very important to count the fat added because it will contribute to your total fat for the day."

Cooking High-Fat, Ethnic Dishes in a Low-Fat Manner

Some clients have a problem combining the low-fat diet with their past high-fat, ethnic eating patterns.

> *Client:* "I have a difficult time avoiding fried foods. They have become such an important part of my usual eating habits."
> *Counselor:* "Martha, what food in particular are you concerned about?"
> *Client:* "I mostly miss fried potatoes."
> *Counselor:* "Let's try using PAM spray and frying your potatoes with very little fat. Would you be willing to try that?"
> *Client:* "I hadn't thought of that. It's a great idea."

Eating in Restaurants

Eating in restaurants forces the client to make many decisions. Initially choosing the restaurant can be a problem. Controlling the amount of food eaten, making changes at the table, and making low-fat requests are all important when eating out (see Adherence Tool 9–1).

Applying Other Strategies To Deal with Lack of Knowledge

Knowledge about how to deal with low-fat substitutions when eating can be valuable in beginning a low-fat diet (see Adherence Tools 9–2 to 9–5).

Knowledge is seldom enough to increase motivation or adherence, but misinformation can definitely undermine success. If a client is motivated but doesn't understand a correct procedure, simply providing the appropriate information can make a great difference. It is important to provide information on what to do, how to do it, and why it should be done. **The tips below are ways to be sure clients understand information adequately:**

- Knowing the rationale for the new eating pattern helps the client remember what information has been provided.
- Asking the client to repeat information can help in knowledge retention.
- Adding new information on the low-fat eating pattern to what the client already knows helps retention.
- Using language the client understands is important.
- Reemphasizing the benefits of the new low-fat eating pattern can help clear up the client's misunderstandings about the regimen and increase the client's involvement in active change.
- Providing information slowly over time helps eliminate overloading the client with too much information at one time.
- Practicing use of information in an actual or simulated situation helps the client retain information.
- Providing identical written information that supports verbally presented material can help the client retain information.

Strategies To Deal with Forgetfulness

Cues to help remind a client to plan to eat a low-fat diet can be very important. Some occasions that call for cueing a client are: vacations, parties, holiday meals, and birthdays.

> *Client:* "I forgot to ask the waitress to give me salad dressing on the side, and I know I ate too much on the salad."
> *Counselor:* "What might you have done to avoid this situation?"
> *Client:* "Sometimes I just need help remembering."
> *Counselor:* "Who might help remind you?"
> *Client:* "My husband might remind me."
> *Counselor:* "That's a great idea. Sometimes reminders from a spouse can turn into nagging. Has that ever happened to you?"
> *Client:* "Yes, it has. How can I avoid that?"
> *Counselor:* "One way is to provide your husband with a few specific things of which to help remind you. The salad dressing on the side might be one of three or four specific reminders. This will eliminate constant general nagging."

Parties, holiday meals, and birthdays may be made easier by preplanning. For example, by calling the hostess ahead of time, clients can check out all items on the menu to determine fat content. By preplanning, the client can choose those items lowest in fat and lessen the temptation just to forget about the diet during the special event.

Aids for remembering can also point to the client's achievements, which are also frequently forgotten. One woman keeps a list of all of those tasks she must do in a day (see Adherence Tool 9–6). A check when each task is completed helps clients feel they have accomplished something.

A sign on the refrigerator with fat scores (tally of total fat eaten in a day) for each day of the week serves as a reminder to strive for a fat score goal.

Strategies To Deal with Lack of Commitment

Three factors contribute to lack of commitment to following a low-fat diet: a history of defeats, a negative attitude, and self-doubts.

A History of Defeats

A client with a history of poor adherence to other diets may have problems following the low-fat eating pattern. Many clients begin a new eating pattern expecting to fail. This type of person needs a great deal of support and encouragement. Counselors should encourage the attitude that success *is* possible, even though it may not have been previously. They can emphasize a break from the old habit of going on and off a diet, stressing instead the idea of a lifestyle change. The client should know that lapses will occur. Building new skills from past problems is important.

Negative Attitude

Some clients who have watched family members die of cancer may be very afraid of its consequences. They may feel that nothing can really help them. Following an eating pattern that may reduce risk is at least one way of easing a troubled mind. Counselors can discuss the goal of the new eating pattern with such clients and emphasize that the eating plan is a healthy one.

Self-Doubts

For some clients, self-doubts can begin to creep into thoughts. Counselors can help clients focus on their successes.

> *Client:* "Life isn't spontaneous anymore. I always have to think about what I'm eating. I'm not sure this new eating plan is worth the trouble."
>
> *Counselor:* "Look at the successes you have already had. Have you ever done anything that you were proud of or successful at in the past? How did you feel

at that time? Did it become easier as time went on? Let's try to build on those past efforts and be successful with this diet also."

This is an example of a client who has reverted to the precontemplation stage. The counselor doesn't give advice, but rather tries to involve the client in looking back over past successes.

Counselors should assist the client in tearing down blocks to adherence, for example, by helping clients develop short-term goals that they can easily achieve. This technique allows for positive self-rewards. By shaping behavior in this way, the counselor helps the client develop a more positive outlook. Counselors can also guide clients in practicing positive self-talk to help identify negative monologues and change them to positive. Positive self-talk can lead to positive changes in eating patterns (see Appendixes F and G).

Some clients may benefit from assertiveness training. Feeling confident enough to ask the ingredients of a dish ordered in a restaurant can be a step toward successfully following the low-fat eating pattern.

What a client believes is true can help or hinder success. Following are some examples. Some clients have misconceptions about a low-fat eating pattern:

Client: "I've been reading that diets too low in fat can be bad for you."
Counselor: "What is your source of information?" [Explain misconceptions]

Some clients have unrealistic beliefs about the low-fat eating style:

Client: "I already eat a low-fat diet. This will be easy."
Counselor: "Your diet diaries show that your current eating pattern is low in visible fat but high in hidden fat. Let me show you what I mean."
Client: "Wow, my diet is high in fat. I'd better start cutting back."

Some clients may begin by being unnecessarily fearful.

Client: "Life will never be the same. I can never again eat just what I want."
Counselor: "If you feel like forgetting the new eating plan, give yourself a controlled 'day off.' By that I mean increase your fat intake but in a controlled fashion. For example, set aside one meal a week as a higher-fat meal."

Many clients find that the higher-fat foods are not so terrific and that, indeed, they have lost their taste for them.

Some behavioral strategies that help increase commitment are:

1. shaping of behaviors
2. self-monitoring
3. contracts
4. self-reward
5. group support networks.

Shaping behavior requires a gradual, stepwise process toward change that helps build success in stages, which promotes further success.

> *Client:* "I know skim milk is lowest in fat, but I grew up on a farm where skim milk was given to livestock. I will never be able to give up whole milk."
>
> *Counselor:* "Would you be willing to try a gradual movement to skim milk?"
>
> *Client:* "I guess I can try."
>
> *Counselor:* "First try using 2 percent milk. You can begin by mixing 2 percent and whole milk and then moving solely to 2 percent. You could then mix 2 percent and 1 percent milk and eventually move to only 1 percent. The same combination of 1 percent and skim would then end in eventual use of only skim milk."

Self-monitoring, another important strategy, encourages self-reliance, provides immediate feedback, shows behavior patterns that undermine or build success, and provides a means of planning for future problems so that they can be minimized. Examples of self-monitoring tools include Adherence Tool 9–7, which records grams of fat consumed in a day, and Adherence Tool 9–8, which allows weekly budgeting, or eating a little more fat one day and a little less the following day. Adherence Tool 9–9 provides a list of low-fat eating behaviors along with a check-off system to determine success. Adherence Tool 9–10 is a form for recording accomplishments in switching to low-fat foods over one week. Adherence Tool 9–11 is a meal planning chart.

> *Client:* "Most of my problem eating times seem to be when I am alone and my husband is out of town."
>
> *Counselor:* "Are there others with whom you can eat when your husband is away to help eliminate boredom?"
>
> *Client:* "Yes, I have a close friend who might go to the movies with me."

Contracts may work well when nothing seems to help the client achieve the adherence goal of a set number of grams of fat per day. In a contract, the client and counselor write down the goal in a very specific manner, along with some reward. **Specific tips on developing contracts include the following:**

- Be sure the contract includes automatic self-rewards such as reading a book, sewing, or anything already available so that extensive shopping or time is not required to obtain the reward.
- Be sure the client is involved in planning and has responsibility for the outcome.
- Be sure the client signs the contract to indicate formal commitment.
- Be sure that rewards are self-administered when goals are achieved.

The counselor provides the support and encouragement while the client plans and carries out the terms of the contract. The client must be involved in making major decisions and striving to fulfill the contract. Adherence Tool 9–11 allows the client to take an active role in meal planning. The contract might specify this as a task instead of eating.

Although nutrition counselors can provide a great deal of reinforcement, teaching the client to provide self-administered rewards can be helpful. An example is a verbal pat on the back: "You followed your exact grams of fat today without going over your prescription. That's great!" For some clients, verbal rewards may be less important than tangible rewards such as spending the weekend alone with a friend, buying clothes, having hair styled, going to a movie, or reading a book.

Positive thinking as a part of rehearsing what will happen can be beneficial. For example, if following the new eating pattern during a party is the goal, a client can imagine standing before the buffet table making only low-fat choices. This behavior can then be followed by a reinforcing outcome, like feeling healthy or taking a pleasant two-mile walk.

Support from groups can help to increase commitment to following a new, low-fat eating pattern. Support can come from others who are following the diet, fellow workers, friends, or family. The group, which can have three or four members or be a buddy system, can offer empathy for similar problems, provide helpful ideas for solving problems, give positive reinforcement when a goal is met, serve as role models, and help to minimize stress.

When goals are not met, reestablishing goals that are easily attainable is important. While a long-term goal may be to lower total fat to 20 percent of total calories, that goal does not tell the client how to develop realistic steps toward that goal.

> *Client:* "I love meat. Since it is my major problem, I should probably set my goal at cutting back drastically on it. I really worry about being able to follow this diet."
>
> *Counselor:* "Just because you see meat as a major barrier to following your new eating plan doesn't mean that you have to tackle it first. What other foods do you eat that are high in fat?"
>
> *Client:* "I still use whole milk, but I don't use a lot of it and it won't be that difficult to switch to skim."
>
> *Counselor:* "Let's start with that area first. It sounds as though you are confident that changes in that area won't be too burdensome."

Waning commitment to an eating pattern can begin with lack of support from a spouse, family members, a housemate, or friends. An otherwise supportive spouse may become unsupportive when faced with a rival, the low-fat diet. A spouse may become jealous, threatened, or hurt by the demands of a new eating style.

> *Client:* "My husband is not supportive. This is an example of how he feels about my new eating style: 'This diet is all yours. I'm not joining you in a feast of rabbit food!' "
>
> *Counselor:* "Have you ever asked how he feels about the low-fat eating pattern?"
>
> *Client:* "No, but I think he is hurt that I no longer pay attention to him but devote all my energy to the new eating pattern."

Counselor: "How have you coped with problems like this in the past?"
Client: "We have always talked through our problems."
Counselor: "What might you say now? Perhaps being honest about your feelings would help. For example, 'It makes me feel angry and hurt when you make fun of my eating habits. You don't have to eat my 'rabbit food,' but your support of my new habits would be appreciated.' "

Sometimes children in a family make it difficult to change eating patterns. Children can also have many different feelings: jealousy, neglect, and deprivation of their favorite foods.

Client: "My children are so negative sometimes. They say things like 'Why do we have to eat this awful, low-fat stuff? We are playing basketball and need some good food.' "
Counselor: "What do you think your children would accept as a compromise?"
Client: "They might appreciate a homemade snack that is lower in fat."
Counselor: "That's a great idea. You might also tell them to eat their favorite high-fat meals or snacks at school."

Some children may not take efforts to follow a low-fat diet seriously: "This is just another crazy diet." The family should know that the new, low-fat eating pattern may be effective in preventing a disease and that it is very important to be supportive. Clients should involve children in meal planning, calculating a fat score, and helping to avoid temptations.

Here are several ways to help increase the support of family members:

- It is important to discuss openly feelings about the new, low-fat eating pattern. If the client tells the family the importance of avoiding high-fat snacks, they will be more likely to comply.
- It is best to be patient. A family needs time to go through changes.
- The client must try to provide reinforcement when support is offered, no matter how minor the support.

Holidays, stressful periods, and eating out are all potential challenges to adherence. Adherence Tool 9–12 provides a way to plan ahead for a special event. Never going off the new, low-fat eating pattern is a very unrealistic expectation and should be avoided as a written goal. Adherence Tool 9–13 lists a variety of strategies to minimize difficult eating situations during vacations and holidays. Here are several suggestions for participants who have trouble during these times:

- Do not be afraid to ask for help from friends or relatives prior to a special holiday. If the request is made early, the hostess will appreciate having low-fat dishes for the client's benefits.
- View following the diet as a series of corrections, not as an undeviating straight line.
- Expect and predict setbacks in a holiday season.
- Practice saying "no."

Stressful periods can cause changes in strict observance of a dietary pattern. Adherence Tool 9–14 provides a few strategies to help save time and thus reduce stress associated with meal preparation. During stressful periods, it is important to identify the cause of the change and the emotion associated with it.

> *Client:* "When I am depressed, tired, or in general under a lot of pressure at work, I turn to my favorite high-fat foods for comfort."
> *Counselor:* "When eating is a way of consoling yourself, you might make a list of those things that provide comfort or positive reinforcement. These should be things that do not involve eating. Can you think of some things now?"
> *Client:* "I like to jog. Sometimes just going to talk with a friend boosts my spirits."

When clients need comfort, other activities that give reinforcement might be taking a bubble bath, listening to music, or calling a friend.

Tension or anxiety may also cause a lapse in adherence. Exercise, like walking or swimming, may relieve stress. Making a list of things to do, and then delegating and prioritizing this list can help manage stress.

When boredom causes the problem, keeping busy may be the answer. Clients can write a list of tasks to be completed or volunteer for an organization, take a class, learn a craft, or participate in any number of other activities.

Eating out is frequently a problem when others make the majority of the decisions. For example, a German meal served family style may lead to eating more than intended. A special occasion on which food is ordered for the client may result in eating inappropriately large amounts of fat. Many occasions call for spontaneity, such as beer and pizza after a bowling game or an office party.

Many options are available to help with social occasions:

- The client can call the restaurant ahead of time to determine what is on the menu and eliminate surprises.
- The client can bring in menus from favorite restaurants for review, and role play with the counselor in selecting from a menu in a safe environment.
- By saving all of the fat for the day and using it only at the special restaurant meal, clients can eat without worrying whether they are adhering to the low-fat eating plan.
- Positive monologues can help clients work through an adherence-challenging situation.
- Sometimes making a compromise can help the client through a difficult situation. For example, "I will order the cheese cake, but only eat one-third of it."
- Eating slowly allows for eating less and prevents others from offering second servings.

Lapses in following the new, low-fat eating pattern should not lead to feelings of guilt or anger. Deviation from the new eating pattern is a way to make corrections; past actions are something to forget. Clients can start anew with more appropriate eating behaviors, viewing the setback as temporary or short-lived ("a bad day") rather than a forecasting of "never" getting better.

When commitment to the study begins to wane, a specific plan of action to help cope with adherence-challenging situations helps clients achieve goals in spite of the barriers. The following are two examples of plans to help eliminate barriers to adherence:

> *Client:* "I find that I go overboard when I attend parties with my husband."
> *Counselor:* "What are some preliminary planning steps that might help you?"
> *Client:* "I suppose I could do what I've done on other days and save my fat for the cocktail party. This means all of my other meals are virtually fat free."
> *Counselor:* "Are there ways to minimize your feelings of hunger during the party?"
> *Client:* "I could snack on low-fat snacks at home. This might prevent eating on a whim during the party."
> *Counselor:* "Great! One suggestion I might give is to avoid alcohol at the party. It can make you careless and less aware of what you are eating."

A second example of overcoming barriers to success in the new eating pattern follows:

> *Client:* "I frequently eat more when I'm under stress."
> *Counselor:* "Can you describe in detail when stresses occur and what causes them?"
> *Client:* "Usually a hectic day at work when someone is on vacation is stressful."
> *Counselor:* "What can you do in advance to avoid these situations?"
> *Client:* "I could plan ahead by bringing a sack lunch on days when I know the potential for stress is greatest."
> *Counselor:* "Great idea!"

To be effective, a strategy should include the following:

- a description of strategy A to be taken, plus an alternative strategy B if A does not work
- rehearsals of specific strategies through role playing or reviewing mentally
- application of these strategies to specific, predictable stressful situations.

Stressful life events, including death or illness in the family, divorce, marriage, or retirement, can cause major changes in commitment. During these times, it is best to maintain changes and avoid making others. Even if a lapse in following an eating pattern occurs at this time, it should be viewed as temporary (one week) with the plan of renewing efforts the next week and maintaining good adherence.

Some clients may feel discouraged at times. The counselor can remind them of how much progress they have already made, focus on these positive changes (such as coming to appointments), and let clients know that others experience this same discouragement.

At times, clients whose commitment wavers can be encouraged by being asked to use their talents to show they are accomplished in areas other than eating. For example, a client can bring in a favorite recipe to share with others, or an artistic client might help design a handout with patient information.

Counseling on a low-fat eating pattern involves knowledge of the fat content of food and an ability to use that knowledge in designing individualized eating patterns. Knowledge can provide assistance in making social eating more pleasant. Reminders to avoid high-fat foods can be beneficial in maintaining good dietary adherence. When commitment wanes, the counselor's ability to deal with goal setting, positive self-talk, assertiveness training, shaping, self-monitoring, contracts, self-rewards, and group support is extremely important

Review of Chapter 9
(Answers in Appendix H)

1. List two problems associated with inappropriate eating behaviors when following a fat-controlled eating pattern.

    a. _____

    b. _____

2. List two dietary components to assess in modifying a diet for possible cancer risk prevention.

    a. _____

    b. _____

3. List three strategies that might help the client follow a fat-controlled eating pattern.

    a. _____

    b. _____

    c. _____

4. The following describes a problem situation with a client who has been instructed on a fat-controlled eating pattern to reduce risk of breast cancer.

    Mrs. B is trying to follow a low-fat diet. During an assessment of her current eating habits, it was apparent that most difficulties occur with the evening meal, which is traditionally high fat (potatoes with gravy, high-fat meat, buttered vegetable, and high-fat dessert). Mrs. B's family loves these high-fat meals. (a) What additional information might you request regarding current eating habits? (b) What strategies would you use to help alleviate the problem? (c) Why did you choose these strategies?

    a. _____

    b. _____

    c. _____

NOTES

1. M.J. Hill, "Diet and Human Cancer: A New Era for Research," in *Diet and Human Carcinogenesis*, ed. J.V. Joossens et al. (New York: Elsevier Science Publishers, 1985), 3–12.

2. R. Doll and R. Peto, "Avoidable Risks of Cancer in the United States Today," *Journal of the National Cancer Institute* 66 (1981): 1226–1238.

3. E.L. Wynder and G.B. Gori, "Contribution of the Environment to Cancer Incidence: An Epidemiologic Exercise," *Journal of the National Cancer Institute* 58 (1977): 825–831.

4. G.M. Williams, "Food: Its Role in the Etiology of Cancer," in *Food and Cancer Prevention: Chemical and Biological Aspects*, eds. K.W. Waldron (Cambridge, U.K.: The Royal Society of Chemistry, 1993), 3.

5. A.B. Miller, "Diet in the Aetiology of Cancer: A Review," *European Journal of Cancer* 30 (1994): 207.

6. J.H. Weisburger and G.M. Williams, "Causes of Cancer," in *American Cancer Society Textbook of Clinical Oncology*, eds. G.P. Murph et al. (Atlanta, GA: American Cancer Society, 1995), 10.

7. G.M. Williams and E.L. Wynder, "Diet and Cancer: A Synopsis of Causes and Prevention Strategies," in *Nutrition and Cancer Prevention*, ed. R.R. Watson and S.I. Mufti (Boca Raton, FL: CRC Press, 1996), 1–2.

8. J.T. Dwyer, "Dietary Fat and Breast Cancer: Testing Interventions To Reduce Risk," *Advances in Experimental Medical Biology* 322 (1992): 155–183.

9. K.K. Carroll and H.R. Khor, "Dietary Fat in Relation to Tumorigenesis," *Progress in Biochemical Pharmacology* 10 (1975): 308–353.

10. J.W. Weisburger and E.L. Wynder, "Dietary Fat Intake and Cancer," *Hematology/Oncology Clinics of North America* 5 (1991): 7.

11. L.A. Cohen et al., "Modulation of N-Nitrosomethylurea Induced Mammary Tumor Promotion by Dietary Fiber and Fat," *Journal of the National Cancer Institute* 83 (1991): 496.

12. R.L. Prentice and L. Sheppard, "Dietary Fat and Cancer: Consistency of the Epidemiologic Data and Disease Prevention That May Follow from a Practical Reduction in Fat Consumption," *Cancer Causes and Control* 1 (1990): 81.

13. R.L. Prentice and L. Sheppard, "Dietary Fat and Cancer: Rejoinder and Discussion of Research Strategies," *Cancer Causes and Control* 2 (1990): 53.

14. W.C. Willett and M. Stampfer, "Dietary Fat and Cancer: Another View," *Cancer Causes and Control* 1 (1990): 103.

15. G.R. Howe, "Dietary Fat and Cancer," *Cancer Causes and Control* 1 (1990): 99.

16. J.E. Hiller and A.J. McMichael, "Dietary Fat and Cancer: A Comeback for Etiological Studies?" *Cancer Causes and Control* 1 (1990): 101.

17. L.N. Kolonel et al., "Association of Diet and Place of Birth with Stomach Cancer Incidence in Hawaii, Japanese and Caucasians," *American Journal of Clinical Nutrition* 34 (1981): 2478–2485.

18. G.B. Gori, "Dietary and Nutritional Implications in the Multifactorial Etiology of Certain Prevalent Human Cancer," *Cancer* 43 (1979): S2151–S2161.

19. A.B. Miller, "A Study of Diet and Breast Cancer," *American Journal of Epidemiology* 107 (1978): 499–509.

20. J.H. Lubin et al., "Role of Fat, Animal Protein, and Dietary Fiber in Breast Cancer Etiology: A Case-Control Study," *Journal of the National Cancer Institute* 77 (1986): 605–611.

21. S. Graham, "Diet in the Epidemiology of Breast Cancer," *American Journal of Epidemiology* 116 (1982): 68–75.

22. W.C. Willett, "Implications of Total Energy Intake for Epidemiologic Studies of Breast and Large-Bowel Cancer," *American Journal of Clinical Nutrition* 45 (1987): 354–360.

23. W.C. Willett et al., "Dietary Fat and the Risk of Breast Cancer," *New England Journal of Medicine* 316 (1987): 22–28.

24. Willett, "Implications of Total Energy Intake for Epidemiologic Studies of Breast and Large-Bowel Cancer."

25. J.R. Hebert and E.L. Wynder, "Letter to the Editor," *New England Journal of Medicine* 317 (1987): 165–166.

26. E.L. Wynder, et al., "Dietary Fat and Breast Cancer: Where Do We Stand on the Evidence?" *Journal of Clinical Epidemiology* 47 (1994): 217–222.

27. S. Self et al., "Statistical Design of the Women's Health Trial," *Controlled Clinical Trials* 9 (1988): 1–18.

28. F. Kakar and M. Henderson, "Diet and Breast Cancer," *Clinical Nutrition* 4 (1985): 119–130.

29. L.N. Kolonel and L. Le Marchand, "The Epidemiology of Colon Cancer and Dietary Fat," in *Dietary Fat and Cancer*, ed. C. Ip et al. (New York: Liss, 1986), 69–91.

30. E.L. Wynder et al., "Nutrition and Metabolic Epidemiology of Cancers of the Oral Cavity, Esophagus, Colon, Breast, Prostate and Stomach," in *Nutrition and Cancer: Etiology and Treatment*, ed. G.R. Newell and N.M. Ellison (New York: Raven Press, 1981), 11–48.

31. D.P. Rose, "The Biochemical Epidemiology of Prostatic Carcinoma," in *Dietary Fat and Cancer,* ed. C. Ip et al. (New York: Liss, 1986), 43–68.

32. B. Armstrong and R. Doll, "Environmental Factors and Cancer Incidence and Mortality in Different Countries, with Special Reference to Dietary Practices," *International Journal of Cancer* 15 (1975): 617–631.

33. D.P. Rose et al., "International Comparisons of Mortality Rates for Cancer of the Breast, Ovary, Prostate, and Colon, and Per Capita Food Consumption," *Cancer* 58 (1986): 2363–2371.

34. E. Mahboubi et al., "Epidemiology of Cancer of the Endometrium," *Clinical Obstetrics and Gynecology* 25 (1982): 5–17.

35. J.R. Hebert et al., "Natural Killer Cell Activity in a Longitudinal Dietary Fat Intervention Trial," *Clinical Immunology and Immunopathology* 54 (1989): 103.

36. J. Barone et al., "Dietary Fat and Natural Killer Cell Activity," *American Journal of Clinical Nutrition* 50 (1989): 861.

37. Subcommittee on Nutritional Surveillance, Committee on Medical Aspects of Food Policy, "The Diet of British School Children," *Reports on Health and Social Subjects* 36 (1989): 1–293.

38. H.P. Lee et al., "Dietary Effects on Breast Cancer Risk in Singapore," *Lancet* 337 (1991): 1197.

39. L.D. Byham, "Dietary Fat and Natural Killer Cell Function," *Nutrition Today* 31 (1991): 31–36.

40. Women's Health Initiative, *Protocol for Clinical Trial and Observation Components*. Seattle, Washington: WHI Clinical Coordinating Center, 1994. NIH Publication No 1-WH-2-2110.

41. K. Glanz, "Nutrition Education for Risk Factor Reduction and Patient Education: A Review," *Preventive Medicine* 14 (1985): 721–752.

42. R.E. Patterson et al., "Low-Fat Diet Practices of Older Women: Prevalence and Implications for Dietary Assessment," *Journal of the American Dietetic Association* 96 (1996): 670–676, 679.

43. Ibid.

44. Glanz, "Nutrition Education."

45. J.S. Carson, "Nutrition in a Team Approach to the Rehabilitation of the Patient with Cancer," *Journal of the American Diabetic Association* 72 (1978): 407–409.

46. D.F. Campbell et al., "Relaxation: Its Effect on the Nutrition Status and Performance Status of Clients with Cancer," *Journal of the American Dietetic Association* 84 (1984): 201–204.

47. Glanz, "Nutrition Education."

Adherence Tool 9–1: Eating Out
(Informational Device)

WHERE YOU EAT

- Choose restaurants with low-fat choices.
- Stay away from all-you-can-eat places.
- Avoid restaurants that serve only fried foods.

HOW MUCH YOU EAT

- Order small servings.
- Select from the appetizer list, not the main dish list.
- Share your meal.

WHAT CHANGES YOU CAN MAKE

- Trim fat from meat.
- Remove skin from chicken.
- Dip your fork into salad dressing and then eat your lettuce.

WHAT REQUESTS YOU CAN MAKE

- Request salad dressing on the side.
- Ask for broiled, poached, or steamed rather than fried foods.
- Ask to have the cheese removed.
- Ask for all foods to have the fat left off (e.g., vegetables and meats with high-fat sauces, burgers with mayonnaise).

Adherence Tool 9–2: Make Your Desserts
Low in Fat (Informational Device)

- Add fresh fruits to all main dishes and desserts.
- Choose ice milk, sherbert, sorbets, fruit ices, nonfat yogurt, and fat-free puddings.
- Choose angel food cake, gingersnaps, fig bars, apple and strawberry bars, vanilla wafers, and animal crackers.
- Select hard candy, licorice, jelly beans, and gumdrops.

Adherence Tool 9–3: Make Your Dairy Food Choices Low in Fat (Informational Device)

- Gradually change your milk from whole to skim.
- Chill your skim milk on ice.
- Use evaporated skim milk for cooking and baking.
- Try part-skim mozzarella and low- or fat-free cheese.
- Eat smaller servings of ice cream less often.
- Choose ice milk, sherbert, or the new fat-free frozen desserts.
- Use fat-free sour cream.
- Use fat-free cream cheese.
- Use low-fat or fat-free frozen whipped toppings.

Adherence Tool 9–4: Ways To Cut Down on Fat (Informational Device)

- Spread margarine thin.
- Use honey or jam, not margarine or butter.
- Do not set butter or margarine on the table.
- Use a tomato sauce for a gravy.
- Choose "light" mayonnaise.
- Stir-fry in broth, flavored vinegar, or wine.

Adherence Tool 9–5: Spicing Low-Fat Foods (Informational Device)

- Try barbeque, Tabasco, catsup, or Worcestershire sauce to season chicken, turkey, and lean meats.
- Try oriental sauces such as hoisin, oyster, or sweet and sour sauce on stir-fry vegetables.
- Use dijon mustard and other hot mustards to add flavor to marinades and sauces.
- Use seasoned rice vinegar as a dressing.
- Try flavored vinegars such as raspberry, balsamic, or herbed.
- Experiment with herbs and spices.

Adherence Tool 9–6: Stress Management Chart (Informational and Cueing Device)

When you feel overwhelmed, make a "to do" list of everything you need to get done.

Date   Item To Do

_____

_____

_____

_____

When you have finished the list, ask yourself the following questions:
1. Can I delete anything from this list that might be classified as unnecessary?
2. What can I delegate to a relative or friend?
3. What can I pay someone else to do?
4. What is the most important task? Now begin by doing it first.

Courtesy of Laura Coleman, Joanne Csaplar, Johanna Dwyer, Carole Palmer, and Molly Holland.

Adherence Tool 9–7: Fat Grams for One Day (Monitoring Device)

Meal or Snack	*Grams of Fat*
Breakfast	Total _____
Snack	Total _____
Lunch	Total _____
Snack	Total _____
Dinner	Total _____
Snack	Total _____
	TOTAL _____

Adherence Tool 9–8: Budgeting for Fat in a Two-Day Period (Monitoring Device)

Day	Grams of Fat
1 _____	_____
_____	_____
_____	_____
_____	_____
_____	_____
	Total _____
2 _____	_____
_____	_____
_____	_____
_____	_____
_____	_____
	Total _____

Adherence Tool 9–9: Low-Fat Action List for a Day (Monitoring Device)

Make a list of specific types of eating behaviors involving low-fat eating that you wish to accomplish:

	Check off when accomplished
1.	( )
2.	( )
3.	( )
4.	( )
5.	( )

Examples: 1. Switch from high-fat wieners to lower-fat turkey franks.
2. Use skim milk instead of 1 percent milk.
3. Have fruit compote for dessert instead of a high-fat fruit cobbler.

Courtesy of Laura Coleman, Joanne Csaplar, Johanna Dwyer, Carole Palmer, and Molly Holland.

Adherence Tool 9–10: Low-Fat Eating Accomplishments (Monitoring and Cueing Device)

Sunday	Monday	Tuesday	Wednesday	Thursday	Friday	Saturday

Courtesy of Laura Coleman, Joanne Csaplar, Johanna Dwyer, Carole Palmer, and Molly Holland.

Adherence Tool 9–11: Client Planning Chart (Informational Device)

Meal planning can help you keep your total fat intake low. Before your next visit, plan three days of meals in which you avoid foods high in fat.

Meal	Day 1	Day 2	Day 3
Breakfast			
Snack			
Lunch			
Snack			
Dinner			
Snack			

Adherence Tool 9–12:   Planning for a Special Event or Occasion (Informational Device)

- Where will I stay?
- What activities will I do?
- Who can help or hinder me in following my diet?
- How do I feel about this occasion, and how will these feelings affect what I eat?
- What foods will be available, and what specific foods do I want to eat?
- How long will I be in this situation, and what can I do to eat less fat before and after it?

Adherence Tool 9–13:   Strategies To Minimize Difficult Eating Situations During Vacations and Holidays (Informational Device)

- Find new recipes or lower the fat in old favorites.
- Plan to eat less fat on days before and after the holidays.
- Plan fun activities that don't involve eating.
- Eat before you go, so that you are not so hungry.
- Prepare a low-fat or fat-free food to bring to the occasion.
- Fill most of your plate with low-fat foods or a salad.
- Plan to spend most of your time talking not eating.
- Eat only high-fat foods that are your favorites.

Adherence Tool 9–14: How To Save Time (Informational Device)

- Plan meals ahead of time.
- Have low-fat and fat-free foods in your pantry and refrigerator.
- Keep a low-fat shopping list.
- Use time-saving equipment to make your meals (pressure cooker, microwave, electric skillet, etc.).
- Use leftovers.
- Use a file of quick and easy recipes.
- Use time-saving ingredients (precut vegetables; boned, skinless chicken; cubed turkey; precut fruits, etc.).
- Use convenience foods (frozen, canned, instant, etc.).
- Make double quantities and freeze part for a later meal.
- Use quick-cooking methods (microwave, stir-fry, poach, broil, etc.).

PART III

Ending Counseling Sessions

This section describes techniques for assessing each counseling session and gives suggestions for client follow-up.

CHAPTER 10

Evaluation and Follow-Up

CHAPTER OBJECTIVES

1. Identify elements necessary for evaluating both client and counselor.

2. Identify strategies to ensure dietary adherence after ceasing reinforcement.

3. Generate the reinstitution of an intervention or treatment plan.

4. Identify elements of the termination process.

EVALUATION OF COUNSELOR PROGRESS

Evaluation of the counselor's individual progress forms an important part of the client's success. A counselor can be ineffective in facilitating client success for a variety of reasons. The questions below are a way to begin defining potential problems.

1. Did the counseling session address the client's major problem?
2. Was assessment prior to designing a modified eating pattern adequate to prepare a dietary regimen compatible with the client's lifestyle?
3. Did the client's goal appear to have been achieved?
4. Were the strategies for altering eating behaviors carried out efficiently?
5. Did the counselor use appropriate verbal and nonverbal communication skills? Where might changes have been made?
6. Did the counselor use appropriate counseling skills? Where might changes have been made?

7. What general changes might the counselor make in the next counseling interview with a similar client?

Each list of questions should be made more specific as the situation requires and can be adapted, depending on answers given during the interview.

EVALUATION OF CLIENT PROGRESS

Evaluating the client's progress is crucial to maintenance of a modified eating pattern. Booster sessions to assist in solving problems may be a direct result of careful evaluation.

Following each session, the counselor can appraise the client's success. **Below is a list of questions the client might ask to determine whether behavior has changed successfully:**

1. Are my dietary patterns different but still compatible with my lifestyle?
2. Have my misconceptions about foods and what they contain been replaced with factual information?
3. Are social occasions less of a problem now than when I first began my diet?
4. Is my family providing needed positive reinforcement?

These very general questions provide insight into potential problems with dietary adherence. Evaluation of client progress is an ongoing process that should be a part of all client counseling sessions. The client should feel a sense of control in changing inappropriate eating behaviors. Self-management of problem eating behaviors is crucial to eventual maintenance of dietary goals.

STRATEGIES TO MAINTAIN DIETARY ADHERENCE

Follow-up interviewing sessions are extremely important to counseling on nutrition-related issues. The number of return visits depends on the success of efforts in following a diet. There is always a point at which the nutrition counselor and client must end a set of counseling sessions. This is the point at which the counselor must be sure that the client can follow the diet without continued help. At that time, the goal of the counseling session is tested: Can the client function adequately in the real world?

Counselors must be sure that their clients are given ample opportunity during the sessions to practice eating behaviors, and these new behaviors must be reinforced in the natural environment. This can be done by asking clients for records of foods consumed, times eating takes place, persons present during the meal or snack, and the type of situation (where and what type of function). These records should be discussed thoroughly with the clients, and problem areas and their solutions noted.

To help with reinforcement in the natural setting, clients are asked to list times and places where their eating behaviors can be supported. The counselors then help them plan for natural situations that reinforce the new eating pattern. If new behaviors are really adjustive, clients should find natural support and natural reinforcements.

In early stages of termination, counselors should help clients identify chains of events that bolster behavior. A woman who had succeeded in losing 10 pounds found that her colleagues at work responded very warmly to her. She was asked out more often and spent more time in discussions with colleagues. She eliminated her clothes-buying reinforcement and instead posted a sign on her refrigerator door: "Dieting keeps the telephone ringing!"

After an eating behavior has been solidified in relation to one antecedent condition, clients can make that behavior even more frequent by gradually increasing the range of situations in which reinforcement occurs. They should test for generalization by looking at how reinforcement can be a part of many situations. By keeping a list of all situations in which either appropriate or inappropriate eating behaviors occur, nutritionists can work on problem situations before counseling is terminated.

An important issue to address before termination is building in resistance to extinction. The best way to ensure that an appropriate eating behavior continues is to develop an intermittent reinforcement schedule. A treatment plan should never be stopped abruptly.

Once an acceptable upper level of behavior has been established, the ratio of its reinforcement can be reduced. Instead of clients' always buying presents for themselves (such as clothing) after eating an appropriate, meal, sporadic buying can be used as a reinforcement, (e.g., 75 percent of the time, then 50 percent, then 25 percent, and so on).

During this gradual reduction in positive reinforcement, both counselors and clients must continue to count the frequency of the appropriate behaviors. There is some danger that these will decline. Alternating between periods of 0 percent and 100 percent reinforcement can keep their frequency at an acceptably high level if the natural supporters are slow to evolve.

Counselors should ensure that adequate practice of the reinforcement has occurred during intervention or treatment. In general, acceptable behaviors are made more probable by providing a certain number of trials on a reinforcement schedule. Practice is important.

This need for practice implies, correctly, that nutrition counselors should not terminate the program as soon as the goal is reached. Instead, it would be wise to continue the plan for a week or two, or perhaps more, depending on the frequency of the opportunities to practice. The number of practices depends on many factors in the intervention plan. For example, a more complicated dietary regimen may require division of practice into small segments, each focusing on one exchange category or a single nutrient counting system.

However, a trial at reducing reinforcement is a good test of the degree to which an eating behavior can be maintained after termination. If the frequency of the targeted behavior drops alarmingly as soon as a reduction in reinforcement begins, it means more practice is necessary. In that case, the 100 percent reinforcement schedule should be resumed, along with more practice. For this reason, the frequency of an eating behavior should be recorded after termination of reinforcement until the rate has stabilized.

REINSTITUTION OF INTERVENTION OR TREATMENT

Nutrition counselors may find that an intervention plan must be restarted if gradually decreasing reinforcement seems to be causing an appropriate eating behavior to decrease. At that point, practitioners must be closely attuned to client needs.

Because clients must deal with many life stresses, their attention to an intervention strategy of gradually decreasing reinforcement may be diverted, resulting in total lack of support. By working with clients' significant others, practitioners can suggest persons who are aware of the importance of reinforcing good eating behaviors in the absence of nutrition counseling sessions. Chapter 3 provides many ideas on how to move from contemplation to action and focuses on the importance of goal setting.

THE TERMINATION PROCESS

The algorithm in Figure 10–1 indicates a step procedure to use in terminating nutrition counseling. Termination should always be approached gradually. The algorithm indicates four possible situations:

1. Some clients begin having negative thoughts. The algorithm suggests listing those thoughts and working on them.
2. Some clients may refuse to discuss their thoughts, in which case they should be asked to record both negative and positive monologues for discussion later.
3. Some other clients may admit to having a drastic change in their lifestyles. Those changes may be temporary. In that case, the intervention plan is reinstituted and reinforcements decreased gradually.

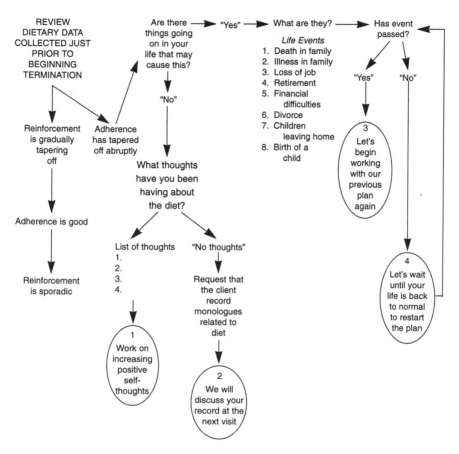

Figure 10–1 Algorithm for Nutrition Counseling Termination

4. Clients in some cases may be in the midst of a change in lifestyle. If so, counselors should wait until clients seem ready to restart the intervention plan, meanwhile keeping in close contact so that the diet is not totally forgotten.

Termination is different for each client. Counselors should be prepared to restart a strategy to help ensure adherence to the diet over long periods. They might call or write to the client periodically to check on progress. Such attention to the client's needs after the counseling has ended will show a sense of caring and may help maintain the individual's motivation.

A gradual fading process of termination rather than an abrupt "goodbye" is essential. If clients are to be successful on their own, they must prove that success is possible. Nutrition counselors can help clients find this success on their own. A gradual termination can prevent regression to problem eating behaviors.

Review of Chapter 10
(Answers in Appendix H)

1. Identify questions you might ask to evaluate counselor progress.

    a. _____

    b. _____

    c. _____

    d. _____

    e. _____

    f. _____

    g. _____

    h. _____

    i. _____

2. Identify questions you might ask to evaluate client progress.

    a. _____

    b. _____

    c. _____

    d. _____

3. Identify five ways in which you as a counselor might facilitate the continuation of appropriate dietary behaviors in clients who no longer will be coming in for interviews and must live with the regimen in the real world.

    a. _____

    b. _____

    c. _____

    d. _____

    e. _____

4. Mr. Y. has been slipping in his adherence to the low-sodium regimen he was following so well when counseling sessions were frequent. What questions might you use to determine exactly what has happened to the reinforcement schedule?

    _____

    _____

    _____

5. What intervention plan can you recommend to help clients maintain dietary adherence?

_____

_____

_____

Checklist of Nutrition Counselor Self-Image

Check the items that are most descriptive of you.

COMPETENCE ASSESSMENT

_____ 1. Constructive negative feedback about myself doesn't make me feel incompetent or uncertain of myself.

_____ 2. I tend to put myself down frequently.

_____ 3. I feel fairly confident about myself as a helper.

_____ 4. I often am preoccupied with thinking that I'm not going to be a competent nutrition counselor.

_____ 5. When I am involved in a conflict, I don't go out of my way to ignore or avoid it.

_____ 6. When I get positive feedback about myself, I often don't believe it's true.

_____ 7. I set realistic goals for myself as a helper that are within reach.

_____ 8. I believe that a confronting, hostile client could make me feel uneasy or incompetent.

_____ 9. I often find myself apologizing for myself or my behavior.

_____ 10. I'm fairly confident I can or will be a successful counselor.

_____ 11. I find myself worrying a lot about "not making it" as a counselor.

_____ 12. I'm likely to be a little scared by clients who would idealize me.

_____ 13. A lot of times I will set standards or goals for myself that are too tough to attain.

Source: From _Interviewing Strategies for Helpers: Fundamental Skills and Cognitive Behavioral Interventions_ by W.H. Cormier and L.S. Cormier. Copyright © 1991, 1985, and 1975 Brooks/Cole Publishing Company, Pacific Grove, California 93950, a division of International Thomson Publishing Inc. By permission of the publisher.

_____ 14. I tend to avoid negative feedback when I can.

_____ 15. Doing well or being successful does not make me feel uneasy.

POWER ASSESSMENT

_____ 1. If I'm really honest, I think my counseling methods are a little superior to other people's.

_____ 2. A lot of times I try to get people to do what I want. I might get pretty defensive or upset if the client disagreed with what I wanted to do or did not follow my direction in the interview.

_____ 3. I believe there is (or will be) a balance in the interviews between my participation and the client's.

_____ 4. I could feel angry when working with a resistant or stubborn client.

_____ 5. I can see that I might be tempted to get some of my own ideology across to the client.

_____ 6. As a counselor, "preaching" is not likely to be a problem for me.

_____ 7. Sometimes I feel impatient with clients who have a different way of looking at the world than I do.

_____ 8. I know there are times when I would be reluctant to refer my clients to someone else, especially if the other counselor's style differed from mine.

_____ 9. Sometimes I feel rejecting or intolerant of clients whose values and lifestyles are very different from mine.

_____ 10. It is hard for me to avoid getting in a power struggle with some clients.

INTIMACY ASSESSMENT

_____ 1. There are times when I act more gruff than I really feel.

_____ 2. It's hard for me to express positive feelings to a client.

_____ 3. There are some clients I would really like to be my friends more than my clients.

_____ 4. It would upset me if a client didn't like me.

_____ 5. If I sense a client has some negative feelings toward me, I try to talk about it rather than avoid it.

_____ 6. Many times I go out of my way to avoid offending clients.

_____ 7. I feel more comfortable maintaining a professional distance between myself and the client.

_____ 8. Being close to people is something that does not make me feel uncomfortable.

_____ 9. I am more comfortable when I am a little aloof.

_____ 10. I am very sensitive to how clients feel about me, especially if it is negative.

____ 11. I can accept positive feedback from clients fairly easily.
____ 12. It is difficult for me to confront a client.

LEARNING ACTIVITY REACTION: APPLICATIONS TO YOUR COUNSELING

____ 1. For each of the three assessment areas above, look over your responses and determine the areas that seem to be OK and the areas that may be a problem for you or something to watch out for. You may find more problems in one area than another.

____ 2. Do your "trouble spots" seem to occur with mostly everyone, or just with certain types of people? In all situations or some situations?

____ 3. Compare yourself now to where you might have been four years ago or where you may be four years from now.

____ 4. Identify any areas you feel you could use some help with, from a colleague, a supervisor, or a counselor.

Checklist of Nutrition Counselor's Nonverbal Behavior

Instructions: Determine whether the counselor did or did not demonstrate the desired nonverbal behaviors listed in the right column. Check "yes" or "no" in the left column to indicate your judgment.

	Demonstrated Behaviors	
Desired Behaviors	*Yes*	*No*
Eye contact—Maintained persistent eye contact without gazing or staring.	———	———
	1. Eyes	
Facial expression—Punctuated interaction with occasional head nods.	———	———
	2. Head Nods	
Mouth—Punctuated interaction with occasional smiles.	———	———
	3. Smiles	
Body orientation and posture—Faced the other person, slight lean forward (from waist up), body appeared relaxed.	———	———
	4. Facing client	
	———	———
	5. Leaning forward	
	———	———
	6. Relaxed body	

Source: From *Interviewing Strategies for Helpers: Fundamental Skills and Cognitive Behavioral Interventions* by W.H. Cormier and L.S. Cormier. Copyright © 1991, 1985, and 1975 Brooks/Cole Publishing Company, Pacific Grove, California 93950, a division of International Thomson Publishing Inc. By permission of the publisher.

Desired Behaviors	Demonstrated Behaviors	
	Yes	No
Paralinguistics—Completed sentences without "who" or hesitations in delivery, asked one question at a time, did not ramble.		
	7. Completed sentences	
	8. Smooth delivery—no speech errors	
Distance—Seats of counselor and client were between 3 feet, or 1 meter, and 5 feet or 1½ meters apart.		
	9. Distance	

APPENDIX C

Measures of Nutritional Status

ANTHROPOMETRY

Elbow breadth, upper arm circumference, and three skinfold thicknesses—triceps, biceps, and subscapular—are described below. The purpose of the elbow breadth measurement is to classify the subject's frame size according to the appropriate column of the standard weight tables. The skinfold and arm circumference measures are used to determine body fatness and arm muscle area. The repeated measurements are used to assess change in body fat and muscle mass.

Preparation

The skinfold calipers must measure accurately at different thicknesses of skinfolds. Use the calibration block to check the caliper calibration before measuring each client. A constant error of 1 millimeter is acceptable and should be added to or subtracted from the actual reading. A greater error requires repair *or* replacement of the calipers.

Measurement

Elbow Breadth

The client extends the right arm forward, perpendicular to the body, with the arm bent so the angle at the elbow measure 90 degrees and with the fingers pointing up and the dorsal part of the wrist toward the measurer. Apply the sliding caliper across the greatest breadth of the elbow joint (at the medial and lateral condyles of the humerus) along the axis of the upper arm. Approximate the arms of the caliper with firm pressure and read the breadth in millimeters.

Have the client repeat the arm maneuver and remeasure. Repeat the reading aloud and record. If the two measurements are within 1 millimeter, use the second measurement as the elbow breadth for the weight table. If the second measure differs by more than one millimeter from the first, repeat until two consecutive measures are within one millimeter. Use the last of the measures as the elbow breadth. Table C–1 gives frame size from height and elbow breadth.

Table C–1 Frame Size from Height and Elbow Breadth[1]

	Men Elbow Breadth		
Height* (centimeters)	Small Frame (millimeters)	Medium Frame (millimeters)	Large Frame (millimeters)
150–154	<62	62–71	>71
155–158	<64	64–72	>72
159–168	<67	67–74	>74
169–178	<69	69–76	>76
179–188	<71	71–78	>78
189–190	<74	74–81	>81
191–194	<76	76–82	>82
195–199	<78	78–83	>83
200–204	<79	79–85	>85
205–209	<80	80–88	>89

	Women Elbow Breadth		
Height* (centimeters)	Small Frame (millimeters)	Medium Frame (millimeters)	Large Frame (millimeters
145–148	<56	56–64	>64
149–158	<58	58–65	>65
159–168	<59	59–66	>66
169–178	<61	61–68	>68
179–180	<62	62–69	>69
181–184	<63	63–70	>70
185–189	<64	64–71	>71
190–194	<65	65–72	>72
195–199	<66	66–73	>73

*Without shoes.

[1]The medium frame elbow breadths for men, <155 cm or ≥ 191 cm, and women, ≥ 181 cm, were determined by extrapolation on a semilog graph.

Courtesy of *Statistical Bulletin*, Metropolitan Life Insurance Company, 1983, New York, New York.

Upper Arm Circumference

The client flexes the right arm to 90 degrees at the elbow. Use the steel tape to measure the distance from the acromion to the end of the humerus. Mark the lateral part of the arm at the midpoint with a pen or skin marker. With the arm hanging freely, place the lower edge of the tape at skin mark and measure the circumference. The tape should fit snugly to the arm without compressing tissue. State the reading in millimeters and record. Repeat the maneuver. Successive measures should be within 5 millimeters. Record the last measure as the midarm circumference.

Skinfolds

Pick up a fold of skin and subcutaneous tissue between the thumb and index finger of the left hand and lift it firmly away from the underlying muscle. Hold the fold between the fingers throughout the time the measurement is being taken. Apply the calipers to the fold 1 centimeter below the fingertip so that pressure on the fold at the point measured is exerted by the caliper faces only, and not by the fingers. The calipers are applied to the skinfold by removing the thumb of the right hand from the trigger lever of the caliper.

The value registered on the calipers sometimes decreases as one watches the pointer of the dial. This decrease can usually be stopped by taking a firmer pinch with the left hand; if it continues, the reading must be taken immediately after application of the spring pressure.

All measurements are read to the nearest 1 millimeter. Obtain two measurements at each site. If the two measures are within 5 percent, record the last measure as the skinfold thickness. If the difference between the measures exceeds 5 percent, repeat the maneuver until two successive measures are within 5 percent.

Most skinfolds are measured in the vertical plane except when the Lines of Linn (natural skinfold lines) result in torsion of the skinfold, in which case the skinfold is taken along these lines.

Triceps skinfold. The client should be standing with right arm relaxed and suspended along midaxillary line. The point of measurement is at the skin mark made for arm circumference measurement. Pinch the skin and subcutaneous tissue (do not include muscle) between the thumb and index finger of your left hand. The pinch should be 1 centimeter above the skin mark and parallel to the long axis of the arm. The jaws of the calipers are placed perpendicular to the fold at the marked level.

Biceps skinfold. The client should be standing with right arm relaxed and suspended along midaxillary line. Pick up the skinfold on the front of the right arm directly above the center of the cubital fossa at the same level as that at which the triceps skinfold is measured.

Subscapular skinfold. The client should be standing and relaxed. Grasp the skin and subcutaneous tissue just below the inferior angle of the right scapula between your left thumb and index finger. Lines of Linn will determine the angle of the skinfold.

CALCULATION OF PERCENT BODY FAT

Percent body fat is determined from (1) a regression equation for the prediction of body density from the triceps, biceps, and subscapular skinfolds and (2) an equation using the known relationship between body density and the proportion of fat in the body.[1]

1. Body density (Y) is calculated as follows:

$$Y = C - M \text{ (log of the sum of the skinfolds)}$$

The coefficients C and M are obtained from Table C–2 for the appropriate age and sex group.

2. Percent body fat is calculated as follows:

$$\% \text{ Fat} = (\frac{4.95}{Y} - 4.5)(100)$$

3. Example: A 45-year-old female has a sum of the three skinfolds of 50 millimeters.

Table C–2 Linear Regression Coefficients for the Estimation of Body Density $\times 10^3$ (kg/m^3) from the Logarithm of the Skinfold Thickness (Biceps + Triceps + Subscapular)

Age (Years) Age Categories	Males		Females	
	C	M	C	M
17–19	1.1643	0.0727	1.1509	0.0715
20–29	1.1593	0.0694	1.1605	0.0777
30–39	1.1213	0.0487	1.1385	0.0654
40–49	1.1530	0.0730	1.1303	0.0635
50+	1.1569	0.0780	1.1372	0.0710
Overall				
17–72	1.1689	0.0793	1.1543	0.0756

Source: Reprinted from "Body Fat Assessment from Total Body Density and Its Estimation from Skinfold Thickness: Measurements on 481 Men and Women Aged from 16 to 72 Years," by J. Durnin and J. Wormersley, in *British Journal of Nutrition*, Vol. 32, p. 77, with permission of Cambridge University Press, © 1974.

$$Y = 1.1303 - 0.0635 \, (\log 50)$$
$$= 1.0224$$

$$\% \text{ Fat} = (\frac{4.95}{1.0224} - 4.5)\,(100)$$

$$= 34.1$$

ARM MUSCLE AREA

The arm muscle area (AMA) is determined by two measurements: (1) triceps skinfold (TSF) in millimeters and (2) midarm circumference (MAC) in milli-meters.[2] The following formula is used to calculate arm muscle area:

$$\text{AMA} = \frac{(\text{MAC} - \text{II} \times \text{TSF})^2}{4\,\text{II}}$$

A corrected AMA_c ("available" arm muscle area) is then calculated separately for men and women as follows:

$$\text{Men AMA}_c = \text{AMA} - 19$$
$$\text{Women AMA}_c = \text{AMA} - 15.5$$

EVALUATION

Continued decreases in arm muscle area may indicate early signs of malnutri-tion. Large decreases in weight to less than 75 percent of standard body weight (as indicated in height and weight Table C–3) should prompt the nutritionist to look at change in arm muscle area. In the weight-loss client, a decrease in body fat as opposed to muscle area is preferable.

NOTES

1. J.V.G.A. Durnin and J. Wormersley, "Body Fat Assessment from Total Body Density and Its Esti-mation from Skinfold Thickness: Measurements on 481 Men and Women," *British Journal of Nutrition* 32 (1974): 77–97.
2. Steven B. Heymsfield et al., "Anthropometric Measurements of Muscle Mass: Revised Equations for Calculating Bone-Free Arm Muscle Area," *American Journal of Clinical Nutrition* 36 (1982): 680–690.

Table C-3 Height and Weight Tables+

	Men Weight in Kilograms				Women Weight in Kilograms		
Height[1] (cm)	Small Frame[2]	Medium Frame[2]	Large Frame[2]	Height[1] (cm)	Small Frame[2]	Medium Frame[2]	Large Frame[2]
153	59.0	61.2	64.7	145	48.5	52.4	56.8
154	59.3	61.5	65.2	146	48.8	52.8	57.2
155	59.7	61.9	65.6	147	49.0	53.1	57.7
156	60.0	62.2	66.0	148	49.3	53.6	58.1
157	60.4	62.6	66.5	149	49.6	54.1	58.6
158	60.7	62.9	66.9	150	50.0	54.5	59.0
159	61.1	63.3	67.4	151	50.4	55.0	59.6
160	61.4	63.7	67.8	152	50.9	55.4	60.2
161	61.8	64.1	68.4	153	51.3	55.9	60.7
162	62.2	64.6	68.9	154	51.7	56.4	61.2
163	62.5	65.0	69.4	155	52.3	57.0	61.9
164	62.9	65.5	70.0	156	52.8	57.5	62.5
165	63.2	66.0	70.6	157	53.3	58.1	63.1
166	63.7	66.6	71.2	158	53.8	58.6	63.7
167	64.1	67.1	71.8	159	54.4	59.1	64.3
168	64.6	67.6	72.4	160	54.9	59.6	64.9
169	65.0	68.1	73.0	161	55.5	60.2	65.5
170	65.5	68.7	73.7	162	56.0	60.7	66.1
171	65.9	69.2	74.3	163	56.6	61.3	66.8
172	66.3	69.7	74.9	164	57.1	61.9	67.5
173	66.8	70.3	75.5	165	57.6	62.4	68.1
174	67.3	70.8	76.2	166	58.2	62.9	68.7
175	67.7	71.3	76.8	167	58.7	63.4	69.3

continues

Height			
168	59.2	63.9	69.9
169	59.7	64.5	70.5
170	60.3	65.0	71.2
171	60.8	65.5	71.7
172	61.3	66.0	72.2
173	61.9	66.6	72.6
174	62.5	67.2	73.3
175	63.0	67.7	73.8
176	63.5	68.3	74.4
177	64.0	68.9	74.9
178	64.6	69.3	75.5
179	65.1	69.8	76.0
180	65.6	70.3	76.5
181	66.1	70.8	77.0
182	66.6	71.3	77.5
183	67.1	71.8	78.0
184	67.6	72.3	78.5
185	68.1	72.8	79.0
186	68.6	73.3	79.5
187	69.1	73.9	80.0
188	69.6	74.4	80.5
189	70.1	75.0	81.0
190	70.6	75.5	81.5

Height			
176	68.1	71.9	77.4
177	68.6	72.4	78.1
178	69.1	73.0	78.7
179	69.6	73.6	79.3
180	70.2	74.3	80.0
181	70.8	74.9	80.7
182	71.4	75.5	81.4
183	72.0	76.2	82.1
184	72.7	76.9	82.9
185	73.3	77.6	83.7
186	73.9	78.2	84.5
187	74.5	78.8	85.3
188	75.3	79.6	86.2
189	76.0	80.4	87.1
190	76.7	81.2	88.0
191	77.3	81.8	88.9
192	78.1	82.6	89.9
193	78.9	83.5	91.0
194	79.7	84.3	92.0
195	80.5	85.1	93.0
196	81.1	85.7	94.0
197	81.9	86.6	95.2
198	82.8	87.5	96.4
199	83.7	88.4	97.6
200	84.6	89.3	98.8

+Weights for heights in men below 155 cm and over 190 cm and in women over 180 cm estimated by extrapolation.

1. Height without shoes.
2. Frame size from Table C–1.

Source: Reprinted with permission from Metropolitan Life Foundation, "Height and Weight Tables," *Statistical Bulletin* (January–June 1983).

Behavioral Chart

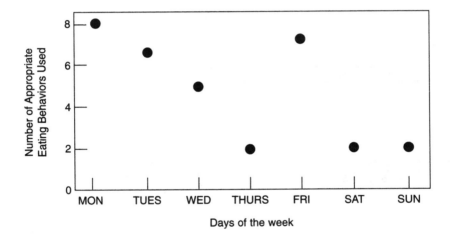

APPENDIX E

Behavioral Log

Date	Time	Setting	Event	Actual Reaction	Desired Reaction

Logs of Thoughts Related to Food

BASELINE LOG

Time	Thoughts
7:30	"I'd really like a doughnut but I'm not going to blow my day."
8:15	"It's not fair, I'm really trying and I haven't lost anything."
9:10	"Wish I had a doughnut or something. I'm hungry."
10:00	"It's not fair, it's snack time and all I get is water."
11:30	"Nothing tastes as good when I know there's no dessert."
12:10	"Look at them. They stuff themselves with sweets and stay skinny."
1:15	"Maybe I could have just a couple of cookies after school. I've earned them."
2:30	"Look at them running off to their afternoon snacks. It's not fair."
3:15	"I don't care if I'm fat. I'll never lose anyway. It's not worth it."
4:30	"I might as well eat and enjoy it. I'll never lose anyway. It's not worth it."
5:45	"You pig. Now you feel stuffed and you've ruined your day."
7:30	"What a failure I am. I don't deserve to be thin."
9:00	"I'll never learn, will I? It's no use."
10:30	"I feel hopeless. I've tried everything and I always blow it."

Source: From *Permanent Weight Control: A Total Solution to the Dieter's Dilemma* by Michael J. Mahoney, PhD, and Kathryn Mahoney, MSW, MS. Copyright © 1976 by W.W. Norton & Company, Inc. Reprinted by permission of W.W. Norton & Company, Inc.

REPLACEMENT LOG

Problem Category	Negative Monologues	Appropriate Monologues
Pounds Lost	"I'm not losing fast enough." "I've starved myself and haven't lost a thing." "I've been more consistent than Mary and she is losing faster than I am. It's not fair."	"Pounds don't count. If I continue my eating habits, the pounds will be lost." "Have patience—those pounds took a long time to get there. As long as they stay off permanently, I'll settle for any progress." "It takes a while to break down fat and absorb the extra water produced. I'm not going to worry about it."
Capabilities	"I just don't have the willpower." "I'm just naturally fat." "Why should this work—nothing else has." "I'll probably just regain it." "What the heck—I'd rather be fat than miserable. Besides, I'm not that heavy."	"There's no such thing as lack of willpower—just poor planning." "If I make a few improvements here and there and take things one day at a time, I can be very successful." "It's going to be nice to be permanently rid of all this extra baggage. I'm starting to feel better already."
Excuses	"If it weren't for my job and the kids, I could lose weight." "It's just impossible to eat right with a schedule like mine." "I'm just so nervous all the time—I have to eat to satisfy my psychological needs." "Maybe next time. . . . "	"My schedule isn't any worse than anyone else's. What I need to do is be a bit more creative in how to improve my eating." "Eating doesn't satisfy psychological problems—it creates them." "Job, kids, or whatever, I'm the one in control."

continues

REPLACEMENT LOG—continued

Problem Category	Negative Monologues	Appropriate Monologues
Goals	"Well, there goes my diet. That coffee cake probably cost me two pounds, and after I promised myself—no more sweets." "I always blow it on the weekends." "Fine—I start the day off with a doughnut. I may as well enjoy myself today."	"What is this—the Olympics? I don't need perfect habits, just improved ones." "Why should one sweet or an extra portion blow it for me? I'll cut back elsewhere." "Those high standards are unrealistic." "Fantastic—I had a small piece of cake and it didn't blow the day."
Food Thoughts	"I can't stop thinking about sweets." "I had images of cakes and pies all afternoon—it must mean that I need sugar." "When we order food at a restaurant, I continue thinking about what I have ordered until it arrives."	"Whenever I find myself thinking about food, I quickly change the topic to some other pleasant experience." "If I see a magazine ad or commercial for food and I start thinking about it, I distract my attention by doing something else (phoning a friend, getting the mail, etc.)."

Daily Record of Cognitive Restructuring

Date:_____		Record of: _____	
Description of Situation	*Coping Thoughts Used*	*Positive Self-Statements Used*	*Date and Time*

Source: From *Interviewing Strategies for Helpers: Fundamental Skills and Cognitive Behavioral Interventions* by W.H. Cormier and L.S. Cormier. Copyright © 1991, 1985, and 1975 Brooks/Cole Publishing Company, Pacific Grove, CA 93950, a division of International Thompson Publishing Inc. By permission of the publisher.

Answers to Chapter Reviews

Each answer should be discussed in depth. The responses provided here are intended only as general suggestions to help initiate discussion.

Answers to Review of Chapter 4

1. a. "I'm off that rotten diet now" syndrome.
   b. "I'm such a rotten person, what's the use" syndrome.
2. a. Identify the general problem.
   b. Collect data.
   c. Identify inappropriate eating pattern and possible ways toward improvement.
3. a. Substituting non–food-related activities.
   b. Interposing time.
   c. Eliminating cues.
   d. Involving spouse, family, and friends.
   e. Thinking positively.
   f. Engaging in physical activity.
4. For the client who has a very negative self-concept, use the positive thinking strategy. By substituting positive thoughts for negative, self-concepts may become more positive.

Answers to Review of Chapter 5

1. a. "Any vegetable oil is OK on a fat-modified diet."
   b. "One single food will lower my cholesterol so I really don't need to worry about eating other foods."
   c. "My family makes me eat high-fat crackers."
   d. "I can't get by on only six ounces of meat. It's not healthy."

e. "That low-fat cheese is terrible!"

f. "I practically drink vegetable oil because I know it will lower my cholesterol level."

2. a. Cholesterol.

b. Saturated fat.

c. Polyunsaturated fat.

d. Monounsaturated fat.

3. a. Tailor the diet to take past eating habits into consideration.

b. Stage the diet instruction.

c. Clear up misconceptions about fat and cholesterol.

	Choles-terol	*Total Fat*	*Saturated Fat*	*Poly-unsaturated Fat*	*Mono-unsaturated Fat*
0 egg/week	0	0	0	0	0
5 oz meat/day (med. fat beef)	129	21.10	9.15	.74	10.95
0 dairy	0	0	0	0	0
4 tsps Fleischmann's Regular, Tub, margarine/day	0	12.00	2.00	5.34	3.34
3 tsps Mazola oil/day	0	11.20	1.90	3.90	5.20
	181	44.30	13.05	9.98	19.49
		P/S = .83			
(% of 2,400 calories)		(17%)	(5%)	(4%)	(7%)

Strategies: Jim might tell his friends how important it is to his health to eat foods low in cholesterol and fat. He also might ask his family to help by positively reinforcing his efforts on social occasions. Supplements would provide needed calcium.

Answers to Review of Chapter 6

1. a. Social pressures.

b. Giving up old eating habits.

c. Avoiding unpalatable commercial substitutes.

2. a. Complex carbohydrates.

b. Simple carbohydrates.

3. a. Tailoring the eating pattern.

b. Staging the diet instruction.

c. Changing behaviors for social occasions.

d. Involving the family.

4. a. Ask questions to elicit thought patterns surrounding the problem.
    b. Encourage food substitutes and positive thinking.
    c. The goal in using these strategies is to (1) provide added dietary informa-
       tion and (2) help in beginning a program of positive thinking when un-
       planned and unrecommended eating is avoided.

Answers to Review of Chapter 7

1. a. Too many changes at one time.
    b. Social pressures.
    c. Giving up old eating habits.
    d. Unpalatable commercial substitutes.
2. a. Protein.
    b. Phosphorus.
    c. Potassium.
    d. Sodium.
    e. Fluid.
3. a. Tailoring.
    b. Staging.
    c. Behavior change for social occasions.
    d. Family involvement.
4. a. There are many correct answers to this question. One basic strategy is to
       initiate added spouse involvement in the interview. If the wife is given a
       sense of belonging to the dietary change process, she may become a more
       positive influence on her husband. The dietary changes can be approached
       in small steps with subgoals so that the new eating pattern seems less over-
       whelming.
    b. The goal in using these strategies is to: (1) focus on increasing spouse sup-
       port and (2) assist in making dietary changes more manageable by setting
       subgoals.

Answers to Review of Chapter 8

1. a. Loss of familiar flavors.
    b. Limited food choices.
    c. Changing old habits.
    d. Unpalatable commercial substitutes.
2. a. Collect data on the sodium content of the baseline diet.
    b. Identify the general problem.
    c. Identify inappropriate eating patterns and possible solutions.
3. a. Tailoring.
    b. Staging.

c. Flavoring substitutes.

d. Altering eating style through family involvement.

4. a. One of many areas to assess is family involvement. If the family members' attitudes toward the sodium restriction are negative, an increase in their involvement is a possible first step. By reviewing baseline information, it may be possible to substitute foods low in sodium for cheese and cold cuts. The client and counselor can build a self-reward system when low-sodium foods are eaten and high-sodium foods avoided.

b. The goal in using these strategies is to: (1) provide necessary dietary information and (2) design a system of self-rewards to help in maintaining good adherence.

Answers to Review of Chapter 9

1. a. Lack of math skills.

b. Familiar high-fat eating pattern.

2. a. Fat.

b. Calories (for persons at ideal body weight, nonfat sources of calories will need to be substituted in the new eating pattern).

3. a. Providing information gradually.

b. Posting fat scores for the day on the refrigerator.

c. Recording positive monologues.

4. a. Ask questions to elicit current successes with changing this high-fat meal. Inquire about family response to these efforts to change.

b. Organize a session in which the family is told how important they are to Mrs. B's success and provide tips on how to be supportive. Ask Mrs. B to keep a list for the week of her low-fat accomplishments in changing foods eaten in this meal.

c. The goals in using these strategies were to: (1) focus on increasing family support and (2) focus on the positive by listing accomplishments in modifying the meal to be lower in total fat.

Answers to Review of Chapter 10

1. a. Did the counseling session address the client's major problem?

b. Was assessment prior to designing a modified eating pattern adequate to prepare a dietary regimen compatible with the client's lifestyle?

c. Did the client's goal appear to have been achieved?

d. Were the strategies for altering eating behaviors carried out efficiently?

e. Did I use appropriate verbal and nonverbal interviewing skills?

f. Where might changes have been made?

g. Did I use appropriate counseling skills?

    h. Where might changes have been made?

    i. What general changes would I make in the next counseling interview with a similar client?

2. a. Have my dietary patterns changed and remained compatible with my life-style?

    b. Have my misconceptions about foods and what they contain been replaced with factual information?

    c. Are social occasions less of a problem now than when I first began my diet?

    d. Is my family providing needed positive reinforcement?

3. a. Reinforce and practice in the new environment.

    b. Promote generalization to many situations.

    c. Build in resistance to extinction.

    d. Practice new behaviors sufficiently.

    e. Promote social support.

4. a. Are there things going on in your life that may cause this?

    b. If "yes," what are they?

    c. Has the intervening event passed?

5. Check with the client to determine the most useful strategy used in the past to maintain adherence. Reinstitute that plan and monitor behavior.

Index

Page numbers in *italics* denote figures and exhibits; those followed by "t" denote tables.

About the Author

LINDA G. SNETSELAAR, PhD, graduated from Iowa State University with a Bachelor of Science Degree in Food and Nutrition in 1972. She did a dietetic internship at the University of Iowa and became a registered dietitian in 1973. Dr. Snetselaar received a Master of Science Degree from the University of Iowa in Nutrition in 1975, and a Doctor of Philosophy Degree in Instructional Design (Health Sciences Education) in 1983.

She has worked as a clinical dietitian instructing patients on modified diets, and as a research nutritionist counseling cardiovascular patients on diet and medication. As head research nutritionist she directed the Foods and Nutrition Resource Center for Lipid Research Clinic's Coronary Primary Prevention Trial (a clinical trial funded by the National Institutes of Health).

She is now involved in three studies funded by the National Institutes of Health. Each involves dietary modification to prevent disease and its complications: the Diabetes Control and Complications Trial, the Modification of Diet in Renal Disease, and Dietary Intervention Study in Children with elevated low-density lipoprotein levels. Currently she is co-principal investigator in the Women's Health Initiative, a National Cancer Institute funded clinical trial.

Dr. Snetselaar is an assistant professor in the Department of Preventive Medicine and an assistant research scientist in the Department of Internal Medicine at the University of Iowa. She team teaches courses in dietetics, chronic disease and nutrition epidemiology, and behavior modification.

She has directed seven workshops funded by the National Institutes of Health on counseling skills applied to nutrition. She has also given numerous talks on the topic. In 1978 Dr. Snetselaar was named Recognized Young Dietitian of the Year in Iowa and received the honor of being named an Outstanding Young Woman in America for 1982. In 1996 she received an award from the National Cancer Institute for her work in the Women's Health Initiative Study.